R. Hofmann • A. Heidenreich • J.W. Moul

Prostate Cancer

Springer-Verlag Berlin Heidelberg GmbH

R. HOFMANN • A. HEIDENREICH
J.W. MOUL (EDS.)

Prostate Cancer

Diagnosis and Surgical Treatment

With Contributions by

R.R. Berges, D. Böhmer, L. Boccon-Gibod, H. Bonkhoff, M.K. Brawer, L. Bubendorf, D. Brandt, S. Deger, B. Djavan, R. Engenhart-Cabillic, A. Erbersdobler, S. Fernandez, R.S. Foster, M. Graefen, A. Haese, P.G. Hammerer, A. Heidenreich, R.-P. Henke, W. Höltl, R. Hofmann, E. Huland, H. Huland, H. Lilja, S.A. Loening, M. Marberger, A. S. Merseburger, J. W. Moul, J. Noldus, P. Olbert, J. Palisaar, D. Paulson, U. Pichlmeier, D. Raghavan, V. Ravery, J. Roigas, F. Schreiter, T. Senge, V. Srikantan, S. Srivastava, I. Türk, Z. Varga, R. v. Knobloch, P. Vacha, S. Wille

With 88 Figures and 36 Tables

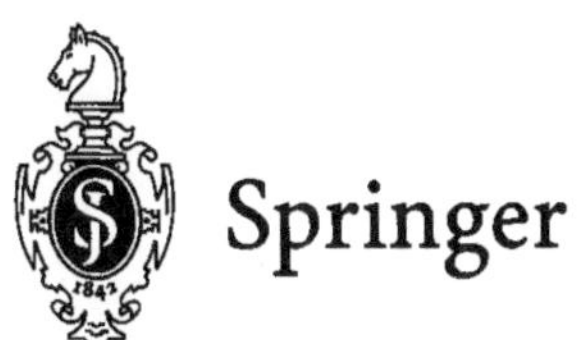

Springer

Prof. Dr. med. REINER HOFMANN
Department of Urology and Pediatric Urology
Philipps Universität Marburg
Baldingerstrasse 3
35043 Marburg/Lahn, Germany

Priv.-Doz. Dr. med. AXEL HEIDENREICH
Department of Urology and Pediatric Urology
Philipps Universität Marburg
Baldingerstrasse 3
35043 Marburg/Lahn, Germany

JUDD W. MOUL, M.D.
Professor of Urology
Department of Surgery
USUHS 430 I Jones Bridge Road
20814-4799 Bethesda, MD
USA

Additional material to this book can be downloaded from http://extras.springer.com.

ISBN 978-3-642-62643-2 ISBN 978-3-642-56321-8 (eBook)
DOI 10.1007/978-3-642-56321-8

Library of Congress Cataloging-in-Publication Data
Prostate cancer : diagnosis and surgical treatment / R. Hofmann, A. Heidenreich, J.W. Moul (eds.). p. cm. Includes bibliographical references and index.
ISBN 3-540-42019-3 (hardcover : alk. paper)
1. Prostate-Cancer-Diagnosis. 2. Prostate-Cancer-Surgery. I. Hofmann, R. (Reinhardt), 1954- II. Heidenreich, A. (Axel), 1964- III. Moul, Judd W.
RC280.P7 P75924 2002 616.99'463--dc21

Springer-Verlag Berlin Heidelberg New York

http://www.springer.de/medicin

Production editor: W. Bischoff, Heidelberg
Layout: W. Bischoff, Heidelberg
Cover design: deblik, Berlin
Medical illustrations: J. Kühn, Heidelberg
Data conversion and page make up: Fotosatz-Service Köhler GmbH, Würzburg
Printing and binding: H. Stürtz AG, Würzburg

Printed on acid-free paper SPIN: 10793312 22/BF3130 - 5 4 3 2 1 0 -

Foreword

Prostate cancer is not only the most common genitourinary tumor but, according to the tumor registry of Munich, the male tumor with the highest incidence. The wide range of information concerning this important disease has been dealt with comprehensively . In a time when interested urologists can surf in the internet to find an article they are looking for, they usually get lost because of the flood of papers covering the same subject. Furthermore, they are still alone in deciding which scientific contribution to believe and which will serve their patients best. A well-edited book such as this, however, provides quick access to all pertinent questions. These renowned authors have taken on the responsibility of writing a balanced report and producing a sort of a guideline, i.e., a diagnostic or therapeutic standard.

The editors are to be congratulated on mastering such a formidable task, bringing together the leading names in prostate cancer to present their views on all the questions one might have about this disease. I trust that this book will serve urologists in practice and their patients well.

J.E. Altwein
München

Contents

Pathology and Molecular Biology of Prostate Cancer

Diagnosis and Staging of Prostate Cancer

Operative Therapy of Clinically Localized Prostate Cancer

Radiotherapy for Localized Prostate Cancer

Complications Following Radical Prostatectomy

List of Contributors

R. Berges, MD
Associate Prof. of Urology,
Department of Urology,
Ruhr-Universität Bochum,
Marienhospital,
Widumer Strasse 8,
44627 Herne, Germany

D. Böhmer, MD
Associate Prof. of
Radiotherapy,
Department of Radiotherapy,
Humboldt University,
Campus-Charité-Mitte,
Schumannstrasse 20-21
10117 Berlin, Germany

L. Boccon-Gibod, MD
Prof. and Chairman,
Department of Urology,
Service d'Urologie,
Hospital Bichat,
46 Rue H. Hichard,
75018 Paris, France

H. Bonkhoff, MD
Prof. of Pathology,
Institute of Pathology,
University of the Saarland,
Kirrbergstrasse 1,
66421 Homburg/Saar,
Germany

M.K. Brawer, MD
Prof. of Urology,
Northwest Prostate Institute,
Northwest Hospital,
1560 N, 115th Street, Ste 209,
Seattle, WA 98133, USA

L. Bubendorf, MD
Associate Prof. of Pathology,
Institute for Pathology,
University of Basel,
Schönbeinstrasse 40,
4003 Basel, Switzerland

D. Brandt, MD
Assistant Prof. of Radiology,
Department
of Nuclear Medicine,
Philipps University Marburg,
Baldingerstrasse 3,
5043 Marburg, Germany

S. Deger, MD
Associate Prof. of Urology,
Department of Urology,
Humboldt University,
Campus-Charité-Mitte,
Schumannstrasse 20–21
10117 Berlin, Germany

B. Djavan, MD PhD
Prof. of Urology,
Department of Urology,
University of Vienna,
Währinger Gürtel 18–20,
1090 Vienna, Austria

R. Engenhart-Cabillic, MD
Prof. and Chair
Department of Radiotherapy,
Philipps-University Marburg,
Baldingerstrasse 3,
35043 Marburg, Germany

A. Erbersdobler, MD
Associate Prof. of Pathology,
Department of Pathology,
University of Hamburg,
Martinistrasse 52,
20246 Hamburg, Germany

S. Fernandez, MD
Associate Prof. of Urology,
Department of Urology,
University of Hamburg,
Martinistrasse 52,
20246 Hamburg, Germany

R.S. Foster, MD
Prof. of Urology,
Department of Urology,
Indiana University Medical
Center,
Indianapolis, IN 46202,
USA

M. Graefen, MD
Assistant Prof. of Urology,
Department of Urology,
University of Hamburg,
Martinistrasse 52,
20246 Hamburg, Germany

A. Haese, MD
Department of Urology,
University of Hamburg,
Martinistrasse 52,
20246 Hamburg, Germany

P. Hammerer, MD
Associate Prof. of Urology,
Department of Urology,
University of Hamburg,
Martinistrasse 52,
20246 Hamburg,
Germany

A. Heidenreich, MD
Associate Prof. of Urology,
Department of Urology and
Pediatric Urology,
Philipps-University Marburg,
Baldingerstrasse 3,
5043 Marburg,
Germany

R.P. Henke, MD
Associate Prof. of Pathology,
Department of Pathology,
University of Hamburg,
Martinistrasse 52,
20246 Hamburg,
Germany

W. Höltl, MD
Prof. and Chairman,
Department of Urology,
Kaiser Franz-Josef-Spital,
Kundratstrasse 3,
1100 Wien, Austria

E. Huland, MD
Prof. of Immunology,
Department of Urology,
University of Hamburg,
Martinistrasse 52,
20246 Hamburg,
Germany

H. Huland
Prof. and Chairman,
Department of Urology,
University of Hamburg,
Martinistrasse 52,
20246 Hamburg,
Germany

R. v. Knobloch, MD
Associate Prof. of Urology,
Department of Urology and
Pediatric Urology,
Philipps-University Marburg,
Baldingerstrasse 3,
5043 Marburg,
Germany

H. Lilja, MD
Prof. and Chair
Department of Clinical Chemistry,
Lund University,
University Hospital Malmö,
20502 Malmö, Sweden

S. Loening, MD
Prof. and Chairman,
Department of Urology,
Humboldt University,
Campus-Charité-Mitte,
Schumannstrasse 20–21
10117 Berlin, Germany

M. Marberger, MD
Prof. and Chairman,
Department of Urology,
University of Vienna,
Währinger Gürtel 18–20,
1090 Vienna, Austria

A. Merseburger, MD
Assistant Professor of Urology,
Center for Prostate Disease Research,
130 East Jefferson Street,
Rockville, MD 20852,
USA

J.W. Moul, MD
Professoer of Urology,
Center for Prostate Disease Research,
130 East Jefferson Street,
Rockville, MD 20852,
USA

J. Noldus, MD
Associate Prof. of Urology,
Department of Urology,
University of Hamburg,
Martinistrasse 52,
20246 Hamburg,
Germany

P. Olbert, MD
Assistant Prof. of Urology,
Department of Urology and Pediatric Urology,
Philipps-University Marburg,
Baldingerstrasse 3,
5043 Marburg,
Germany

J. Palisaar, MD
Department of Urology,
University of Hamburg,
Martinistrasse 52,
20246 Hamburg, Germany

D.F. Paulson, MD
Prof. and Chairman,
Division of Urology,
Duke University Medical Center,
P.O. Box 2977,
Durham, NC 27710,
USA

U. Pichlmeier, MD
Associate Prof.,
Department of Biostatistics,
University Hamburg-Eppendorf,
Martinistrasse 52,
20246 Hamburg,
Germany

D. Raghavan, MBBS, PhD
Prof. of Medicine and Urology, Chief,
Division of Medical Oncology,
University of Southern California,
Norris Comprehensive Cancer Center,
1141 East Lake Ave.,
Los Angeles, CA 90033,
USA

V. Ravery, MD
Prof. of Urology,
Department of Urology,
Service d'Urologie,
Hospital Bichat,
46 Rue H. Hichard,
75018 Paris, France

J. Roigas, MD
Associate Prof. of Urology,
Department of Urology,
Humboldt University,
Campus-Charité-Mitte,
Schumannstrasse 20-21
10117 Berlin, Germany

F. Schreiter, MD
Prof. and Chairman
Department of urology and Pediatric Urology,
Allgemeines Krankenhaus Hamburg,
Eissendorfer Pferdeweg 52,
21075 Hamburg, Germany

Th. Senge, MD
Prof. and Chairman,
Department of Urology,
Ruhr-Universität Bochum,
Marienhospital,
Widumer Strasse 8,
44627 Herne, Germany

V. Srikantan, PhD
Center for Prostate Disease Research,
Department of Surgery,
Uniformed Services University of the Health Sciences,
4301 Jones Bridge Road,
Bethesda, MD 20814-4799,
USA

S. Srivastava, PhD
Center for Prostate Disease Research,
Department of Surgery,
Uniformed Services University of the Health Sciences,
4301 Jones Bridge Road,
Bethesda, MD 20814-4799,
USA

T. Sulser, MD
Prof. and Chairman,
Department of Urology,
University of Basel,
4003 Basel, Switzerland

I. Türk, MD
Associate Prof. of Urology,
Department of Urology,
Humboldt University,
Campus-Charité-Mitte,
Schumannstrasse 20–21
10117 Berlin, Germany

P. Vacha, MD
Assistant Prof. of Radiotherapy,
Department of Radiotherapy,
Philipps-University Marburg,
Baldingerstrasse 3,
5043 Marburg,
Germany

Z. Varga, MD
Assistant Prof. of Urology,
Department of Urology and Pediatric Urology,
Philipps-University Marburg,
Baldingerstrasse 3,
5043 Marburg,
Germany

S. Wille, MD
Assistant Prof. of Urology,
Department of Urology and Pediatric Urology,
Philipps-University Marburg,
Baldingerstrasse 3,
5043 Marburg,
Germany

Pathology and Molecular Biology of Prostate Cancer

1 Morphogenetic Aspects of Prostate Cancer

H. Bonkhoff

1.1 Introduction

Prostate cancer is a complex disease process, involving genetic, hormonal, and other epigenetic factors. Despite its clinical magnitude and the recent progress made in molecular biology, the pathogenesis of prostate cancer remains poorly understood. This reflects a number of factors including:

1. The complex composition of the prostate gland by different anatomic, cellular, and functional compartments
2. The heterogeneous and multifocal nature of prostate cancer
3. The limited number of established cell lines for in vitro studies
4. The lack of suitable animal models that faithfully recapitulate all stages of disease progression [39]

The present review focuses on current morphogenetic factors implicated in the development of prostate cancer and tumor progression. The concepts discussed below refer to recent data obtained in human prostate tissue.

1.2 The Cellular Biology of the Prostatic Epithelium

The prostatic epithelium has a complex composition by three cell types differing in their hormonal regulation and marker expression (Fig. 1.1). The most prevalent phenotype consists of secretory luminal cells expressing prostate-specific antigen (PSA) and cytokeratins 8 and 18 [35, 41]. Basal cells, the second most important phenotype, mediate attachment to the stroma and express high molecular weight cytokeratins [2, 39, 40]. The third phenotype shows neuroendocrine (NE) differentiation. NE cells express chromogranins and secrete a number of neurosecretory products which may have growth promoting properties [26, 27]. Although these basic cell types clearly differ in their marker expression and biological functions, they obviously share a common origin from pluripotent stem cells located in the basal cell layer [2, 6, 7]. This concept is based on the occurrence of intermediate differentiation among the three basic cell types making up the prostatic epithelium [13, 41] and the biological properties of basal cells [2, 6, 7]. Cell kinetic studies indicate that the proliferation compartment of the normal or hyperplastic epithelium is located in the basal cell layer [14]. Seventy percent of proliferating epithelial cells express basal cell specific cytokeratins, while the remaining 30% of cycling cells are identified in secretory luminal cell types [14]. Chromogranin A positive NE cells lack proliferative activity and represent a terminal differentiated cell population within the prostatic epithelial cell system [8, 16]. It is therefore most unlikely that NE cells present in the normal or dysplastic epithelium are precursors of prostate cancer cells, even those with NE features [4]. In benign

This work was supported by the Deutsche Forschungsgemeinschaft.

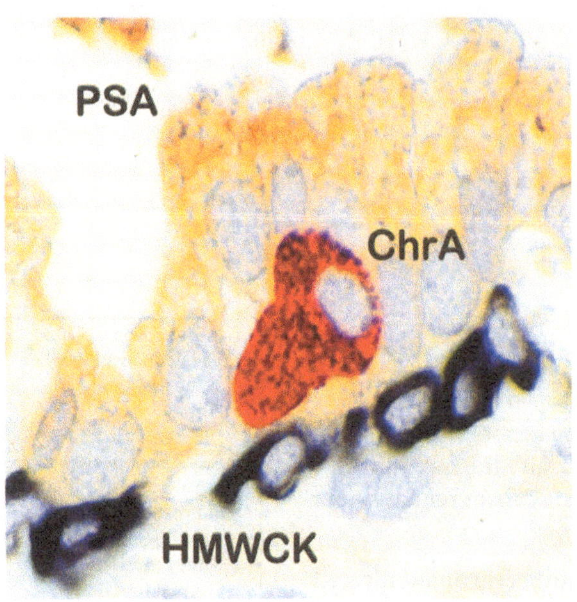

Fig. 1.1.
Cellular composition of the prostatic epithelium. Simultaneous demonstration of PSA (secretory luminal cells), high molecular weight cytokeratins, HMWCK (basal cells) and Chromogranin A (endocrine cells)

prostate tissue, apoptotic cell death mainly occurs in secretory luminal cells, while basal cells uniformly express the apoptosis-suppressing Bcl-2 oncoprotein which obviously protects the proliferation compartment from programmed cell death [18].

The cellular diversity of the prostatic epithelium is maintained through a network of hormonal controls, growth factors, and adhesive interactions with the underlying basement membrane. Secretory luminal cells are androgen dependent and require circulating androgens for their growth and maintenance. It is not surprising that these cells strongly express the nuclear androgen receptor (AR). Conversely, basal cells are androgen independent, but remain androgen responsive in vivo. In human prostate tissue, subsets of basal cells express the nuclear AR at high levels [5]. Basal cells also contain the 5α-reductase isoenzyme 2 which is crucial for the dihydrotestosterone forming process [17]. It is likely that androgen-responsive basal cells are committed to differentiate toward luminal cells under appropriate androgen stimulation [2, 6]. This differentiation process is balanced by estrogens. In benign prostate tissue, expression of the classical estrogen receptor (ERα) is restricted to stromal and basal cells [20]. Estrogen treatment leads to atrophy of luminal cells and basal cell hyperplasia by preventing basal cells from differentiating toward luminal cells [2, 6].

A number of nonsteroidal growth factors are involved in the regulation of benign glandular growth. Basal cells express growth factor receptors (e.g. EGF-R), oncogenes (erbB-2, erbB-3, c-met, Bcl-2) and tumor suppressor genes (nm-23-H1) [7, 34]. The interplay between these factors may ultimately determine the growth fraction within the basal cell layer. Alternatively, differentiation processes within the prostatic epithelial cell system most likely depend on a hormonal balance between circulating androgens and estrogens [2, 6, 7].

Another important factor implicated in benign prostatic growth is concerned with adhesive interactions between basal cells and epithelial basement membranes (BM) [3]. Prostatic epithelial cells require BM components for their in vitro growth and differentiation [29]. In human prostate tissue, basal cells exhibit polarized distribution of integrin receptors ($\alpha6\beta1$, $\alpha2\beta1$, $\alpha6\beta4$) and hemidesmosome-associated proteins (BP180, BP220, HD1) [11, 31, 36]. It seems likely that formation of stable hemidesmosomes and adhesive interactions with the BM contribute significantly to the integrity and biological functions of basal cells. Based on the present information, basal cells play a pivotal role in benign prostate growth. The basal cell layer houses pluripotent stem cells and maintains cell proliferation and normal epithelial-stromal relations (Fig. 1.2). Genetic and epigenetic factors interfering with the normal function of basal cells are therefore crucial for the development of prostate cancer.

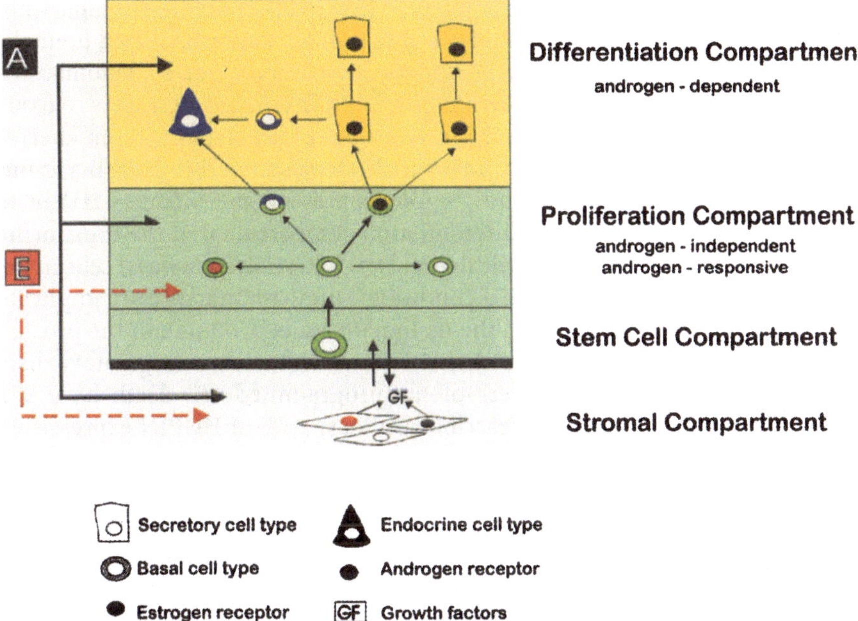

Fig. 1.2. Stem cell model for the organization of the prostatic epithelium. Two functional compartments can be identified within the complex prostatic epithelial cell system. The differentiation compartment consists of secretory luminal cells which are androgen-dependent but have a limited proliferative capacity. The basal cell layer is androgen-independent and makes up the proliferation compartment. The proliferation function of basal cells is maintained by a number of growth factors (e.g. EGF), oncogenes (erbB-2, erbB-3, c-met) and tumor suppressor gene products (nm23-H1), while Bcl-2 protects basal cells from apoptotic cell death. The basal cell layer houses a small stem cell population which gives rise to all epithelial cell types through a process of intermediate differentiation. These differentiation processes depend on a delicate balance between androgens and estrogens. Androgens are likely to induce basal cell differentiation towards secretory luminal cells, while estrogens prevent this process leading to atrophy of luminal cells and basal cell hyperplasia. Thus, the turnover of luminal cells may depend on the number of androgen-responsive basal cells in the proliferation compartment. It is conceivable that the age-related decrease of circulating androgens hypersensitize basal cells to the reduced level of bioavailable androgens, thus leading to glandular hyperplasia by accelerating the differentiation process from basal cells to luminal cells

1.3 Differentiation and Proliferation Disorders in Early Phases of Prostatic Cancerogenesis

High grade prostatic intraepithelial neoplasia (HGPIN) is the most likely precursor of prostate cancer [23]. This lesion usually arises in preexisting ducts and duct-acinar units of the peripheral zone and shares cytological features with intermediate and high grade carcinoma, but retains basal cell differentiation [23]. Autopsy studies indicate that PIN precedes carcinoma by ten years and more. HGPIN is currently the most significant risk factor for prostate cancer. Its identification in prostatic biopsy specimens warrants further searches for concurrent cancer [23].

Several morphogenetic factors are involved in the malignant transformation of the prostatic epithelium. In HGPIN, the basal cell layer (proliferation compartment) loses its proliferation function, whereas secretory luminal (dysplastic) cells acquire increased proliferative activity [14]. Less than 10% of cycling cells detected in HGPIN belong to what had previously been the proliferation compartment [14] (Fig. 1.3). Extension of the proliferative zone to

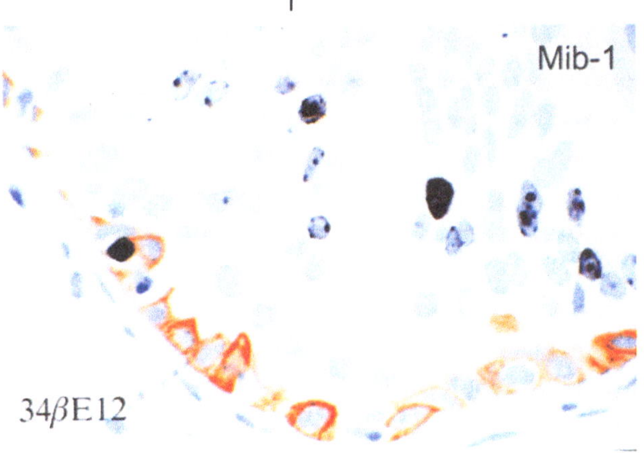

Fig. 1.3. Proliferation abnormalities detected in HGPIN. The proliferation zone of the prostatic epithelium extends to secretory luminal cells (differentiation compartment). Less than 10% of cycling cells are identified in the basal cell layer, the proliferation compartment of the normal prostatic epithelium. Simultaneous demonstration of the proliferation marker Mib-1 and basal cells specific cytokeratins (34βE12) in HGPIN

luminal cells in the differentiation compartment is a typical feature of well established premalignant lesions such as colorectal adenomas. The premalignant proliferation disorders encountered in HGPIN are associated with an aberrant expression of oncogenes (erbB-2, erbB-3, c-met) and tumor suppressor genes (nm23-H1) in the differentiation compartment of the transformed epithelium [7, 34]. Restricted to basal cells in normal conditions, these biomarkers are implicated in the malignant transformation of the prostatic epithelium. In addition, severe regulatory disorders of the programmed cell death have been described. At least 20% of HGPIN expresses the apoptosis-suppressing Bcl-2 oncoprotein in the differentiation compartment of the transformed epithelium [18]. This abnormal Bcl-2 expression pattern may induce severe differentiation disorders by preventing cells of the differentiation compartment from apoptotic cell death. The resulting prolonged life-span of transformed cells, together with their high proliferation rate, provides an excellent environment in which genetic instability can occur. The most common genetic alterations in HGPIN include:

a) Gain of chromosome 7, particularly 7q31
b) Loss of 8p and gain of 8q
c) Loss of 10q, 16q, and 18q.

The overall frequency of numeric chromosomal anomalies reported is remarkably similar in HGPIN and invasive cancer, suggesting that they have a similar pathogenesis [30, 38].

Clinical studies have shown that HGPIN generally regresses after androgen deprivation, while a minority persists even after neoadjuvant total androgen blockade [23]. This observation obviously reflects the fact that most of HGPIN lesions express the nuclear AR and Bcl-2 as described in benign acini. Conversely, HGPIN with aberrant expression of Bcl-2 in the differentiation compartment tends to downregulate the AR, as documented by markedly reduced levels of detectable receptor proteins [18]. It is likely that such premalignant lesions escape the androgen-dependent programmed cell death. Accordingly, Bcl-2 may be a promising biomarker to define the virulence of HGPIN.

The role of estrogens in the malignant transformation of the prostatic epithelium remains controversial, although a number of epidemiological and experimental data suggests that estrogens are involved in prostatic cancerogenesis. In human prostate tissue, ERα mRNA expression is restricted to basal cells in normal conditions, but shifts to luminal cells in HGPIN [20]. At least 10% of HGPIN expresses the ERα protein in the dysplastic epithelium [20]. The estrogen - inducible PS2 protein has been identified in a significant number of benign and dysplastic prostate tissues from patients with locally advanced prostate cancer, but not in prostate tissue from patients without evidence of malignant disease [15]. These data suggest that estrogens can affect early phases of prostatic cancerogenesis through an ERα-mediated process.

In summary, virtually all phenotype and genotype data amassed in recent years support the concept that HGPIN is the precursor of intermediate and high grade cancer arising in the peripheral zone [23, 30, 33]. Conversely, the significance of atypical adenomatous hyperplasia (AAH) as a precursor of low grade transition zone cancer is not well established [33]. Although the proliferative activity of AAH is increased, comparing with hyperplastic lesions, the proliferation zone and Bcl-2 expression are restricted to basal cells as described in benign prostate tissue [7, 14]. Thus, AAH does not reveal typical premalignant proliferation and differentiation abnormalities as found in HGPIN. Nevertheless, allelic imbalance may occur, indicating a genetic link between AAH and prostatic adenocarcinoma [24]. Much more work is needed to define the morphogenesis of low grade transition zone cancer.

1.4 Pathogenesis of Stromal Invasion

Adhesive interactions in premalignant lesions do not differ significantly from those encountered in benign prostate tissue. Dramatic changes occur during early stromal invasion when the transformed epithelium loses basal cell differentiation [3]. This process is associated with the loss of a number of hemidesmosome-forming proteins and associated adhesive molecules, including collagen VII, $\beta 3$ and $\gamma 2$ subchains of laminin 5, and $\alpha 6\beta 4$ integrins [31, 36]. It is quite clear that benign acini and HGPIN require these adhesive elements to maintain basal cell differentiation. Alternatively, the inability of transformed cells to express hemidesmosome-associated proteins obviously presents a key step in the neoplastic progression of HGPIN to early invasive cancer. Another important event in early stromal invasion refers to the synthesis of tumor-associated basement membranes (BM) [9, 10]. Invasive prostate cancer cells produce BM-like matrices and express associated integrins ($\alpha 6\beta 1$, $\alpha 2\beta 1$) that mediate attachment to this newly formed matrix [9, 10, 11] (Fig. 1.4). This particular tumor-host relation encountered in prostate cancer is maintained through the various stages of the disease, including high grade, metastatic and recurrent lesions [9, 10, 11]. Recent in situ hybridization analyses show that these BMs are produced by tumor cells and not by the host tissue [37]. High steady state levels of laminin and type IV collagen mRNA are detected in metastatic lesions when compared with primary tumors [37]. This indicates that the BM-forming process increases with tumor progression.

Neoplastic BMs differ from their normal counterparts in their differential susceptibility to pepsin treatment, and lack hemidesmosome-associated laminin 5, collagen VII, and type IV collagen $\alpha 5$ and $\alpha 6$ chains [9, 31, 36]. Their functional significance for the process of stromal invasion has also been demonstrated in vitro, showing that prostate cancer cell lines generally require reconstituted BMs (Matrigel) to be tumorigenic in athymic mice [3]. In summary, de novo synthesized BMs and adhesion via specific receptors significantly contribute to the ability of prostate cancer to penetrate the extracellular matrix during stromal invasion and metastasis [3].

Fig. 1.4. Epithelial-stromal relation in prostate cancer. Invasive tumor cells are separated from the host tissue by pericellular and periacinar basement membranes (BM) expressing laminin (*red*) and other BM components. Pertinent receptors such as $\alpha 6\beta 1$ integrins (*blue*) mediate attachment to these newly formed matrices. Computer-assisted double staining reveals coordinate expression of the extracellular receptor domain and its corresponding ligand in basement membranes (*shown in yellow*)

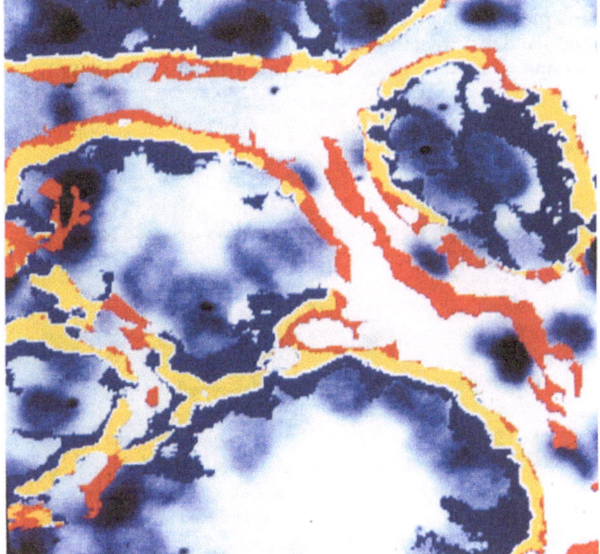

1.5 Morphogenetic Factors Implicated in Prostate Cancer Progression and Hormone Therapy Failure

Common prostatic adenocarcinoma is mainly composed of exocrine tumor cells expressing PSA and cytokeratins 8, 18, and share phenotype similarity with secretory luminal cells of the normal prostatic epithelium [35, 39]. These exocrine tumor cells generally express the nuclear AR and 5α reductase 1 and 2 in primary, metastatic and recurrent lesions [12, 17]. This observation suggests that exocrine tumor cells are androgen-responsive, and maintain the dihydrotestosterone-forming process even in hormone refractory stages of the disease. The continuous expression of the nuclear AR in androgen-insensitive carcinomas is surprising, and involves a high level of AR gene amplification identified in at least 30% of recurrent lesions [32]. The presence of the nuclear AR in prostate cancer tissue, however, does not imply androgen dependence. Point mutations in the steroid binding domain of the AR gene can seriously interfere with the normal function of the receptor protein [25, 32]. It has been shown that mutated AR bind estrogens and other steroids in the absence of androgens [25]. However, such point mutations could not be identified in a substantial number of recurrent lesions, indicating that other factors are involved in the multifactorial process of androgen insensitivity. Alternative pathways by which prostate cancer cells escape androgen deprivation refer to their ability to acquire neuroendocrine (NE) features [4] or to use estrogens for their own growth [20, 21, 22].

1.5.1 Neuroendocrine Differentiation

The second most prevalent phenotype encountered in prostate cancer shows neuroendocrine (NE) differentiation [26, 27]. Virtually all prostatic adenocarcinomas reveal at least focal NE features as assessed by immunohistochemical markers such as Chromogranin A (ChrA). Tumors with extensive and multifocal NE features (accounting for approximately 10% of all prostatic malignancies) tend to be poorly differentiated, more aggressive and resistant to hormonal therapy [26, 27]. Several pathways have been described showing how NE differentiation can affect tumor progression and hormone therapy failure [4]. It has been shown that prostate cancer cells expressing ChrA consistently lack the nuclear androgen receptor (AR) in primary, metastatic, and recurrent lesions [12] (Fig. 1.5). This clearly indicates that NE phenotypes constitute an androgen-insensitive cell population in all stages of the disease. NE tumor cells most likely derive from exocrine phenotypes through a process of intermediate differentiation, which obviously reflects the differentiation repertoire of prostatic stem cells. In fact, NE foci frequently harbor amphicrine cell types expressing both endocrine (ChrA) and exocrine (PSA) markers [13]. It has been shown that NE differentiation predominantly occurs in the Go phase of the cell cycle, and is lost when tumor cells reenter the cell cycle [8, 16]. Although NE tumor cells lack proliferative activity, they exert growth-promoting effects on adja-

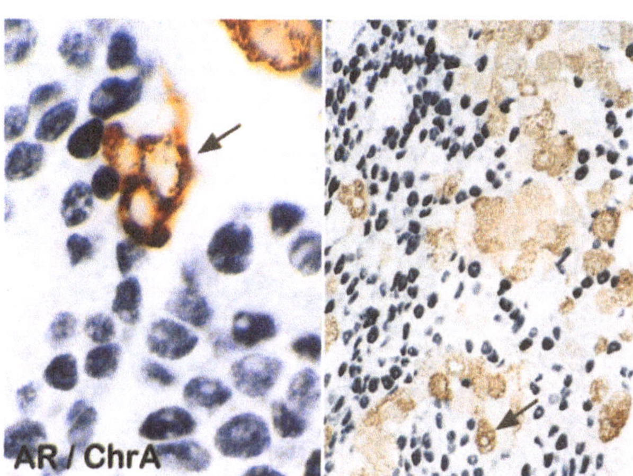

Fig. 1.5. Androgen receptor status in endocrine and exocrine prostate cancer cells. Androgen receptor expression is restricted to exocrine tumor cells. Neuroendocrine tumor cells identified by Chromogranin A (*arrows*) consistently lack the nuclear androgen receptor in both primary (*left*) and recurrent (*right*) lesions

cent (exocrine) tumor cells. A growing number of neurosecretory products with growth-promoting properties in vitro, including bombesin, calcitonin, and parathyroid hormone related peptides has been identified in NE phenotypes of prostate cancer [26, 27]. It is likely that these NE growth factors can maintain cell proliferation in adjacent (exocrine) tumor cells through a paracrine (androgen-independent) mechanism. Recent studies also indicate that NE (ChrA positive) tumor cells escape the apoptotic cell death as assessed by DNA fragmentation assays [19, 28]. The absence of proliferative and apoptotic activity in NE phenotypes may have some therapeutic implications, knowing that radiation therapy and other cytotoxic drugs mainly affect cycling cells. Given their cell kinetic features, it will be very difficult to kill prostate cancer cells with NE features by endocrine and other cytotoxic treatments currently available. Recent clinical studies lend credence to this concept. Elevated serum levels of ChrA in patients with prostate cancer correlate with poor prognosis and are scarcely influenced by either endocrine therapy or chemotherapy [1].

1.5.2 Role of Estrogens in Androgen-Insensitive Prostatic Growth

Since the time of Higgins, estrogens have been widely used in the medical treatment of advanced prostate cancer to reduce the testicular output of androgens. The recent discovery of the classical estrogen receptor alpha (ERα) and estrogen-regulated proteins such as the progesterone receptor (PR) and the heat shock protein HSP27 clearly shows that prostate cancer cells can use estrogens for their own growth [20, 21, 22]. In contrast with breast cancer, the presence of the ERα and the estrogen-inducible PR and HSP27 is a late event in prostate cancer progression. The most significant levels of these markers are detectable in recurrent and metastatic lesions [20, 21, 22] (Fig. 1.6). This indicates that metastatic and androgen-insensitive tumors are estrogen-responsive and can use estrogens for their maintenance and growth to survive in an androgen-deprived milieu. The progressive emergence of the ERα and PR during tumor progression provides a theoretical background for studying the efficiency of antiestrogens and antigestagens in the medical treatment of advanced prostate cancer. The current morphogenetic factors implicated in prostate cancer development and progression are summarized in Fig. 1.7.

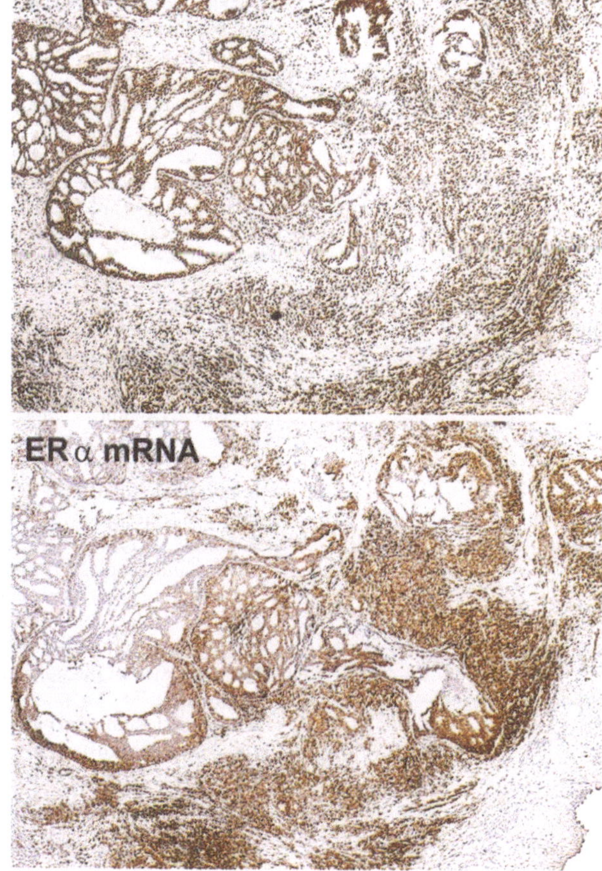

Fig. 1.6. Estrogen (ER) and progesterone (PR) receptor expression in recurrent prostatic adenocarcinoma. High levels of estrogen receptor α mRNA and the progesterone receptor are detected in androgen-insensitive prostate cancer, indicating that such lesions can use estrogens through a receptor-mediated process

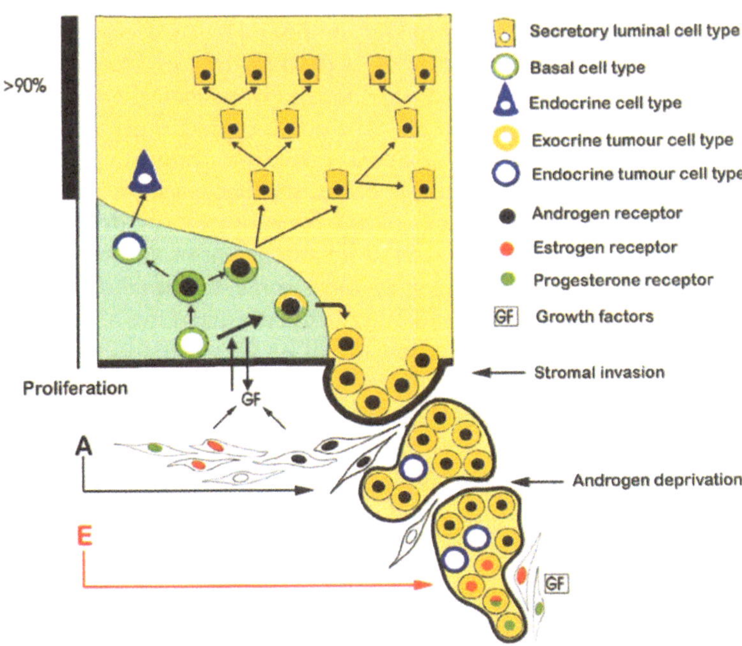

Fig. 1.7. Morphogenetic pathways implicated in prostate cancer development and tumor progression. Preinvasive phases of prostatic cancerogenesis are characterized by severe differentiation and proliferation disorders within the prostatic epithelial cell system (see text). Transformed precursor cells originating from the basal cell layer acquire exocrine features and produce an altered extracellular matrix. These newly formed (tumor-associated) basement membranes provide a supporting scaffold for penetration of the host tissue during stromal invasion and metastasis. Exocrine tumor cells (the most prevalent phenotype of prostatic adenocarcinoma) remain androgen-responsive even in hormone refractory stages of the disease. Point mutations in the steroid binding domain of the AR gene, however, can seriously interfere with the normal function of the receptor protein. The progressive emergence of neuroendocrine (NE) tumor cells during tumor progression obviously reflects the differentiation potency of prostatic stem cells. Devoid of the nuclear AR, NE tumor cells are androgen-insensitive but produce NE growth factors which can exercise growth promoting effects on adjacent exocrine tumor cells. The lack of proliferative and apoptotic activity in NE tumor cells further contribute to their drug resistance. After androgen deprivation prostate cancer cells acquire the ability to use estrogens and gestagens through a receptor-mediated process. The presence of ERα and PR in metastatic and recurrent lesions provides a novel target for antiestrogens and antigestagens in the medical treatment of advanced prostate cancer

References

1. Berruti A, Dogliotti L, Mosca A, Bellina M, Mari M, Torta M, Tarabuzzi R, Bollito E, Fontana D, Angeli A (2000) Circulating neuroendocrine markers in patients with prostate carcinoma. Cancer 88:2590–2597
2. Bonkhoff H (1996) Role of the basal cells in premalignant changes of the human prostate: a stem cell concept for the development of prostate cancer. Eur Urol 30:201–205
3. Bonkhoff H (1998) Analytical molecular pathology of epithelial-stromal interactions in the normal and neoplastic prostate. Anal Quant Cytol Histol 20:437–442
4. Bonkhoff H (1998) Neuroendocrine cells in benign and malignant prostate tissue: morphogenesis, proliferation, and androgen receptor status. Prostate Suppl 8:18–22
5. Bonkhoff H, Remberger K (1993) Widespread distribution of nuclear androgen receptors in the basal layer of the normal and hyperplastic human prostate. Virchows Arch A Pathol Anat 422:35–38
6. Bonkhoff H, Remberger K (1996) Differentiation pathways and histogenetic aspects of normal and abnormal prostatic growth: a stem cell model. Prostate 28:98–106
7. Bonkhoff H, Remberger K (1998) Morphogenetic concepts of normal and abnormal growth of the human prostate. Virchows Arch 433:195–202
8. Bonkhoff H, Wernert N, Dhom G, Remberger K (1991) Relation of endocrine-paracrine cells to cell proliferation in normal, hyperplastic and neoplastic human prostate. Prostate 18: 91–98

9. Bonkhoff H, Wernert N, Dhom G, Remberger K (1991) Basement membranes in fetal, adult normal, hyperplastic and neoplastic human prostate. Virchows Archiv A Pathol Anat 418:375– 381
10. Bonkhoff H, Wernert N, Dhom G, Remberger K (1992) Distribution of basement membranes in primary and metastatic carcinomas of the prostate. Hum Pathol 23:934–939
11. Bonkhoff H, Stein U, Remberger K (1993) Differential expression of α-6 and α-2 very late antigen integrins in the normal, hyperplastic and neoplastic human prostate. Simultaneous demonstration of cell surface receptors and their extracellular ligands. Hum Pathol 24: 243–248
12. Bonkhoff H, Stein U, Remberger K (1993) Androgen receptor status in endocrine-paracrine cell types of the normal, hyperplastic, and neoplastic human prostate. Virchows Arch A Pathol Anat Histopathol 423:291–294
13. Bonkhoff H, Stein U, Remberger K (1994) Multidirectional differentiation in the normal, hyperplastic and neoplastic human prostate. Simultaneous demonstration of cell specific epithelial markers. Hum Pathol 25:42–46
14. Bonkhoff H, Stein U, Remberger K (1994) The proliferative function of basal cells in the normal and hyperplastic human prostate. Prostate 24:114–118
15. Bonkhoff H, Stein U, Welter C, Remberger K (1995) Differential expression of the pS2 protein in the human prostate and prostate cancer: association with premalignant changes and neuroendocrine differentiation. Hum Pathol 26:824–828
16. Bonkhoff H, Stein U, Remberger K (1995) Endocrine-paracrine cell types in the prostate and prostatic adenocarcinoma are postmitotic cells. Hum Pathol 26:167–170
17. Bonkhoff H, Stein U, Aumüller G, Remberger K (1996) Differential expression of 5 α-reductase isoenzymes in the human prostate and prostatic carcinoma. Prostate 29:261–267
18. Bonkhoff H, Fixemer T, Remberger K (1998) Relation between Bcl-2, cell proliferation and the androgen receptor status in prostate tissue and precursors of prostate cancer. Prostate 1;34: 251–258
19. Bonkhoff H, Fixemer T, Hunsicker I, Remberger K (1999) Simultaneous detection of DNA fragmentation (apoptosis), cell proliferation (MIB-1), and phenotype markers in routinely processed tissue sections. Virchows Arch 434:71–73
20. Bonkhoff H, Fixemer T, Hunsicker I, Remberger K (1999) Estrogen receptor expression in prostate cancer and premalignant prostatic lesions. Am J Pathol 155:641–647
21. Bonkhoff H, Fixemer T, Hunsicker I, Remberger K (2000) Estrogen receptor gene expression and its relation to the estrogen-inducible HSP27 heat shock protein in hormone refractory prostate cancer. Prostate 45:36–41
22. Bonkhoff H, Fixemer T, Hunsicker I, Remberger K (2001) Progesterone receptor expression in human prostate cancer. Correlation with tumor progression. Prostate 15: 285-291
23. Bostwick DG (1996) Prospective origins of prostate carcinoma. Prostatic intraepithelial neoplasia and atypical adenomatous hyperplasia. Cancer 78:330–336
24. Cheng L, Shan A, Cheville JC, Qian J, Bostwick DG (1998) Atypical adenomatous hyperplasia of the prostate: a premalignant lesion? Cancer Res 1;58:389–391
25. Culig Z, Hobisch A, Bartsch G, Klocker H (2000) Androgen receptor – an update of mechanisms of action in prostate cancer. Urol Res 28:211–219
26. Di Sant'Agnese PA (1992) Neuroendocrine differentiation in carcinoma of the prostate: diagnostic, prognostic and therapeutic implications. Cancer 70:254–268
27. Di Sant'Agnese PA, Cockett AT (1996) Neuroendocrine differentiation in prostatic malignancy. Cancer 15;78:357–361
28. Fixemer T, Remberger K, Bonkhoff H Apoptotic status of neuroendocrine phenotypes in prostatic adenocarcinoma. Prostate (submitted)
29. Fong C, Sherwood E, Sutkowski D, Abu-Jawdeh G, Yokoo H, Bauer K, Kozlowski J, Lee C (1991) Reconstituted basement membrane promotes morphological and functional differentiation of primary human prostatic epithelial cells. Prostate 19:221–235
30. Foster CS, Bostwick DG, Bonkhoff H, Damber JE, van der Kwast T, Montironi R, Sakr WA (2000) Cellular and molecular pathology of prostate cancer precursors. Scand J Urol Nephrol Suppl 205:19–43
31. Knox JD, Cress AE, Clark V, Manriquez L, Affinito KS, Dalkin BL, Nagle RB (1994) Differential expression of extracellular matrix molecules and the alpha 6-integrins in the normal and neoplastic prostate. Am J Pathol 145:167–174
32. Koivisto P, Kolmer M, Visakorpi T, Kallioniemi OP (1998) Androgen receptor gene and hormonal therapy failure of prostate cancer. Am J Pathol 152:1–9
33. Montironi R, Bostwick DG, Bonkhoff H, Cockett A, Helpap B, Troncoso P, Waters D (1996) Origins of prostate cancer. Cancer 78:362–365
34. Myers RB, Grizzle WE (1996) Biomarker expression in prostatic intraepithelial neoplasia. Eur Urol 30:153–166
35. Nagle RB, Brawer MK, Kittelson J, Clark V (1991) Phenotypic relationship of prostatic intraepithelial neoplasia to invasive prostatic carcinoma. Am J Pathol 138:119–128
36. Nagle RB, Hao J, Knox JD, Dalkin BC, Clark V, Cress AE (1995) Expression of hemidesmosomal and extracellular matrix proteins by normal and malignant human prostate tissue. Am J Pathol 146:1498–1507

37. Pföhler C, Fixemer T, Jung V, Dooley S, Remberger K, Bonkhoff H (1998) In situ analysis of genes coding collagen IV a1 chain, laminin b1 chain, and S-laminin in prostate tissue and prostate cancer. Increased basement membrane gene expression in high grade and metastatic lesions. Prostate 36:143–150
38. Qian J, Jenkins RB, Bostwick DG (1998) Determination of gene and chromosome dosage in prostatic intraepithelial neoplasia and carcinoma. Anal Quant Cytol Histol 20:373–380
39. Ware JL (1994) Prostate cancer progession. Implications of histopathology. Am J Pathol 145:983–993
40. Wernert N, Seitz G, Achtstätter T (1987) Immunohistochemical investigations of different cytokeratins and vimentin in the prostate from fetal period up to adulthood and in prostate carcinoma. Pathol Res Pract 182:617–626
41. Xue Y, Smedts F, Debruyne FM, de la Rosette JJ, Schalken JA (1998) Identification of intermediate cell types by keratin expression in the developing human prostate. Prostate 34:292–301

2 Cytogenetics of Prostate Cancer

L. Bubendorf

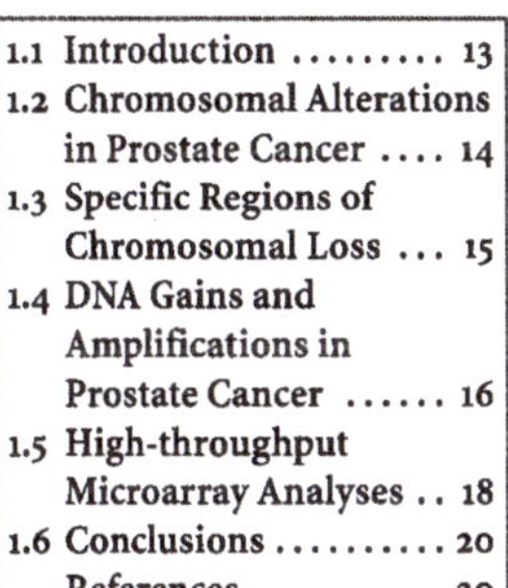

1.1 Introduction

The biological behavior of prostate cancer is highly unpredictable. While some patients die with rather than of prostate cancer, others succumb rapidly progressive disease. Although most advanced prostate cancers respond favorably to androgen withdrawal therapy, they eventually recur after a few months or years. There is still no efficient second-line therapy for recurring prostate cancer [29]. There is a need for molecular markers to better predict the biological behavior and guide therapy decisions in individual patients. Altered expression of cancer-related genes is often linked to chromosomal changes. Inactivation of tumor-suppressor genes can be associated with chromosomal deletion, whereas oncogenes are often activated through increased gene copy numbers. Therefore, the identification of chromosomal alterations can be a first step for the identification of previously unknown genes. Different techniques have been used to analyze chromosomal alterations in cancer. Conventional cytogenetic analysis always includes a short-term culturing of tumor cells, which are subsequently arrested in metaphase or prometaphase. After dropping these cells on glass slides, the chromosomes are spread and can be analyzed after Giemsa staining. Major limitations of classical cytogenetics are the need for fresh tissue and the risk of selecting non-representative clones (neoplastic or non-neoplastic) during cell culture. The simultaneous analysis of the entire genome and the ability to detect structural changes (translocations, inversions) are the strongest advantages of cytogenetics, which has recently been further improved by the ability to simultaneously identify all chromosomes in different colors [69]. This has resulted in a better understanding of the complex translocations occurring in prostate cancer cell

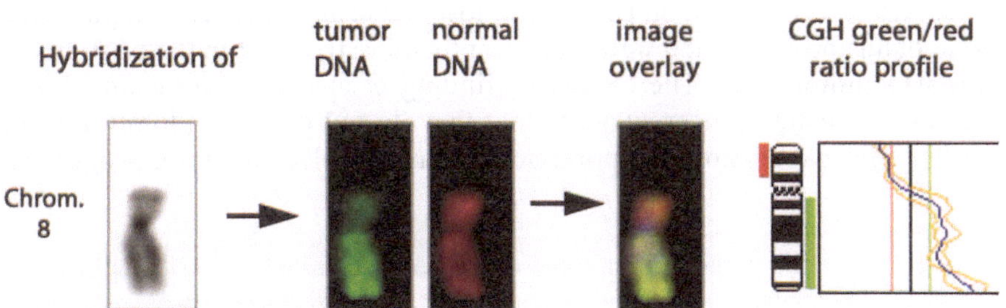

Fig. 2.1. Comparative genomic hybridization (*CGH*). Example of hybridization images and a corresponding green:red ratio profile for chromosome 8 with typical DNA sequence alterations. Tumor DNA was labeled with Spectrum green, and normal reference DNA with Spectrum Red. The mean green:red fluorescence ratio profile are shown as a *blue curve* and its standard deviation (SD) as *orange curves* . The *black vertical line* indicates the baseline ratio (1.0); the *red* and *green* vertical lines indicate the threshold ratio values of 0.8 (*red*) and 1.2 (*green*). Red bars on the left of the chromosome indicate DNA loss, and bars on the right indicate DNA gains. The profile shows loss of 8p, gain of 8q, and high-level amplification at 8q24-ter (Figure modified from [28], with permission)

lines [3]. Unfortunately, prostate cancer belongs to those tumor types that are difficult to culture. Therefore, the number of prostate cancers analyzed by cytogenetics is limited. Molecular cytogenetic techniques such as comparative genomic hybridization (CGH) and fluorescence in situ hybridization (FISH) are applicable to archival tissue and have substantially improved our understanding of the genetic changes in prostate cancer. CGH is based on the simultaneous hybridization of differentially labeled tumor and normal DNA of normal metaphase chromosomes (Fig. 2.1). CGH allows the detection of all amplifications and deletions in a single examination [26, 36]. FISH allows visualization (and therefore quantitation) of individual chromosomes and genes on a cell-by-cell basis by using chromosome-specific or locus-specific DNA probes [57, 79]. In this review, the current knowledge about chromosomal alterations in prostate cancer is summarized, and an outlook is given on the impact of new technologies that are likely to accelerate the discovery of new genes and therapeutic modalities.

1.2 Chromosomal Alterations in Prostate Cancer

Studies by CGH have shown recurrent chromosomal alterations in prostate cancer, including frequent losses of 8p, 6q, 10q, and 13q, and gains of 8q, 7q, and Xq [12, 13, 21, 28, 34, 49, 63, 65, 75]. Most of these changes have also been observed by conventional cytogenetics (http://cgap.nci.nih.gov/Chromosomes/Mitelman), although this technique has been difficult to carry out in clinical prostate cancer because of the preferential growth of non-malignant cells. In our previous CGH studies, we explored the chromosomal aberrations that occur during the progression of prostate cancer [21, 28]. Different stages of progression were analyzed in our laboratory, including 28 tumors that were still organ-confined at the time of radical prostatectomy (stage pT2), 28 tumors with infiltration of the seminal vesicles (pT3b), and 27 advanced, clinically not organ confined, mostly hormone-refractory tumors. Most of the chromosomal changes found in our studies have previously been described in prostate cancer, but were not systematically analyzed across different stages of tumor progression [2, 13, 14, 34, 49, 63, 65, 75]. Several chromosomal changes were significantly more frequent in the 27 advanced tumors as compared to our 56 clinically localized tumors (pT2-pT3b). They included loss of 6q, 8p, 10q, 13q, 16q, and 18q, and gain of 8q, suggesting that genes with a role in prostate cancer progression are located on these chromosomal arms (Table 2.1). In particular, gain of 8q and loss of 18q were significantly more frequent in the pT3b than in the pT2 tumors [28]. The consistent finding of specific chromosomal alterations in prostate cancer suggests that they do not occur randomly, but may rather reflect activation or suppression of genes involved in tumor progression.

Table 2.1. Significant chromosomal alterations during the progression of prostate cancer (CGH analysis, from [28] and [21])

	n=	6q-	8p-	8q+	10q-	13q-	16q-	18q-
pT2	28	14%	11%	0%	0%	21%	0%	4%
pT3b	28	14%	32%	18%	7%	21%	4%	21%
hr recurr.	27	48%	52%	48%	19%	52%	26%	37%
P-value		0.004	0.0045	0.0001	0.045	0.02	0.002	0.009

hr recurr., hormone-refractory local recurrences.

1.3 Specific Regions of Chromosomal Loss

Given the low resolution of CGH and the fact that each chromosome contains approximately 1,500 genes on average, it is almost impossible to identify individual target genes based on gross chromosomal alterations. The identification of target genes based on chromosomal gains or losses is greatly facilitated in case of small overlapping regions of gains or deletions after analysis of many different tumors. Techniques of mapping discrete loci of allelic imbalance include loss of heterozygosity (LOH) analysis and FISH. LOH or FISH studies often show a higher prevalence of specific alterations than expected from CGH studies. An underestimate of specific DNA copy number changes by CGH can be explained by the limited resolution of CGH, which precludes the identification of short deletions and gains (<5–10 Mb).

1.3.1 Loss of Chromosome 8p

Loss of 8p is one of the most frequent chromosomal alterations in prostate cancer and has been narrowed down by FISH and LOH analysis to a preferentially deleted region encompassing 8p21-p22. Loss of 8p21-p22 has been found in up to 86% of prostate cancers and was associated with advanced disease and adverse prognosis [32, 35, 51, 77]. Identification of separate discrete regions of loss suggests the presence of at least two different tumor-suppressor genes on 8p21-p22 [35, 77]. Loss of 8p21 was not only found in advanced tumors but also in a subset of high-grade prostatic intraepithelial neoplasia (PIN) [23], indicating that 8p loss is not only important for tumor progression, but is also associated with early development of prostate cancer. We recently found that NKX3.1, a prostate-specific gene with growth suppressing effects, might be one of the tumor-suppressor genes at 8p21, since its expression is frequently lost in advanced prostate cancer [6].

1.3.2 Loss of Chromosome 10q

Deletion of 10q was found in up to 40% of advanced prostate cancers by CGH [21, 49]. Phosphatase and tensin homologue, mutated in multiple advanced cancers 1 (PTEN/MMAC1) at 10q23.3 has been suggested as a target tumor-suppressor gene on 10q. PTEN/MMAC1 is lost and/or mutated in up to 60% of advanced prostate cancers [11, 76], and loss of protein expression is associated with a high Gleason score and an advanced pathological stage [45]. MAX-interacting protein 1 (MXI1) is another putative tumor-suppressor gene that is frequently lost and mutated in prostate cancers showing 10q deletions [60]. MXI1, which is located telomeric to PTEN/MMAC1 at 10q24-q25, negatively regulates MYC oncoprotein activity, further supporting its tumor-suppressor function.

1.3.3 Loss of Chromosomes 6q, 13q, 16q, and 18q

Deletions of *chromosome 6q* are more prevalent in advanced than in clinically localized tumors (48% versus 14%, respectively), suggesting that it contains genes that are associated with tumor progression [21, 28]. A minimal overlapping region has been located at 6q14-q16 [2, 14, 16, 21, 28, 49, 63, 65, 71, 75], but no candidate tumor-suppressor genes have been identified so far.

Chromosome 13q is a frequently deleted region in prostate cancer using CGH (20%–70%) [2, 13, 14, 21, 49, 63, 65, 75]. Several deleted regions have been identified on 13q by LOH studies, including 13q14 and 13q21-q22, which were preferentially altered in metastatic lesions [19, 31]. Deletions on 13q have been shown to involve the retinoblastoma (Rb) gene and the BRCA-2 locus [46]. However, the biological role of Rb or BRCA2 in prostate cancer has not yet been determined, and other genes on 13q may be more important targets [40, 42].

Deletion of *chromosome 16q* has been found in a high fraction of advanced tumors including local recurrences and distant metastases. DNA sequences on 16q23-q24 were lost in up to 83% of metastases [21, 22, 39, 43], and loss of 16q24 was also shown to be a predictor of poor patient survival [22]. Introduction of human chromosome 16 into the highly metastatic Dunning rat prostate cancer cell line led to a markedly decreased metastatic ability of the resultant hybrid clones, further emphasizing an important role of genes on 16q for metastasis formation in prostate cancer [44]. Although decreased protein expression of the E-cadherin gene at 16q22.1 is associated with invasion and metastasis in prostate cancer [18, 62], E-cadherin does not map to the most commonly deleted regions, suggesting other genes on 16q23-q24 as the frequent targets of deletions in prostate cancer [43].

Loss of *chromosome 18q* has been found in 19%–45% of prostate cancers by CGH and was associated with an advanced tumor stage [21, 28, 32, 73, 75]. The most commonly deleted region locates to 18q21.1 [73], but the tumor-suppressor gene(s) on 18q in prostate cancer also remain unknown [52].

1.4 DNA Gains and Amplifications in Prostate Cancer

It has been shown that low-level copy number gains of whole chromosome arms can lead to an increased expression of a high number of different genes [24, 30]. It is unclear, however, whether and, if so, to what extent such gene overexpression provides a growth advantage to affected cells. The impact of high-level amplifications is more obvious. High-level amplifications, which represent narrow chromosomal regions with a highly increased copy number of DNA sequences (at least three-fold), often lead to a dramatic overexpression of genes within the amplified region. Amplified and overexpressed genes can result in a growth advantage of affected tumor cell clones that eventually determine the biological behavior of the tumor. High-level gene amplifications are rare in primary prostate cancer, but have been reported in advanced tumors. Amplification sites that have been found in prostate cancer are listed in Table 2.2.

Table 2.2. Sites of amplifications in prostate cancer and methods used for detection

Technique	Amplification sites (target genes)	References
Southern Blot	INT2/FGF3	[27]
Comparative PCR	SOX2, IL12 A, SLCA2, MDS1	[66]
FISH	AR, MYC, PSCA, eIF3, CCND1	[9, 33, 50, 61, 64, 74]
CGH	1q21–25, 8q21, 10q22, 14q12–24, 17q24	[5, 21, 54]

PCR, polymerase chain reaction; FISH, fluorescence in situ hybridization; CGH, comparative genomic hybridization.

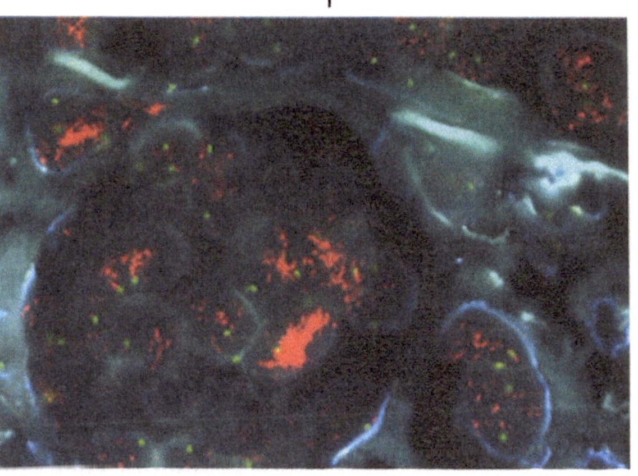

Fig. 2.2. Hormone-refractory prostate cancer with androgen receptor (AR) amplification by fluorescence in situ hybridization (magnification × 630). Many clustered AR gene signals (*red*) as compared to few centromere X reference signals (*green*)

The most frequent high-level amplification in prostate cancer was found at Xq11.2–12 [21, 49, 75]. This amplification is present in 20%–30% of hormone-refractory prostate cancers and has never been described in any tumor type other than prostate cancer. The androgen receptor (AR) gene has been identified as the most likely target of this amplification by FISH [9, 37, 74] (Fig. 2.2). AR-amplified tumor cells may become hypersensitive after androgen withdrawal to the remaining low levels of androgen and thereby retain AR-mediated growth signaling. Accordingly, AR-amplified hormone-refractory prostate cancers have been shown to better respond to second-line total androgen blockage than tumors without AR amplification [53]. Other amplifications are less frequent in prostate cancer. However, amplified genes detected in only a small fraction of tumors or in individual tumors may be overexpressed in a much larger fraction of tumors through alternative mechanisms of activation (e.g., mutation, translocation, or posttranslational activation). Even oncogenes that are overexpressed in a small fraction of patients may be clinically relevant, if they can be used as a target for new efficient therapies.

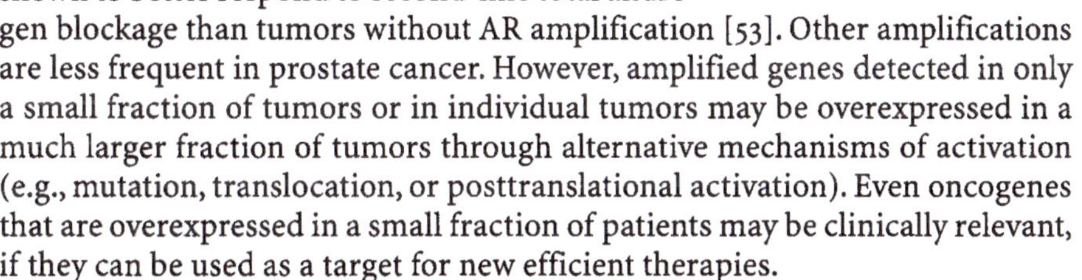

Gain of DNA sequences on *chromosome 8q* is among the most frequent alterations in prostate cancer. The presence of different amplified loci and regional gains suggests that chromosome 8q contains several oncogenes with a role in prostate cancer. MYC is one of the target genes of an amplification at 8q24, which is often present in advanced prostate cancers [33]. MYC amplification has preferentially been found in metastases, suggesting a role in their formation [9, 33]. Other putative oncogenes on 8q include the p40 subunit of eukaryotic translation initiation factor 3 (eIF3) at 8q23 [50] and the prostate stem cell antigen (PSCA) at 8q24 [61], both of which are frequently coamplified with MYC. A frequent minimal overlapping region of DNA sequence copy number gain on 8q was located on 8q21 [13, 21, 49, 65]. Since amplifications were also found at 8q21 in hormone-refractory local recurrences, this site may contain important target gene(s) for prostate cancer progression [21, 49]. Amplifications or regional gains at 8q21 have also been observed in other tumor types such as breast cancer [25], where the transcription factor E2F5 and the tumor protein D52 (TPD52) gene at 8q21 have both been suggested as possible amplification targets [4, 58].

We found regional gain or amplification at *11q13* in 15% of 27 advanced prostate cancers by CGH [21]. Cyclin D1 is the most likely target gene on 11q13. In a previous FISH study with locus specific probes, cyclin D1 amplification was found in a small subfraction of 371 specimens (5%) on a prostate cancer tissue microarray [9]. The biological significance of cyclin D1 amplification in prostate cancer remains to be determined, as well as the role of other possible target genes on 11q13 such as fibroblast growth factor 4 (FGF4) or fibroblast growth factor 3 (FGF3) [27, 41].

The high frequency of amplifications of the *HER2/ERBB2 gene at 17q12* in prostate cancer reported by one group [64] is controversial and has not been confirmed by others [9, 27, 68, 70]. Although HER2 amplifications are unlikely to occur in prostate cancer, Her-2 protein overexpression through other mechanisms than amplification may still be important [17, 67, 70]. Her-2 overexpression has been implicated in the activation of the androgen receptor and in the development of hormone-refractory growth of prostate cancer [17, 70, 78]. Metastatic breast cancers with amplification and overexpression of HER2 respond to treatment with trastuzumab (Herceptin), a therapeutic antibody that is directed against the Her-2 protein [55]. It remains to be shown if the experimental evidence of favorable response of prostate cancer xenograft models holds true in clinical prostate cancers [1]. In our experience, prostate cancers not only lack HER2 amplification, but are also negative with the FDA approved HercepTest kit (Dako, Inc.). The HercepTest has been designed to detect the high levels of Her-2 expression that are required for responsiveness to Herceptin therapy in breast cancer. It is therefore possible that the expression of Her-2 in prostate cancer may not reach the levels that are required for therapy response. This could also explain the lack of objective responses of prostate cancers to Herceptin in a preliminary analysis of an ongoing clinical trial [47].

We also found amplifications at *1q21–25* (3/27 tumors), *10q22*, and *17q24* (2/27 tumors, each) in advanced, mostly hormone-refractory prostate cancers by CGH [21]. These amplification sites have not yet been described in clinical prostate cancer, and the target genes at these loci are unknown. Interestingly, the amplification at 10q22 is also present in the hormone-insensitive prostate cancer cell line PC-3 [5, 54], suggesting that genes involved in hormone-refractory growth may reside at this location.

There is growing evidence that the simple one gene-one amplicon concept does not accurately reflect the biology of tumor progression. Amplification may be a mechanism that is particularly effective in simultaneously overexpressing multiple adjacent genes which may jointly provide a growth advantage to amplified tumor cells [15]. Therefore, rather than exploring one gene at a time, looking at a high number of genes simultaneously increases the chance of finding the relevant target genes within chromosomal regions of interest.

1.5 High-throughput Microarray Analyses

New high-throughput microarray technologies – together with publicly available human genome resources – make it now possible to gain a comprehensive insight into the molecular basis of human diseases, including prostate cancer [7, 80]. The search for genes that are differentially expressed in tumors has been greatly facilitated by the cDNA microarray technology [20]. In cDNA microarray technology, the RNA expression level of hundreds or thousands of genes in a tumor can be surveyed simultaneously. This approach also greatly enhances the chance to identify jointly overexpressed amplification target genes. Furthermore, the same microarrays that are used for expression analyses can also be applied for high resolution analysis of DNA copy numbers on a gene by gene basis, thus allowing a high-resolution analysis of DNA amplifications, which cannot be achieved by traditional CGH because of its limited resolution [59].

To explore the prevalence and clinicopathological associations of molecular alterations such as amplifications, a high number of tumors across various stages of progression need to be analyzed. However, traditional FISH is both labor and cost intensive, making large-scale studies difficult. To facilitate large-scale molecular analyses in hundreds of tumors simultaneously, we have recently developed the tissue microarray (TMA) technology [38]. To construct a tissue microarray, cylinders of tumor tissues measuring 0.6 mm in diameter are punched out of tumor blocks and placed in a defined order in a premade hole in a new “recipient” paraffin block. As a result, defined specimens of as many as 1000 different tumors can be put into one array. These 1000 tumors

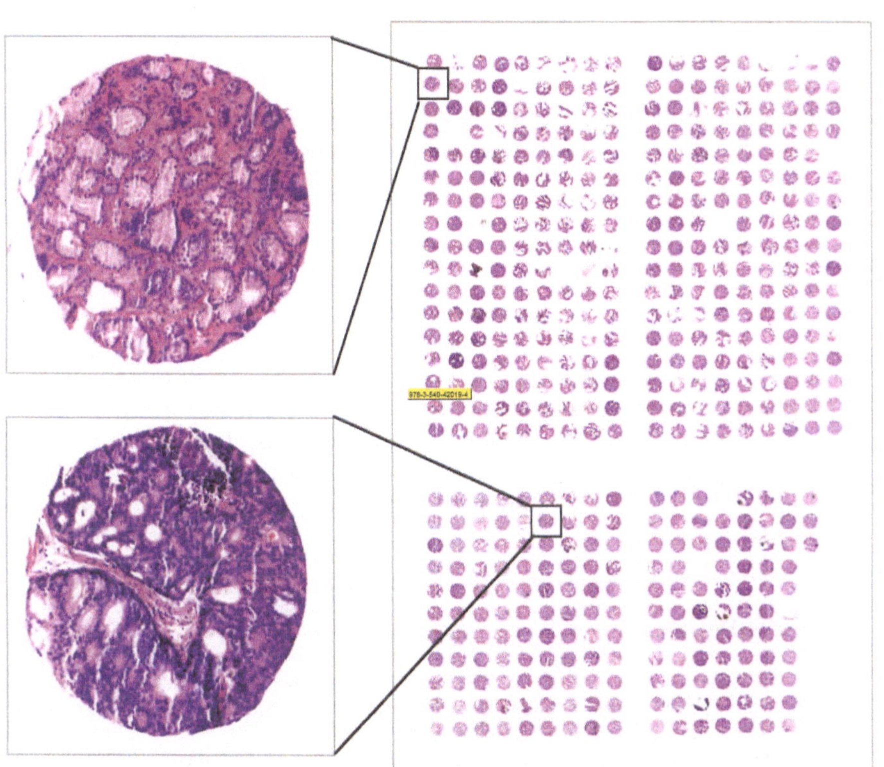

Fig. 2.3.
Section of a prostate cancer tissue microarray containing specimens from 485 tumors and benign controls (hematoxylin-eosin staining)

can then be simultaneously analyzed by immunohistochemistry, RNA in situ hybridization (mRNA ISH) or FISH on consecutive sections. TMAs have many advantages [10]. Importantly, TMAs do not only facilitate efficient large-scale studies, but also preserve precious tissue blocks that would otherwise be used up after only a few studies. Several types of prostate TMAs have been constructed so far. For example, we have generated a prostate progression TMA with >350 specimens across all stages of progression, including benign controls, PIN, primary localized and advanced cancers, hormone-refractory local recurrences, and distant metastases (Fig. 2.3).

Prostate TMAs have already been successfully applied in a number of studies and are likely to become an important standard tool with which to screen for the prevalence and clinical importance of new genes [6, 8, 9, 48, 56, 72]. For example, we used the TMA technology to survey gene amplification during the progression of prostate cancer. Fluorescent probes for five genes, including AR, MYC, Cyclin D1, HER2, and N-MYC, together with the corresponding centromeric probes were applied [9]. High-level amplifications of all of the tested loci were very rare in primary prostate cancer (<2%). In contrast, amplifications were substantially more prevalent in samples from hormone-refractory locally recurrent tumors and metastases. AR amplification was as common in distant metastatic deposits as in local recurrences (22% vs. 23%). In contrast, MYC was more frequently amplified in metastases, supporting its role for metastatic capability in prostate cancer [33]. In addition, we found that also Cyclin D1 can occasionally be amplified in prostate cancer. HER2 and N-MYC amplifications were never detected at any stage of prostate cancer progression and are therefore unlikely to play a significant role in prostate cancer. This example illustrates how one can rapidly explore the prevalence of molecular alterations in a high number of tumors across all stages of progression and establish clinical correlations using TMAs.

1.6 Conclusions

Several non-random chromosomal changes occur during the progression of prostate cancer. This includes frequent loss of regions on 8p, 13q, 16q, and 18q, and gain of regions on 8q, suggesting that genes important for prostate cancer reside in these chromosomal regions. DNA amplifications, which are most likely to contain oncogenes with a profound effect on tumor biology, are preferentially found in advanced prostate cancers. AR amplification at Xq11.2–12 has been identified as a possible mechanism of hormone-refractory growth in a fraction of prostate cancers, but the target genes of other amplifications that have been found at 1q21-q25, 8q21, 10q22, and 17q14 are still unknown. High-throughput microarray technologies such as cDNA microarrays and TMAs are likely to markedly facilitate the identification of critical candidate genes and pathways in prostate cancer, and may thus accelerate the translation of genomic findings to new predictors of prognosis or therapy response, or new therapeutic targets.

References

1. Agus DB, Scher HI, Higgins B, Fox WD, Heller G, Fazzari M, Cordon-Cardo C, Golde DW (1999) Response of prostate cancer to anti-Her-2/neu antibody in androgen-dependent and -independent human xenograft models. Cancer Res 59:4761–4764
2. Alers JC, Krijtenburg PJ, Vis AN, Hoedemaeker RF, Wildhagen MF, Hop WC, van Der Kwast TH, Schroder FH, Tanke HJ, van Dekken H (2001) Molecular cytogenetic analysis of prostatic adenocarcinomas from screening studies: early cancers may contain aggressive genetic features. Am J Pathol 158:399–406
3. Aurich-Costa J, Vannier A, Gregoire E, Nowak F, Cherif D (2001) IPM-FISH, a new M-FISH approach using IRS-PCR painting probes: application to the analysis of seven human prostate cell lines. Genes Chromosomes Cancer 30:143–160
4. Balleine RL, Fejzo MS, Sathasivam P, Basset P, Clarke CL, Byrne JA (2000) The hD52 (TPD52) gene is a candidate target gene for events resulting in increased 8q21 copy number in human breast carcinoma. Genes Chromosomes Cancer 29:48–57
5. Bernardino J, Bourgeois CA, Muleris M, Dutrillaux AM, Malfoy B, Dutrillaux B (1997) Characterization of chromosome changes in two human prostatic carcinoma cell lines (PC-3 and DU145) using chromosome painting and comparative genomic hybridization. Cancer Genet Cytogenet 96:123–128
6. Bowen C, Bubendorf L, Voeller HJ, Slack R, Willi N, Sauter G, Gasser TC, Koivisto P, Lack EE, Kononen J, Kallioniemi OP, Gelmann EP (2000) Loss of NKX3.1 expression in human prostate cancers correlates with tumor progression. Cancer Res 60:6111–6115
7. Bubendorf L (2001) High-throughput microarray technologies-from genomics to clinics. Eur Urol 40:231–238
8. Bubendorf L, Kolmer M, Kononen J, Koivisto P, Mousses S, Chen Y, Mahlamaki E, Schraml P, Moch H, Willi N, Elkahloun AG, Pretlow TG, Gasser TC, Mihatsch MJ, Sauter G, Kallioniemi OP (1999) Hormone therapy failure in human prostate cancer: analysis by complementary DNA and tissue microarrays. J Natl Cancer Inst 91:1758–1764
9. Bubendorf L, Kononen J, Koivisto P, Schraml P, Moch H, Gasser TC, Willi N, Mihatsch MJ, Sauter G, Kallioniemi OP (1999) Survey of gene amplifications during prostate cancer progression by high-throughput fluorescence in situ hybridisation on tissue microarrays. Cancer Res 59:803–806
10. Bubendorf L, Nocito A, Moch H, Kononen J, Kallioniemi OP, Sauter G (2001) Tissue microarray technology: miniaturized pathology archives for high-throughput research. J Pathol 195: 72–79
11. Cairns P, Okami K, Halachmi S, Halachmi N, Esteller M, Herman JG, Jen J, Isaacs WB, Bova GS, Sidransky D (1997) Frequent inactivation of PTEN/MMAC1 in primary prostate cancer. Cancer Res 57:4997–5000
12. Cher ML, MacGrogan D, Bookstein R, Brown JA, Jenkins RB, Jensen RH (1994) Comparative genomic hybridization, allelic imbalance, and fluorescence in situ hybridization on chromosome 8 in prostate cancer. Genes Chromosomes Cancer 11:153–162
13. Cher ML, Bova GS, Moore DH, Small EJ, Carroll PR, Pin SS, Epstein JI, Isaacs WB, Jensen RH (1996) Genetic alterations in untreated metastases and androgen-independent prostate cancer detected by comparative genomic hybridization and allelotyping. Cancer Res 56:3091–3102

14. Cher ML, Lewis PE, Banerjee M, Hurley PM, Sakr W, Grignon DJ, Isaac JP (1998) A similar pattern of chromosomal alterations in prostate cancers from African-Americans and Caucasian Americans. Clin Cancer Res 4:1273–1278
15. Cohen BA, Mitra RD, Hughes JD, Church GM (2000) A computational analysis of whole-genome expression data reveals chromosomal domains of gene expression. Nat Genet 26: 183–186
16. Cooney KA, Wetzel JC, Consolino CM, Wojno KJ (1996) Identification and characterization of proximal 6q deletions in prostate cancer. Cancer Res 56:4150–4153
17. Craft N, Shostak Y, Carey M, Sawyers CL (1999) A mechanism for hormone-independent prostate cancer through modulation of androgen receptor signaling by the HER-2/neu tyrosine kinase. Nat Med 5:280–285
18. De Marzo AM, Knudsen B, Chan-Tack K, Epstein JI (1999) E-cadherin expression as a marker of tumor aggressiveness in routinely processed radical prostatectomy specimens. Urology 53: 707–713
19. Dong JT, Chen C, Stultz BG, Isaacs JT, Frierson HF (2000) Deletion at 13q21 is associated with aggressive prostate cancers. Cancer Res 60:3880–3883
20. Duggan DJ, Bittner M, Chen Y, Meltzer P, Trent JM (1999) Expression profiling using cDNA microarrays. Nat Genet 21:10–14
21. ElGedaily A, Bubendorf L, Willi N, Fu W, Richter J, Moch H, Mihatsch MJ, Sauter G, Gasser TC (2001) Discovery of new amplification loci in prostate cancer by comparative genomic hybridization. Prostate 46:184–190
22. Elo JP, Harkonen P, Kyllonen AP, Lukkarinen O, Vihko P (1999) Three independently deleted regions at chromosome arm 16q in human prostate cancer: allelic loss at 16q24.1-q24.2 is associated with aggressive behaviour of the disease, recurrent growth, poor differentiation of the tumour and poor prognosis for the patient. Br J Cancer 79:156–160
23. Emmert-Buck MR, Vocke CD, Pozzatti RO, Duray PH, Jennings SB, Florence CD, Zhuang Z, Bostwick DG, Liotta LA, Linehan WM (1995) Allelic loss on chromosome 8p12–21 in microdissected prostatic intraepithelial neoplasia. Cancer Res 55:2959–2962
24. Epstein CJ, Epstein LB, Cox DR, Weil J (1981) Functional implications of gene dosage effects in trisomy 21. Hum Genet Suppl 2:155–172
25. Fejzo MS, Godfrey T, Chen C, Waldman F, Gray JW (1998) Molecular cytogenetic analysis of consistent abnormalities at 8q12-q22 in breast cancer. Genes Chromosomes Cancer 22:105–113
26. Forozan F, Karhu R, Kononen J, Kallioniemi A, Kallioniemi OP (1997) Genome screening by comparative genomic hybridization. Trends Genet 13:405–409
27. Fournier G, Latil A, Amet Y, Abalain JH, Volant A, Mangin P, Floch HH, Lidereau R (1995) Gene amplifications in advanced-stage human prostate cancer. Urol Res 22:343–347
28. Fu W, Bubendorf L, Willi N, Moch H, Mihatsch MJ, Sauter G, Gasser TC (2000) Genetic changes in clinically organ-confined prostate cancer by comparative genomic hybridization. Urology 56:880–885
29. Heidenreich A, von Knobloch R, Hofmann R (2001) Current status of cytotoxic chemotherapy in hormone refractory prostate cancer. Eur Urol 39:121–130
30. Hughes TR, Roberts CJ, Dai H, Jones AR, Meyer MR, Slade D, Burchard J, Dow S, Ward TR, Kidd MJ, Friend SH, Marton MJ (2000) Widespread aneuploidy revealed by DNA microarray expression profiling. Nat Genet 25:333–337
31. Hyytinen ER, Frierson HF Jr, Boyd JC, Chung LW, Dong JT (1999) Three distinct regions of allelic loss at 13q14, 13q21–22, and 13q33 in prostate cancer. Genes Chromosomes Cancer 25:108– 114
32. Jenkins R, Takahashi S, DeLacey K, Bergstralh E, Lieber M (1998) Prognostic significance of allelic imbalance of chromosome arms 7q, 8p, 16q, and 18q in stage T3N0M0 prostate cancer. Genes Chromosomes Cancer 21:131–143
33. Jenkins RB, Qian J, Lieber MM, Bostwick DG (1997) Detection of c-myc oncogene amplification and chromosomal anomalies in metastatic prostatic carcinoma by fluorescence in situ hybridization. Cancer Res 57:524–531
34. Joos S, Bergerheim US, Pan Y, Matsuyama H, Bentz M, du MS, Lichter P (1995) Mapping of chromosomal gains and losses in prostate cancer by comparative genomic hybridization. Genes Chromosomes Cancer 14:267–276
35. Kagan J, Stein J, Babaian RJ, Joe YS, Pisters LL, Glassman AB, von Eschenbach AC, Troncoso P (1995) Homozygous deletions at 8p22 and 8p21 in prostate cancer implicate these regions as the sites for candidate tumor suppressor genes. Oncogene 11:2121–2126
36. Kallioniemi A, Kallioniemi OP, Sudar D, Rutovitz D, Gray JW, Waldman F, Pinkel D (1992) Comparative genomic hybridization for molecular cytogenetic analysis of solid tumors. Science 258:818–821
37. Kaltz-Wittmer C, Klenk U, Glaessgen A, Aust DE, Diebold J, Lohrs U, Baretton GB (2000) FISH analysis of gene aberrations (MYC, CCND1, ERBB2, RB, and AR) in advanced prostatic carcinomas before and after androgen deprivation therapy. Lab Invest 80:1455–1464
38. Kononen J, Bubendorf L, Kallioniemi A, Barlund M, Schraml P, Leighton S, Torhorst J, Mihatsch MJ, Sauter G, Kallioniemi OP (1998) Tissue microarrays for high-throughput molecular profiling of tumor specimens. Nat Med 4:844–847

39. Latil A, Cussenot O, Fournier G, Driouch K, Lidereau R (1997) Loss of heterozygosity at chromosome 16q in prostate adenocarcinoma: identification of three independent regions. Cancer Res 57:1058–1062
40. Latil A, Bieche I, Pesche S, Volant A, Valeri A, Fournier G, Cussenot O, Lidereau R (1999) Loss of heterozygosity at chromosome arm 13q and RB1 status in human prostate cancer. Hum Pathol 30:809–815
41. Lese CM, Rossie KM, Appel BN, Reddy JK, Johnson JT, Myers EN, Gollin SM (1995) Visualization of INT2 and HST1 amplification in oral squamous cell carcinomas. Genes Chromosomes Cancer 12:288–295
42. Li C, Larsson C, Futreal A, Lancaster J, Phelan C, Aspenblad U, Sundelin B, Liu Y, Ekman P, Auer G, Bergerheim US (1998) Identification of two distinct deleted regions on chromosome 13 in prostate cancer. Oncogene 16:481–487
43. Li C, Berx G, Larsson C, Auer G, Aspenblad U, Pan Y, Sundelin B, Ekman P, Nordenskjold M, van Roy F, Bergerheim US (1999) Distinct deleted regions on chromosome segment 16q23–24 associated with metastases in prostate cancer. Genes Chromosomes Cancer 24:175–182
44. Mashimo T, Watabe M, Cuthbert AP, Newbold RF, Rinker-Schaeffer CW, Helfer E, Watabe K (1998) Human chromosome 16 suppresses metastasis but not tumorigenesis in rat prostatic tumor cells. Cancer Res 58:4572–4576
45. McMenamin ME, Soung P, Perera S, Kaplan I, Loda M, Sellers WR (1999) Loss of PTEN expression in paraffin-embedded primary prostate cancer correlates with high Gleason score and advanced stage. Cancer Res 59:4291–4296
46. Melamed J, Einhorn JM, Ittmann MM (1997) Allelic loss on chromosome 13q in human prostate carcinoma. Clin Cancer Res 3:1867–1872
47. Morris MJ, Reuter VE, Kelly WK, Slovin SF, Kenneson KI, Osman I, Agus D, Scher HI (2000) A phase II trial of herceptin alone and with taxol for the treatment of prostate cancer [abstract]. Proc ASCO 19:330
48. Mucci NR, Akdas G, Manely S, Rubin MA (2000) Neuroendocrine expression in metastatic prostate cancer: evaluation of high throughput tissue microarrays to detect heterogeneous protein expression. Hum Pathol 31:406–414
49. Nupponen NN, Kakkola L, Koivisto P, Visakorpi T (1998) Genetic alterations in hormone-refractory recurrent prostate carcinomas. Am J Pathol 153:141–148
50. Nupponen NN, Porkka K, Kakkola L, Tanner M, Persson K, Borg A, Isola J, Visakorpi T (1999) Amplification and overexpression of p40 subunit of eukaryotic translation initiation factor 3 in breast and prostate cancer. Am J Pathol 154:1777–1783
51. Oba K, Matsuyama H, Yoshihiro S, Kishi F, Takahashi M, Tsukamoto M, Kinjo M, Sagiyama K, Naito K (2001) Two putative tumor suppressor genes on chromosome arm 8p may play different roles in prostate cancer. Cancer Genet Cytogenet 124:20–26
52. Padalecki SS, Troyer DA, Hansen MF, Saric T, Schneider BG, O'Connell P, Leach RJ (2000) Identification of two distinct regions of allelic imbalance on chromosome 18q in metastatic prostate cancer. Int J Cancer 85:654–658
53. Palmberg C, Koivisto P, Kakkola L, Tammela TL, Kallioniemi OP, Visakorpi T (2000) Androgen receptor gene amplification at primary progression predicts response to combined androgen blockade as second line therapy for advanced prostate cancer. J Urol 164:1992–1995
54. Pan Y, Lui WO, Nupponen N, Larsson C, Ji, Visakorpi T, Bergerheim US, Kytola S (2001) 5q11, 8p11, and 10q22 are recurrent chromosomal breakpoints in prostate cancer cell lines. Genes Chromosomes Cancer 30:187–195
55. Pegram M, Slamon D (2000) Biological rationale for HER2/neu (c-erbB2) as a target for monoclonal antibody therapy. Semin Oncol 27:13–19
56. Perrone EE, Theoharis C, Mucci NR, Hayasaka S, Taylor JM, Cooney KA, Rubin MA (2000) Tissue microarray assessment of prostate cancer tumor proliferation in African-American and white men. J Natl Cancer Inst 92:937–939
57. Pinkel D, Andreev M (eds) (1999) An introduction to fluorescence in situ hybridization. Wiley, New York
58. Polanowska J, Le Cam L, Orsetti B, Valles H, Fabbrizio E, Fajas L, Taviaux S, Theillet C, Sardet C (2000) Human E2F5 gene is oncogenic in primary rodent cells and is amplified in human breast tumors. Genes Chromosomes Cancer 28:126–130
59. Pollack JR, Perou CM, Alizadeh AA, Eisen MB, Pergamenschikov A, Williams CF, Jeffrey SS, Botstein D, Brown PO (1999) Genome-wide analysis of DNA copy-number changes using cDNA microarrays. Nat Genet 23:41–46
60. Prochownik EV, Eagle Grove L, Deubler D, Zhu XL, Stephenson RA, Rohr LR, Yin X, Brothman AR (1998) Commonly occurring loss and mutation of the MXI1 gene in prostate cancer. Genes Chromosomes Cancer 22:295–304
61. Reiter RE, Sato I, Thomas G, Qian J, Gu Z, Watabe T, Loda M, Jenkins RB (2000) Coamplification of prostate stem cell antigen (PSCA) and MYC in locally advanced prostate cancer. Genes Chromosomes Cancer 27:95–103
62. Richmond PJ, Karayiannakis AJ, Nagafuchi A, Kaisary AV, Pignatelli M (1997) Aberrant E-cadherin and alpha-catenin expression in prostate cancer: correlation with patient survival. Cancer Res 57:3189–3193

63. Rokman A, Koivisto PA, Matikainen MP, Kuukasjarvi T, Poutiainen M, Helin HJ, Karhu R, Kallioniemi OP, Schleutker J (2001) Genetic changes in familial prostate cancer by comparative genomic hybridization. Prostate 46:233–239
64. Ross JS, Sheehan C, Hayner BA, Ambros RA, Kallakury BV, Kaufman R, Fisher HA, Muraca PJ (1997) HER-2/neu gene amplification status in prostate cancer by fluorescence in situ hybridization. Hum Pathol 28:827–833
65. Sattler HP, Rohde V, Bonkhoff H, Zwergel T, Wullich B (1999) Comparative genomic hybridization reveals DNA copy number gains to frequently occur in human prostate cancer. Prostate 39:79–86
66. Sattler HP, Lensch R, Rohde V, Zimmer E, Meese E, Bonkhoff H, Retz M, Zwergel T, Bex A, Stoeckle M, Wullich B (2000) Novel amplification unit at chromosome 3q25-q27 in human prostate cancer. Prostate 45:207–215
67. Scher HI (2000) HER2 in prostate cancer – a viable target or innocent bystander? J Natl Cancer Inst 92:1866–1868
68. Schraml P, Kononen J, Bubendorf L, Moch H, Bissig H, Nocito A, Mihatsch MJ, Kallioniemi OP, Sauter G (1999) Tissue microarrays for gene amplification surveys in many different tumor types. Clin Cancer Res 5:1966–1975
69. Schrock E, Padilla-Nash H (2000) Spectral karyotyping and multicolor fluorescence in situ hybridization reveal new tumor-specific chromosomal aberrations. Semin Hematol 37:334–347
70. Signoretti S, Montironi R, Manola J, Altimari A, Tam C, Bubley G, Balk S, Thomas G, Kaplan I, Hlatky L, Hahnfeldt P, Kantoff P, Loda M (2000) Her-2-neu expression and progression toward androgen independence in human prostate cancer. J Natl Cancer Inst 92:1918–1925
71. Srikantan V, Sesterhenn IA, Davis L, Hankins GR, Avallone FA, Livezey JR, Connelly R, Mostofi FK, McLeod DG, Moul JW, Chandrasekharappa SC, Srivastava S (1999) Allelic loss on chromosome 6Q in primary prostate cancer. Int J Cancer 84:331–335
72. Srivastava M, Bubendorf L, Srikantan V, Fossom L, Nolan L, Glasman M, Leighton X, Fehrle W, Pittaluga S, Raffeld M, Koivisto P, Willi N, Gasser TC, Kononen J, Sauter G, Kallioniemi OP, Srivastava S, Pollard HP (2001) ANX7, a candidate tumor suppressor gene for prostate cancer. Proc Nat Acad Sci 98:4575–4580
73. Ueda T, Komiya A, Emi M, Suzuki H, Shiraishi T, Yatani R, Masai M, Yasuda K, Ito H (1997) Allelic losses on 18q21 are associated with progression and metastasis in human prostate cancer. Genes Chromosomes Cancer 20:140–147
74. Visakorpi T, Hyytinen E, Koivisto P, Tanner M, Keinanen R, Palmberg C, Palotie A, Tammela T, Isola J, Kallioniemi OP (1995) In vivo amplification of the androgen receptor gene and progression of human prostate cancer. Nat Genet 9:401–406
75. Visakorpi T, Kallioniemi AH, Syvanen AC, Hyytinen ER, Karhu R, Tammela T, Isola JJ, Kallioniemi OP (1995) Genetic changes in primary and recurrent prostate cancer by comparative genomic hybridization. Cancer Res 55:342–347
76. Vlietstra RJ, van Alewijk DC, Hermans KG, van Steenbrugge GJ, Trapman J (1998) Frequent inactivation of PTEN in prostate cancer cell lines and xenografts. Cancer Res 58:2720–2723
77. Vocke CD, Pozzatti RO, Bostwick DG, Florence CD, Jennings SB, Strup SE, Duray PH, Liotta LA, Emmert BM, Linehan WM (1996) Analysis of 99 microdissected prostate carcinomas reveals a high frequency of allelic loss on chromosome 8p12–21. Cancer Res 56:2411–2416
78. Wen Y, Hu MC, Makino K, Spohn B, Bartholomeusz G, Yan DH, Hung MC (2000) HER-2/neu promotes androgen-independent survival and growth of prostate cancer cells through the Akt pathway. Cancer Res 60:6841–6845
79. Werner M, Wilkens L, Aubele M, Nolte M, Zitzelsberger H, Komminoth P (1997) Interphase cytogenetics in pathology: principles, methods, and applications of fluorescence in situ hybridization (FISH). Histochem Cell Biol 108:381–390
80. Wheeler DL, Church DM, Lash AE, Leipe DD, Madden TL, Pontius JU, Schuler GD, Schriml LM, Tatusova TA, Wagner L, Rapp BA (2001) Database resources of the National Center for Biotechnology Information. Nucleic Acids Res 29:11–16

3 Molecular Dissection of the Prostate Cancer Genome

V. Srikantan, S. Srivastava

3.1 Introduction

Prostate cancer (CaP) is the most common solid malignant tumor in American males [88]. The wide spectrum of biologic behavior [116] exhibited by prostatic neoplasms poses the difficulty of predicting the clinical course in the individual patient [73, 80]. Because of increasing public awareness and screening efforts, the enhanced incidence has translated into a large increase in the use of radical prostatectomy as well as four other treatment modalities for localized disease [89]. With this huge rise in surgical intervention, a frustrating realization of the inability to predict organ-confined disease and clinical outcome for a given patient [89, 119] has emerged. Traditional prognostic markers such as grade, clinical stage, and pretreatment prostate-specific antigen (PSA) are of limited prognostic value for individual men. There is clearly a need to recognize and develop molecular and genetic biomarkers to improve both the prognosis and the management of the patient with clinically localized CaP. As with other common human neoplasms [120], the search for molecular genetic markers to better define the genesis and progression of CaP is the key focus for cancer research investigations worldwide.

A comprehensive study of CaP prone men of predominantly Caucasian origin has actually led to the identification of a familial prostate cancer susceptibility loci *HPC1* on chromosome 1q24–25 [99], *PCAP* on 1q42 [8], *HPCX* on Xq27 [122], *CAPB* on 1p36, [40]. The *ELAC2* gene on chromosome 17p has recently been shown to be linked to familial prostate cancer in a small subset of prostate cancer prone families [110]. Other molecular epidemiologic studies have shown that polymorphisms of the CAG repeats in the AR gene [45] and increased plasma insulin-like growth factor (IGF)-1 levels are indicative of a higher risk for CaP [21]. Methodologies such as fluorescent in situ hybridization (FISH), comparative genomic hybridization (CGH), and, more recently, spectral karyotyping (SKY) are helping to identify candidate genes at specific chromosome loci and break points. Recent advances in the understanding of the role of oncogenes and tumor suppressor genes (TSG) have dominated the research evaluating the biology of human cancer [120]. The evaluation of these genes has provided new prognostic markers as well as the potential targets for new cancer therapies [120]. Despite recent intensive investigations, much remains to be learned about specific molecular defects associated with CaP [51, 58, 69, 82, 98]. This review will focus on consistent genetic alterations and proposed mechanisms that may contribute to our comprehension of prostate tumorigenesis and aid in our battle against the disease.

The opinions and assertions contained herein are the private views of the authors and are not to be construed as reflecting the views of the US Army or the Department of Defense.

3.2 Prostate Cancer Susceptibility Genes

An exciting breakthrough in the context of hereditary or familial CaP, genetic susceptibility, and increased risk in men with relatives having CaP came as a result of a large multicentric genetic analysis of 91 pedigrees in which CaP was present in three or more first-degree relatives [99]. Several studies suggested the familial clustering of the disease. This clustering could be due to two factors: the first and potentially most important one is that there is an inherited genetic risk factor; the second is that there is an environmental carcinogen leading to the exposure of related family members [20, 57]. It has been estimated that high-risk alleles may account for 9% of all prostate cancers and 40% of early onset disease. First linkage studies pointed to a locus on chromosome 1q23–25, which could harbor a hereditary prostate cancer gene.

Since the cancer susceptibility gene in cancer-prone families often plays a significant role in the genesis of the same type of non-familial/sporadic cancers, the observation suggesting the absence of any significant allelic imbalance in the *HPC1* locus in sporadic CaP is intriguing. A gain in the region on 1q has been shown in sporadic prostate cancer by recent CGH studies [24]. Cloning of the HPC1 gene will no doubt provide valuable information with respect to molecular mechanisms of prostatic tumorigenesis. Although some studies have subsequently confirmed the original findings of HPC1 as a CaP locus, other reports did not lend support for the presence of a susceptibility gene at this locus [28, 78]. The two large cohorts of African-American families tested for linkage to the HPC1 locus showed a significant correlation [99]. Other prostate cancer susceptibility genes have also been identified through linkage studies which appear to be involved in hereditary prostate cancer. These include *PCAP* on 1q42.2–43 [8], *CABP* on 1q36 [40], *HPCX* on xq27 [122], and *HPC20* at 20q13 [7]. Recently, a genome-wide scan of high-risk pedigrees from Utah has provided evidence for involvement of a candidate tumor suppressor gene, *ELAC2* on chromosome 17p, in a small subset of familial prostate cancer [110]. It is apparent that no single locus of predisposition mapped so far explains the presence of one prostate cancer susceptibility gene common to a large proportion of familial prostate cancer as has been the case with a number of familial cancers. It appears difficult to identify prostate cancer susceptibility genes due to late age diagnosis, presence of phenocopies within high-risk families, and genetic complexities. The subtleties of the molecular mechanism of CaP susceptibility in the African-American population are also poorly understood [81]. More recently a multigene model of prostate cancer predisposition has also been proposed. Genes involved in androgen signaling may play some role in predisposition of African-Americans to CaP as well (see below); however, more precise information is needed to fully understand the biology of prostate cancer predisposition in high-risk groups.

3.3 Proto-oncogene Alteration in CaP

Proto-oncogenes with established functions in the process of tumorigenesis have been extensively analyzed in CaP. There is exhaustive literature on the subject; summarized in this review are some of the key findings with regard to some of the most-studied gene alterations in CaP. Among the known proto-oncogenes, the *ras* family of genes, and *c-erb-2*, *myc*, and bcl-2 have been widely studied in CaP. In this section we will primarily focus on observations evaluating *c-erb-2*, IGF, myc, and bcl-2 alterations in CaP.

3.3.1 Alterations of the *c-erb-2* Gene in CaP

The *c-erbB-2/neu/HER-2* (hereafter *c-erbB-2*) gene encodes a trans-membrane tyrosine kinase receptor with considerable homology to the epidermal growth factor receptor (EGFR) [63, 97]. Amplification of *c-erbB-2* has been found in a significant number of cell lines derived from human adenocarcinomas, but rarely in cancer cell lines derived from other cell types [75]. Several groups have utilized immunohistochemistry (IHC) to evaluate levels of *c-erbB-2* protein, with conflicting results [82]. While some studies have shown a relationship of *c-erbB-2* protein overexpression with advanced stage and higher Gleason scores, other studies – including ours – have not found any significant relationship between tumor stage or grade and the expression of *c-erbB-2* [68, 79, 95, 114, 118, 126]. However, a trend towards higher recurrence rates or poor prognosis in patients with *c-erbB-2* oncoprotein overexpression was observed [68, 95]. Recent studies by Ross et al. utilizing FISH with a digoxygenin-labeled *c-erbB-2*-unique sequence probe confirmed *c-erbB-2* gene amplification in 27 of 62 cases (44%) [93]. This amplification correlated with a higher tumor grade, non-diploid DNA content, and advanced pathologic stage. A follow-up study by the same group confirmed their original observations and substantiated the potential utility of studying *c-erbB-2* amplification by FISH and its relevance in predicting postoperative disease recurrence [94]. Further validation for these interesting observations is anticipated since large numbers of pathologic specimens can be analyzed using this technique. More recent studies have also measured the levels of *c-erbB-2* protein in serum of CaP patients. Three independent studies have shown elevated serum *c-erbB-2* protein levels in advanced stages of CaP [2, 85]. On the basis of several studies, *c-erbB-2* overexpression/amplification appears relevant in a subset of prostate cancers that evolve as high-grade tumors. Apparent discrepancies in the reported frequency of *c-erbB-2* alterations may reflect the heterogeneous, multifocal nature of CaP.

To evaluate the biologic effects of the *c-erbB-2* by transfection, a mutated rat *neu* oncogene was introduced into a rat ventral prostatic epithelial cell line, NbE, and the human prostate cancer cell line PC3. This helped establish the aggressive metastatic phenotype of *c-erbB-2/neu* transfected cell lines in these orthotopic prostate tumor models [76, 127]. In androgen-responsive LNCaP cells, *c-erbB-2* expression has been shown to be positively regulated by androgen *in vitro* and *in vivo*. When LNCaP tumors were grown in castrated hosts, levels of *c-erbB-2* and PSA expression initially decreased only to reach levels maintained in intact adult males over a period of 3 weeks [127]. A recently characterized androgen-repressed highly metastatic human prostate cancer cell line, ARCaP, also expressed *c-erbB-2* at very high levels, in addition to *c-erbB-3* and EGFR [128]. Recently, overexpression of *c-erbB-2* has been implicated in the androgen-independent growth of prostate cancer cells by activating the protein kinaseB (Akt) pathway [121]. Phosphorylation of Akt has been shown to be negatively regulated by *PTEN1* TSG, which is frequently mutated in advanced prostate cancer (see 3.4). It may very well be that deregulation of Akt phosphorylation plays an important role in the progression of CaP [17].

3.3.2 IGF and Prostate Cancer

IGF plays an important role in the regulation of cell growth. Its components have been evaluated in CaP cell culture models as well as *in vivo* [31]. As noted earlier, increased serum levels of IGF-I may serve as a risk indicator for CaP

[21]. IGF-binding proteins (IGFBPs), the negative regulators of the IGFs, have also been similarly evaluated. It has been suggested that PSA may modulate IGF1 function by degrading IGFBP3 [43]. Growth factors also interact with the AR signaling pathway and IGF1, in particular, may activate AR. The role of growth factors and their receptors in CaP has been extensively reviewed recently [31].

3.3.3 Alterations of the *myc* Gene Family in CaP

The *myc* family of proto-oncogenes belongs to the basic helix-loop-helix leucine-zipper (bHLH2) class of transcription factors, which are involved in regulation of cell proliferation as well as cell death pathways [60]. The *myc* protein functions as a transcriptional activator by binding to other target proteins such as max. *C-myc* in particular has received considerable attention due to a possible role in CaP. Some studies showed that the *c-myc* messenger RNA was elevated in CaP, but was low in benign prostatic hyperplasia (BPH) and normal tissues. There is a trend, moreover, for enhanced expression in tumors of higher grades. However, the heterogeneous nature of CaP complicated the interpretation of data obtained from RNA studies done with homogenized tissue extracts of epithelium and stroma. Precisely, it was not very clear whether *c-myc* alterations were indeed common in CaP [82]. Jenkins et al. recently applied FISH using a region-specific probe for *c-myc* (8q24 region), and combined it with immunostaining for the *myc* protein in matched prostatic intraepithelial neoplasia (PIN), prostatic carcinoma, and lymph node metastases. *C-myc* amplification by FISH strongly complemented the IHC staining profile showing *myc* protein overexpression and correlated this to the grade of the tumor. Foci of carcinoma cells contained more FISH-defined amplifications when compared to areas of PIN. The gain of chromosome 8q and the amplification of *c-myc* demonstrate that they are more likely to be potential markers for CaP progression [60]. However, since the region of amplification of *myc* on 8q was fairly large, the involvement of other genes, such as prostate stem cell antigen (PSCA), which is a prostate tissue-specific gene at 8q24.2, could not be precluded [92].

3.3.4 Alterations of the bcl-2 Gene Family in CaP

Proteins encoded by the bcl-2 gene family play an important role in the regulation of apoptosis. The bcl-2 protein is an inhibitor of apoptosis. Its interaction with the bcl-2 related *bax* gene, which promotes apoptosis, may determine the rate of apoptosis. Other members of the bcl-2 gene family include *bcl-x* and *mcl-1* [65]. Expression of the bcl-2 protein has been evaluated in CaP by several groups [51, 69]. Its overexpression is also a feature of hormone refractory CaP [77, 83]. LNCaP, which overexpresses *bcl- 2*, is protected from apoptosis *in vitro* [91]. In a recently described LUCaP prostate cell line, the emergence of the hormone-refractory phenotype is directly connected with bcl-2 overexpression [72]. Taiguchi et al. analyzed the relationship of bcl-2 expression and intranuclear DNA fragmentation, which is a marker of apoptosis, in radical prostatectomy specimens from patients managed with or without androgen ablation prior to surgery. A reciprocal relationship was established between DNA fragmentation and bcl-2 overexpression. Individuals treated with nonsteroidal anti-androgenic drugs exhibited significant bcl-2 overexpression compare to those receiving other drugs [109]. Apakama et al. studied the hormone-refractory phenotype and bcl-2 expression and noted that a high fraction of CaP exhibiting bcl-2 overexpression failed anti-androgen therapy (20/27 patients – 74%) [1]. Bauer et al. from our group analyzed bcl-2 protein expression in a large series of radical prostatectomy tissue from 175 patients. Twenty-seven percent of tumors showed bcl-2 overexpression. These patients had significantly higher treatment failure rates than those patients who did not overexpress the bcl-2 protein in their tumors. Multivariate Cox regression analysis also established bcl-2 as an independent predictor for shorter disease-free survival [5]. In a recent report, several members of the bcl-2 gene family: bcl-2, *bax*, *bcl-x*, *mcl-1* were assessed in CaP and PIN specimens. The results suggest that the expression of several anti-apoptotic members of the bcl-2 family, including bcl-2, *bcl-x*, and *mcl-1*, were enhanced during the progression of the cancer, but not in PIN [66].

3.4 Tumor Suppressor Gene Alterations in Prostate CaP

Although most of the tumor-suppressor genes (TSGs) involved in human cancer have been identified through the analysis of rare familial cancer syndromes, alterations of some of the TSGs, namely, retinoblastoma (RB), p53, and p16, have been found in a wide variety of sporadic neoplasms [36]. A large number of studies have evaluated the role of p53 in CaP. RB and p16 genes have also received similar attention.

3.4.1 RB Alterations in CaP

The RB gene encodes a 110- to 115-kDa nuclear phosphoprotein that plays a central role in the regulation of the cell cycle [86, 120]. The activity of the RB protein is regulated by phosphorylation mechanisms mediated by cyclin D and cyclin dependent kinases (CDK), such as CDK 4, 6, and their inhibitors, p16 and p27. The unphosphorylated (active) form of RB functions by binding and blocking the action of a number of transcription factors needed for the passage of cells from the G1 to the S phase of the cell cycle. Loss of RB function, therefore, would result in a deregulated cell cycle that promotes uncontrolled cell proliferation.

Analysis of RB alterations in CaP cell lines revealed the presence of a mutated non-functional protein in DU145 [10]. Restoration of normal RB function in DU145 cells via a retrovirus-mediated (wt) RB gene transfer resulted in the loss of tumorigenic properties of DU145 in nude mice [11]. Analysis of seven CaP specimens, including primary and metastatic tissues, revealed RB alterations in one specimen that displayed a loss of protein expression due to a deletion in one RB allele and the loss of the other normal RB allele. Analysis of the RB gene locus using intragenic polymorphic markers shows allelic imbalance (AI) in about 21% (11/46) of CaP tissue specimens [15]. Another study has reported allelic loss of RB in 50% of samples tested. The simultaneous analysis of RB protein by IHC was positive in seven of nine patients with cancer, while nuclear RB staining was observed in areas of BPH [90]. The analysis of the entire coding region (exon 1 to 27) by polymerase chain reaction (PCR), single strand conformation polymorphism (SSCP), and DNA sequencing revealed RB gene alterations in 16% of 25 primary prostate cancers [67]. On the basis of these limited analyses of RB alterations in CaP, it is apparent that only a subset of CaP harbors RB gene defects. Whether RB alterations would serve as an independent prognostic factor in CaP remains to be proven. It is also important to note that the large size of the RB gene imposes a limitation for mutational analysis. However, analysis of RB gene expression at the RNA and protein levels may be more practical. Promising preliminary observations summarized here warrant a more thorough analysis of RB alterations in CaP.

3.4.2 p53 Gene Alterations in CaP

The tumor suppressor gene p53 is one of the most frequently mutated genes in human cancer [47, 70]. The normal function of the p53 protein includes regulation of critical cellular functions involving the G1 and G2 cell-cycle checkpoints in response to DNA damage and of apoptosis induced by certain stimuli such as DNA-damaging agents and hypoxia [49, 53]. It is no wonder that p53 plays a key role in maintaining the integrity of the cellular genome. The inactivation of p53 by mutations or other mechanisms favors genetic instability, which is the hallmark of tumor cells. Mutations of p53 have been found in a variety of cancers, including urologic neoplasms. A recent review of the literature revealed that there are over 150 publications related to p53 alterations in prostate cancer. Several studies conducted on CaP cite the frequency of p53 alterations in localized cancers (ranging from 4% to 80%) and in more advanced hormone-refractory disease (as high as 94%) [44, 48]. We have also recently reviewed the studies of p53 alterations in CaP [51]. Here we provide a few key observations with respect to a possible role for p53 in prostate pathology. The majority of studies have revealed a low percentage of p53 abnormalities in early-stage (clinically organ-confined) CaP. Studies conducted on primary/organ-confined CaP show a wide range of p53 alterations (0% to 80%). IHC was predominantly the tool of choice for detecting p53 status in CaP, but some studies have combined IHC with DNA-based mutation detection assays. Visakorpi et al. [115], Bookstein et al. [12], and Berner et al. [6] showed a 13%–20% frequency for p53 alterations by IHC on a large series of primary CaP. There was good correlation between the IHC results and the presence of p53 mutations in tissues containing more than 20% of p53 positive cells. However, specimens with fewer than 20% p53 positive cells did not yield consistent results with respect to mutations [12].

Although the preponderance of research reveals a low (0% to 25%) frequency of p53 abnormalities in untreated primary CaP, there are some studies that suggest otherwise. Higher frequencies of p53 expression have been independently reported [4, 52, 105, 113]. The fact that the pattern of p53 staining in the tumor was very focal was noted by Henke et al. [52] and Bauer et al. [4]. Previous studies ignored such areas of focal p53 positivity. Interestingly, if focal p53 positivity was ignored, the frequency of p53 protein expression would be more in line with the previously reported rates of 10% to 20% [4]. It could well be that "focal p53 positivity" may serve as an independent prognostic indicator for CaP recurrence after radical prostatectomy. Mutational analysis of a large number of p53 positive clones derived from PCR amplification of p53 exons (paired primary and metastatic tumors) suggested that tissues with heterogeneous focal p53 staining (0% to 14% cells positive by IHC) in the primaries are capable of clonal expansion to distant metastatic sites [103]. In a recent study, Yang et al. showed a significant association of clustered p53 staining in primary CaP and cancer recurrence [125]. In general, mutation detection assays have described low frequencies in primary CaP [51]. However, when tumor RNA is used as the starting material, a rate of 42% overall p53 gene abnormalities (including either lack of expression (6%) or mutation (35%)) was seen in primary CaP [25].

A review of the numerous studies on p53 and CaP revealed that some pathologic parameters correlate with the frequency of p53 protein expression.

High p53 protein levels were found in tumors with a higher Gleason score, nuclear grade, pathologic stage, and cellular proliferation [51]. In summary, previous work with primary tumors from men with early-stage disease showed low levels (10% to 20%) of p53 alteration. When higher numbers of primary tumor samples are taken for IHC assay, the number of patients with heterogeneous focal p53 positivity is also much higher (50% to 80%). Regardless of the exact timing of p53 mutations, a case can be made that mutation is associated with disease progression. Several studies have found that more p53 abnormalities are seen in untreated metastatic tumors than in untreated primary CaP [50, 59]. The nature of p53 alterations in primary CaP appears focal and heterogeneous much like the inherent pathology of the prostate. What is encouraging are the promising results of p53 gene therapy for CaP, both in animal models and *in vitro* [3, 64, 102].

3.4.3 *PTEN1* and Prostate Cancer

PTEN/MMAC1 maps to 10q23 and encodes a dual-specific/phosphatidylinositol-3, 4,5-phosphate (PIP3) phosphatase. *PTEN1* by dephosphorylating phophoinositides negatively controls the phosphoinositide 3-kinase mediated phosphorylation of the Akt. Therefore *PTEN1* may play a role in the negative regulation of cell growth and cell survival [17]. *PTEN1* has been shown to be mutated in diverse cancers including CaP [30, 71, 104]. Furthermore, analysis of a large series of CaP specimens revealed chromosome deletions at 10q23 in 28% (23 of 80) of tumors. DNA sequence analysis of the entire PTEN1 protein coding region in the specimen s showing loss of heterozygosity (LOH) at 10q detected mutations in 43% (10/23) [18]. The inactivation of *PTEN1* by two hits, including loss of wild type (wt) allele and the retention of the mutant (mt) *PTEN1* allele, strongly favors the involvement of the *PTEN1* gene in CaP. Moreover, a higher frequency of *PTEN1* gene alterations has been observed in metastatic CaP and CaP cell lines compared to primary tumors [18, 71]. To study the role of *PTEN1* in the progression of CaP, 50 metastatic CaP tissues from 19 cancer death patients were used. Using SSCP and sequence analysis, deletions or point mutations were observed in at least one metastatic site in 12 of 19 patients, including homozygous deletions [108].

3.4.4 Sites of Putative TSGs in CaP

Allelic losses at 8p are the most frequently noted chromosomal alterations in CaP. Three separate regions between 8p12–22 (8p12, 8p21, and 8p22) have been reported to be involved in CaP, suggesting the presence of more than one TSG at these loci. Several groups have reported 8p22 loss in 30%–100% of CaP utilizing LOH assays [13, 22, 34, 74, 112]. Variations in the reported frequency of 8p22 LOH are most likely due to differences in purity of the tumors sampled and the heterogeneity inherent in multifocal CaP. The analysis of carefully microdissected primary prostate CaP cells has set the overall LOH at 8p12–22 at 86% [34]. A more recent study analyzing 8p12–22 LOH by Southern, microsatellite, and CGH analyses further revealed allelic losses of 80% in metastatic lymph nodes [24]. Furthermore, allelic losses of 8p12–22 loci appear to be an early event in prostate tumorigenesis. A significant proportion (30%–65%) of PIN exhibits LOH at these loci [34]. Comprehensive analyses of 8p loci in prostate tumors strongly suggest the presence of one or more TSGs between 8p12–21, which may represent an early event, and another distinct TSG at the 8p22 locus that is responsible for tumor progression. The fine mapping of a homozygous deletion at 8p22, spanning 730–970 kbp, in a metastatic CaP specimen, has provided the basis for the search in this region. Other candidate genes on 8p21–22 are being simultaneously evaluated for their role in CaP [117]. Introduction of 8p into a rat prostate cancer cell line by microprotoplast-mediated chromosome transfer (MMCT) inhibited the metastatic ability of this cell line, further strengthening the case for the existence of putative TSGs in this chromosomal fragment [56]. Bearing in mind the relevance of 8p12–22 loci in prostate tumorigenesis as well as in other cancers, several molecular approaches are being employed to identify prostate-specific genes in these loci.

Apart from 8p loci, other regions harboring putative TSGs have received attention in CaP. Carter et al. [19] studied the common region of 16q deletions in CaP that included a proposed candidate TSG, E-cadherin, which mapped to 16q22.1. Reduced or lack of expression of the E-cadherin gene has also been noted in about half the tumors studied [42]. The region of minimal deletion was refined and eventually reassigned to 16q24 [23].

There are some groups that have evaluated allelic losses at 6q [27 32, 100]. Cooney et al. [27] and Srikantan et al. [100] have shown allelic losses of 27–33% at 6q16–23 in primary CaP, with a higher frequency of such alterations in non-organ-confined disease [100].

3.4.5 Androgen Receptor Alterations in CaP

The cornerstone of therapy in patients with metastatic disease is androgen ablation, commonly referred to as "hormonal therapy" since Huggins and Hodges' seminal discovery in 1941 [55]. It is well established that androgens play a key role in the growth and differentiation of the prostate gland. Androgen ablation, in response to castration in animal models, results in the degeneration of the prostate gland with extensive apoptosis of prostatic epithelial cells. Androgen-mediated molecular and cellular functions are mediated by the androgen receptor (AR) protein that belongs to the super family of steroid receptors [29]. One of the proposed mechanisms by which CaP cells escape the effects of the androgen ablation may involve constitutive activation of androgen signaling pathways. Constitutive activation of growth factor receptors by mutations/amplification has been amply demonstrated in numerous models of tumorigenesis [87, 120]. Mutational activation of AR, which might accelerate CaP cell proliferation independent of androgens, has been extensively evaluated. CaP-associated alterations of the AR gene have been summarized in a recent review by Hakimi et al. [45].

The first study of AR mutations in CaP specimens revealed a mutation at codon 730 (GTG - ATG; val-met) in one of 26 tumors analyzed [45]. Subsequent reports, including ours, have addressed mutational alterations of AR in advanced stage CaP [37, 106, 107, 111]. There is a general agreement concerning a very low rate of AR gene mutations in early-stage, organ-confined prostate cancer. Most of the reported AR gene mutations were present in the hormone-binding domain of the protein. A significant number of the AR gene mutations has been reported at or around codon 877, which was originally shown to be mutated in LNCaP cells [26, 33]. A recent study has also shown that AR codon 877 mutation may be frequently selected in response to anti-androgen therapy [107]. In addition to mis-sense mutations, other types of AR alterations have also been reported in CaP. Amplifications of the AR gene were shown in 30% (7 of 23) of hormone-refractory tumors. These studies suggested that AR gene amplifications may occur as a result of cell growth selection due to low androgen concentration during ablation therapy. Recurrent therapy-resistant tumors, unlike the primaries, exhibited AR gene amplification. Tumors which recurred early or did not respond to hormonal therapy at all lacked AR amplification. AR amplification correlated well with a better prognosis [62]. Recently, spontaneous AR variants from primary autochthonous prostate tumors have been reported using a transgenic adenocarcinoma of mouse prostate (TRAMP) model that mimics the progressive pathology of CaP [46].

Alterations in the number of trinucleotide repeats (CAG and GGC) in the transcription transactivation domain of the AR have also been suspect [41, 45, 96]. The length of CAG repeats varies in different racial groups and is considered to be a normal polymorphism. The average number of CAG repeats in Caucasians is 21 compared to 18 in African-Americans [46]. Tumor-associated somatic alteration of the CAG repeat has been reported in only one primary CaP specimen [33]. A recent report of a case control study of 587 CaP patients and 588 normal controls showed an association between fewer CAG repeats in the AR gene and a higher risk of CaP (relative risk = 1.52 at 95% confidence interval). Men with shorter AR CAG repeats were at particularly high risk of developing metastatic and fatal prostate cancer [41].

3.4.6 Role of Novel Prostate-Specific Genes in Prostate Biology and Cancer

PSA as a prostate-specific gene has revolutionized the early detection of CaP [38, 39]. The current method of detecting prostate cancer is the serum prostate-specific antigen (PSA) test. Over the past 10 years it has revolutionized the early detection of CaP, and organ-confined disease can be effectively cured by surgical intervention or radiation treatment. Since the introduction of the PSA test, there has been a sharp decline in the incidence of metastatic CaP. However, the PSA blood test is not always entirely accurate. It is not CaP specific. It may identify men with CaP but it is often elevated in men with benign prostatic hyperplasia (BPH), prostatitis (inflammation of the prostate), and other non-malignant, non-life-threatening prostate disorders. Current figures on this common diagnostic test (PSA) show that about 25% of men with cancer will have normal PSA levels and more than half of men with higher PSA may be cancer free. Prostate-specific membrane antigen (PSMA), which has been studied in detail has been correlated with more aggressive CaP [35]. CaP-associated expression of *PSMA* is being evaluated for imaging of CaP by radiolabeled anti-PSMA monoclonal antibodies and for immunotherapy [35, 84]. Human *hK2* is also a prostate-specific gene; it is very similar to *PSA* and has been shown to be elevated in CaP [61].

Recent discovery of several prostate-specific genes has resulted in enthusiasm for evaluating their potential role in CaP. *NKX3.1*, a prostate tissue-specific homeobox gene, maps to 8p21, the chromosomal region frequently deleted in CaP [9]. It has been shown that mice heterozygous for targeted disruption of *NKX3.1* have abnormal prostate growth and disruption of prostate epithelial morphology, which indicates the importance of this gene in prostate development [9]. We have shown tumor-associated overexpression of *NKX3.1* at RNA level in a subset of matched tumor/normal tissues. *NKX3.1* expression in our study correlated with pathologic stage C disease and AR expression [123]. In a recent study of tissue microarrays, loss of NKX3.1 protein expression has been shown to strongly correlate with the cancer progression [14] supporting role of NKS3.1 function loss in CaP. Clearly, future studies should further define the regulation of *NKX3.1* expression in human CaP. More recently discovered prostate-specific genes, *PSCA* [92], *DD3* [16], and *STEAP* [54], have been shown to be overexpressed in CaP. In our laboratory, we have identified two novel prostate-specific genes, namely, *PCGEM1* [101] and *PSGR* [124], which are overexpressed in CaP. It is intriguing to note that there are quite a few genes that are highly prostate specific and are overexpressed in CaP. The roles of these novel genes in prostate biology and cancer remain to be defined. These new prostate-specific genes may provide novel targets for prostate cancer diagnosis and treatment.

3.5 Hypothetical Model for Prostate Tumorigenesis

It is reasonable to propose a model for prostate cancer initiation, nature of differentiation, progression, and metastasis on the basis of a few recognizable molecular profiles for these entities. A hypothetical model (Fig. 3.1) is presented as an interpretation of the several genetic events that are involved in the genesis of the complex phenotype of the malignant prostate. It appears reasonable to believe that organ-confined CaP, with high-grade PIN, carries genetic alterations, which are already quite complex. In other words, non-organ-confined, invasive CaP is a magnification of the genetic events observed in high-grade PIN. It is very likely that there is a precursor or pre-malignant lesion/cell in the

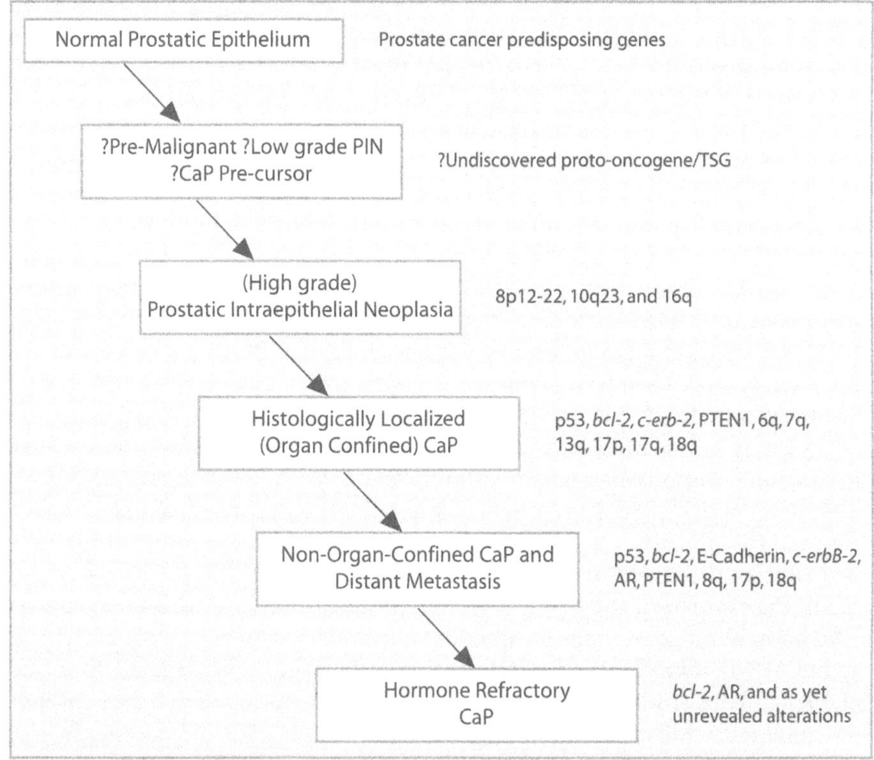

Fig. 3.1. Genetic alterations associated with prostate tumorigenesis. Distinct prostate cancer predisposing genes may associate with subsets of familial prostate cancer. Shorter CAG repeats of the AR gene and IGF-I levels may also confer a high risk of CaP. CaP-associated allelic losses on specific regions of different chromosome loci 6q, 7q, 8p, 13q, 17q, and 18q may harbor TSGs which need to be identified. Gains on 8q, which include *c-myc* have been frequently detected in CaP. Allelic losses of 8p are the most common genetic alterations in CaP. Recent studies have noted frequent PTEN1 (10q) gene mutations in advanced CaP. Alterations of p53, bcl-2 genes are detected in localized CaP and a much higher frequency of bcl-2 and p53 alterations is noted in advanced CaP. A subset of advanced androgen-independent CaP exhibits mutations/amplifications of the AR gene

prostate that carries hitherto unrecognized, novel, or unique prostate-cancer-specific alterations.

As seen, innumerable genetic alterations are described in CaP. The present and future challenges include:

1. Careful clinicopathological documentation and preparation/sampling of tumor tissues by laser capture microdissection or other sophisticated tools for molecular studies
2. Interpretation of these molecular alterations in the context of the multifocal nature and tumor heterogeneity of CaP
3. Development of reproducible immunohistochemistry and in situ hybridization-based high throughput assays for routine multi-parameter analyses of pathologic specimens
4. Identification of genes on chromosome loci frequently altered in CaP
5. Study of the molecular mechanisms and associated gene alterations in low versus high grade PIN, and identifying the "pre-neoplastic" lesion for CaP
6. Investigation of the role of androgen signaling in prostate cancer
7. Institution of larger clinical studies for studying the utility of molecular alterations for early diagnosis and prognostication in CaP
8. Development of novel therapeutics on the basis of gene targeting directed against specific genetic alterations in CaP

Acknowledgements. The authors wish to apologize for omitting many of the references cited in the body of this chapter. This is due to the fact that there is a large volume of references which cannot be cited in their entirety in the space allotted for this information. The authors wish to acknowledge the editorial assistance of Ms. Justine Cowan for her help in the preparation of this chapter.

References

1. Apakama I, Robinson MC, Walter NM, Charlton RG, Royd JA, Fuller CE, Neal DE, Hamdy FC (1996) bcl-2 overexpression combined with p53 accumulation correlates with hormone refractory prostate cancer. Br J Cancer 74:1258–1262
2. Arai Y, Yoskiki T, Yoshida O (1997) *c-erbB*-2 oncoprotein: a potential biomarker of advanced prostate cancer. Prostate 30:195–201
3. Asgari K, Sesterhenn IA, McLeod DG, Cowan K, Moul JW, Seth P, Srivastava S (1997) Inhibition of the growth of pre-established subcutaneous tumor nodules of human prostate cancer cells by single injection of the recombinant adenovirus p53 expression vector. Int J Cancer 71:377–382
4. Bauer JJ, Sesterhenn IA, Mostofi FK, McLeod DG, Srivastava S, Moul JW (1995) p53 nuclear protein expression is an independent prognostic marker in clinically localized prostate cancer patients undergoing radical prostatectomy. Clin Cancer Res 1:1295–1300
5. Bauer JJ, Sesterhenn IA, Mostofi FK, McLeod DG, Srivastava S, Moul JW (1996) Elevated levels of apoptosis regulator proteins p53 and bcl-2 are independent prognostic biomarkers in surgically treated clinically localized prostate cancer patients. J Urol 156:1511–1516
6. Berner A, Harvei S, Treti S, Fossa SD, Nesland JM (1994) Prostate carcinoma: a multivariate analysis of prognostic factors. Br J Cancer 69:924–930
7. Berry R, Schroeder JJ, French AJ, McDonnell SK, Peterson BJ, Cunningham JM, Thibodeau SN, Schaid DJ (2000) Evidence for a prostate cancer-susceptibility locus on chromosome 20. Am J Hum Genet 67:82–91
8. Berthon P, Valeri A, Cohen-Akenine A, Drelon E, Paiss T, Wohr G, et al (1998) Predisposing gene for early onset prostate cancer, localized on chromosome 1q42.2–43. Am J Hum Genet 62:1416–1424
9. Bhatia-Gaur R, Donjacour AA, Sciavolino PJ, Kim M, Desai N, Young P, Norton CR, Gridley T, Cardiff RD, Cunha GR, Abate-shen C, Shen MM (1999) Roles of NKX3.1 in prostate development and cancer. Genes Dev 13:966–977
10. Bookstein R, Rio P, Madreperla SA, Hong F, et al (1990) Promoter deletion and loss of retinoblastoma gene expression in human prostate carcinoma. Proc Natl Acad Sci 87: 7762–7766
11. Bookstein R, Shew JY, Chen PL, Scully P, Lee WH (1990) Suppression of tumorgenicity of human prostate carcinoma cells by replacing a mutated RB gene. Science 247:712–715

12. Bookstein R, MacGrogan D, Hisenbeck SG, Sharkey F, Allred DC (1993) p53 mutated in a subset of advanced stage prostate cancers. Cancer Res 53:3369–3373
13. Bova GS, Carter BS, Bussemakers MJ, Emi M, Fujiwara Y, Kyprianou N, Jacobs SC, Robinson JC, Epstein JI, Walsh PC, et al (1993) Homozygous deletion and frequent allelic loss of chromosome 8p22 loci in human prostate cancer. Cancer Res 53:3869–3873
14. Bowen C, Bubendorf L, Voeller HJ, Slack R, Willi N, Sauter G, Gasser TC, Koivisto P, Lack EE, Kononen J, Kallioniemi OP, Gelmann EP (2000) Loss of *NKX3.1* expression in human prostate cancers correlates with tumor progression. Cancer Res 60:6111–6115
15. Brooks JD, Bova GS, Isaacs WB (1995) Allelic loss of the retinoblastoma gene in primary human prostatic adenocarcinoma. Prostate 26:35–39
16. Bussemakers MJH, Van Bokhoven A, Verhaegh GW, Smitt FP, Karthaus HF, Schalken JA, Debruyne FM, Ru N, Isaacs WB (1999) DD3: a new prostate-specific gene, highly overexpressed in prostate cancer. Cancer Res 59:5975–5979
17. Cantley LC, Neel BG (1999) New insights into tumor suppresssion: *PTEN* suppresses tumor formation by restraining the phosphoinositide 3-kinase/AKT pathway. Proc Natl Acad Sci USA 96:4240–4245
18. Cairns P, Okami K, Halachmi S, Halachmi N, Esteller M, Herman JG, Jen J, Isaacs WB, Bova GS, Sidransky D (1997) Frequent inactivation of PTEN/MMAC1 in primary prostate cancer. Cancer Res 57:4997–5000
19. Carter BS, Ewing CM, Ward WS, Treiger BF, Aalders TW, Schalken JA, Epstein JI, Isaacs WB (1990) Allelic loss of chromosomes 16q and 10q in human prostate cancer. Proc Natl Acad Sci USA 87:8751–8755
20. Carter BS, Bova GS, Beaty TH, Steinberg GD, Childs B, Issacs WB, Walsh PC (1993) Hereditary prostate cancer: epidemiologic and clinical features. J Urol 150:797–802
21. Chan JM, Stampter MJ, Giovannucci E, Gann PH, Ma J, Wilkinson P, Hennekens CH, Pollak M (1998) Plasma insulin-like growth factor-1 and prostate cancer risk: a prospective study. Science 279:563–566
22. Cher ML, MacGrogan D, Bookstein R, Brown JA, et al (1994) Comparative genomic hybridization, allelic imbalance, and fluorescence in situ hybridization on chromosome 8 in prostate cancer. Genes Chromosomes Cancer 11:153–162
23. Cher ML, Ito T, Weidner N, Carroll PR, Jensen RH (1995) Mapping of regions of physical deletion on chromosome 16q in prostate cancer cells by fluorescence *in situ* hybridization (FISH). J Urol 153:249–254
24. Cher ML, Bova GS, Moore DH, Small EJ, Carroll PA, Pinn SS, Epstein JL, Isaacs WB, Jensen RH (1996) Genetic alterations in untreated metastases and androgen-independent prostate cancer detected by comparative genomic hybridization and allotyping. Cancer Res 56:3091–3102
25. Chi S-G, deVere White R, Meyers FJ, Siders DB, Lee F, Gumerlock PH (1994) p53 in prostate cancer: frequent expression transition mutations. J Natl Cancer Inst 86:926–933
26. Coffey DS (1992) The molecular biology, endocrinology and physiology of the prostate and seminal vesicle. In: Walsh PC, Retik AB, Stamey TA, Vaughan ED Jr (eds) Campbell's urology, vol 1. Saunders, Philadelphia, pp 221–266
27. Cooney KA, Wetzel JC, Consolino CM, Wojno KJ (1996) Identification and characterization of proximal 6q deletions in prostate cancer. Cancer Res 56:4150–4153
28. Cooney KA, McCarthy JD, Lange E, Huang L, Miefeldt S, Montie JE, Oesterling JE, Sandler HM, Lange K (1997) Prostate cancer susceptibility locus on chromosome 1q: a confirmatory study. J Natl Cancer Inst 89:955–959
29. Crawford ED, Eisenberger MA, McLeod DG, Spaulding JT, Benson R, Dorr FA, Blumenstein A, Davis MA, Goodman PJ (1989) A controlled trial of leuprolide with and without flutamide in prostatic carcinoma. N Engl J Med 321:419–424
30. Cristofano AD, Pandolfi PP (2000) The multiple roles of PTEN in tumor suppression. Cell 100:387–390
31. Culig Z, Hobisch A, Cronauer MV, Radmayr C, Hittmair A, Zhang J, Thurnher M, Bartsch G, Klocker H (1996) Regulation of prostatic growth and function by peptide growth factors. Prostate 28:392–405
32. Cunningham JM, Shan A, Wick MJ, McDonnell SK, Schaid DJ, Tester DJ, Qian J, Takahashi S, Jenkins RB, Bostwick DG, Thibodeau SN (1996) Allelic imbalance and microsatellite instability in prostate adenocarcinoma. Cancer Res 56:4475–4482
33. Edwards A, Hammond HA, Jin L, Caskey CT, Chakraborty R (1992) Genetic variation at five rimeric and tetrameric tandem repeat loci in four human population groups. Genomics 12: 241–253
34. Emmert-Buck M, Vocke CD, Pozzatti RO, Duray PH, Jennings SB, Florence CD, Zhuang Z, Bostwick DG, Liotta LA, Linehan WM (1995) Allelic loss on chromosome 8p12–21 in microdissected prostatic intraepithelial neoplasia. Cancer Res 55:2959–2962
35. Fair WR, Israeli RS, Heston WD (1997) Prostate-specific membrane antigen. Prostate 32:140–148
36. Fearon ER (1997) Human cancer syndromes: clues to the origin and nature of cancer. Science 278:1043–1050

37. Gaddipati JP, McLeod DG, Heidenberg HB, Sesterhenn IA, Finger MJ, Moul JW, Srivastava S (1994) Frequent detection of codon 877 mutation in the androgen receptor gene in advanced prostate cancer. Cancer Res 54:2861–2864
38. Gao CL, Dean RC, Pinto A, Mooneyhan R, Connelly RR, McLeod DG, Srivastava S, Moul JW (1999) Detection of circulating PSA-expressing prostatic cells in bone marrow of radical prostatectomy patients by sensitive reverse transcriptase-polymerase chain reaction (RT-PCR). J Urol 161:1070–1076
39. Garnick MB, Fair WR (1998) Combating prostate cancer. Sci Am 279:74–83
40. Gibbs M, Stanford JL, Mcindoe TA, Jarvik GP, Kolb S, Goode El, Chakrabarti L, et al (1999) Evidence for a rare prostate cancer-susceptibility locus at chromosome 1p36. Am J Hum Genet 64:776–787
41. Giovannucci E, Stampfer MJ, Kiothivas K, Brown M, Brufsky A, Talcott J, Hennekens CH, Kantoff PH (1997) The CAG repeat within the androgen receptor gene and its relationship to prostate cancer. Proc Natl Acad Sci 94:3320–3323
42. Giroldi LA, Schalken JA (1993) Decreased expression of the intercellular adhesion molecule E. cadherin in prostate cancer: biological significance and implications. Cancer Metastasis Rev 12:29–37
43. Grandori C, Eisenman RN (1997) *myc* target genes. Trends Biochem Sci 22:177–181
44. Greenblatt MS, Bennett, WP, Hollstein M, Harris CC (1994) Mutations in the p53 tumor suppressor gene: clues to cancer etiology and molecular pathogenesis. Cancer Res 54:4855–4878
45. Hakimi JM, Rondinelli RH, Schoenberg MP, Barrack ER (1996) Androgen receptor gene structure and function in prostate cancer. World J Urol 14:329–337
46. Han G, Foster BA, Mistry S, Buchanan G, Harris JM, Tilley WD, Greenberg NM (2000) Hormone status selects for spontaneous somatic androgen receptor variants that demonstrate specific ligand and cofactor dependent activities in autochthonous prostate cancer. J Biol Chem 10:1074
47. Harris CC (1996) Structure and function of p53 tumor suppressor gene: clues for rational cancer therapeutic strategies. J Natl Cancer Inst 88:1442–1455
48. Harris CC, Hollstein M (1993) Clinical implications of the p53 tumor suppressor gene. N Engl J Med 329:1318–1327
49. Hartwell LH, Kastan MD (1994) Cell cycle control and cancer. Science 266:1821–1828
50. Heidenberg HB, Sesterhenn IA, Gaddipati P, Weghorst CM, Buzard GS, Moul JW, Srivastava S (1995) Alterations of the tumor suppressor gene p53 in a high fraction of treatment resistant prostate cancer. J Urol 154:414–421
51. Heidenberg HB, Bauer JJ, McLeod DG, Moul JW, Srivastava S (1996) The role of p53 tumor suppressor gene in prostate cancer: a possible biomarker? Urology 48:971–979
52. Henke RP, Kruger E, Ayhan N, Hubner D, Hammerer P, Huland H (1994) Immunohistochemical detection of p53 protein in human prostatic cancer. J Urol 152:1296–1301
53. Hermeking H, Lengauer C, Polyak K, He T-C, Zhang L, Thiagalingam S, Kinzler KW, Vogelstein B (1997) 14-3-3α is a p53 regulated inhibitor of G2 M progression. Mol Cell 1:3–11
54. Hubert RS, Vivanco I, Chen E, Rastagar S, Leong K, Mitchell SC, Madraswala R, Zhou Y, Ku J, Raitano AB, Jakobovits A, Saffran DC, Afar DE (1999) STEAP: a prostate-specific cell-surface antigen highly expressed in human prostate tumors. Proc Natl Acad Sci USA 96:14523–14528
55. Huggins C, Hodges CV (1941) Studies on prostatic cancer, effects of castration, of estrogens and of androgen injection on serum phosphatase in metastatic carcinoma of the prostate. Cancer Res 1:293–297
56. Ichikawa T, Nihei N, Suzuki H, Oshimura M, Emi M, Nakamura Y, Hayata I, Isaacs JT, Shimazaki J (1994) Suppression of metastasis of rat prostatic cancer by introducing human chromosome 8. Cancer Res 54:2299–2302
57. Issacs SD, Kimeney LALM, Baffoe-Bonnie A, Bety TH, Walsh PC (1995) Risk of cancer in relatives of prostate cancer probands. J Natl Cancer Inst 87:991–996
58. Issacs WB, Bova GS (1998) Prostate cancer. In: Vogelstein B, Kinzler KW (eds) The genetic basis of human cancer. McGraw-Hill, New York, pp 653–660
59. Ittman M, Wieczorek R, Helle P, Dave A, Provet J, Krolewski J (1994) Alterations in the p53 and MDM-2 genes are infrequent in clinically localized, stage B prostate adenocarcinomas. Am J Pathol 145:287–293
60. Jenkins RB, Qian J, Lieber MM, Bostwick DG (1997) Detection of *c-myc* oncogene amplification and chromosomal anomalies in metastatic prostatic carcinoma by fluorescence *in situ* hybridization. Cancer Res 57:524–531
61. Kawakami M, Okaneya T, Furihata K, Nishizawa O, Katsuyama T (1997) Detection of prostate cancer cells circulating in peripheral blood by reverse transcription-PCR for *hKLK2*. Cancer Res 57:4167–4170
62. Kazemi-Esfarjani P, Trifiro MA, Pinsky L (1995) Evidence for a repressive function of the long polyglutamine tract in the human androgen receptor: possible pathogenetic relevance for the $(CAG)_n$ expanded neuronopathies. Hum Mol Genet 4:523–527
63. King CR, Kruas MH, Aaronson SA (1985) Amplification of a novel *c-erbB* related gene in a human mammary carcinoma. Science 229:974

64. Ko SC, Gotoh A, Thalmann GN, Zhau HE, Jhonston DA, Zhang WW, Kao C, Chung LW (1996) Molecular therapy with recombinant p53 adenovirus in androgen independent metastatic human prostate cancer model. Hum Gene Ther 7:1683–1691
65. Korsmeyer SJ (1996) Molecular thanatopsis: discourse on the bcl-2 family and cell death. Blood 88:386–401
66. Krajewska M, Krajewska S, Epstein JL, Shabaik A, Sauvagest J, Song K, Kitada S, Reed C (1996) Immunohistochemical analysis of bcl-2, *bax, bcl-x and mcl-1* expression in prostate cancer. Am J Pathol 148:1567–1576
67. Kubota Y, Fujinamic K, Uemura H, Dobashi Y, Miyamoto H, Iwasaki Y, Kitamura H, Shuin T (1995) Retinoblastoma gene mutations in primary human prostate cancer. Prostate 27: 314–320
68. Kuhn EJ, Kurnot RA, Sesterhenn IA, Chang EH, Moul JW (1993) Expression of the *c-erb*B-2 (HER-2 *neu*) oncoprotein in human prostatic carcinoma: prognostic determinants? J Urol 150:1427–1433
69. Lalani E-N, Laniado ME, Abel PD (1997) Molecular and cellular biology of prostate cancer. Cancer Metastasis Rev 16:29–66
70. Levine A (1997) p53, the cellular gatekeeper for growth and division. Cell 88:323–331
71. Li J, Yen C, Liaw D, Podsypanina K, Bose S, Wang SI, Puc J, Miliaresis C, Rodgers L, McCombie R, Bigner SH, Giovanella BC, Itterman M, Tycko B, Hibshoosh H, Wigler MH, Parsons R (1997) PTEN, a putative protein tyrosine phosphatase gene mutated in human brain, breast and prostate cancer. Science 275:1943–1947
72. Liu AY, Corey E, Bladou F, Lange PH, Vessella RL (1996) Prostatic cell lineage markers: emergence of bcl-2$^+$ cells of human prostate cancer xenograft LuCaP 23 following castration. Int J Cancer 65:85–89
73. Lu-Yao GL, McLerran D, Wasson J, Wennberg JE (1993) An assessment of radical prostatectomy. Time trends, geographical variations and outcomes. JAMA 269:2633–2636
74. Macoska JA, Trybus TM, Benson PD, Sakr WA, Grignon DJ, Wojno KD, Pietruk T, Powell IJ (1995) Evidence for three tumor suppressor gene loci on chromosome 8p in human prostate cancer. Cancer Res 55:5390–5395
75. Maguire HC, Greene MI (1989) The *neu* (*c-erbB-2*) oncogene. Semin Oncol 16:148
76. Marengo SR, Sikes RA, Anezinis P, Chang SM, Chung LW (1997) Metastasis induced by overexpression of p185 *neu*-T after orthotopic injection into a prostatic epithelial cell line (NbE). Mol Carcinog 19:165–175
77. McDonnell TJ, Troncoso P, Brisbay SM, Logothetis C, Chung LW, Hsieh JT, Tu SM, Campbell ML (1992) Expression of proto-oncogene bcl-2 in the prostate and its association with emergence of androgen-independent prostate cancer. Cancer Res 52:1940–1944
78. McIndoe RA, Stanford JL, Gibbs M, Jarvik GP, Brandzel S, Neal CL, Li S, Gammack JT, Gay AA, Goode EL, Hood L, Ostrander EA (1997) Linkage analysis of 49 high-risk families does not support a common familial prostate cancer susceptibility gene at 1q24–25. Am J Hum Genet 61:347–353
79. Mellon K, Thompson S, Charlton RG, et al (1992) p53, *c-erb*-B2 and the epidermal growth factor receptor in the benign and malignant prostate. J Urol 147:496–499
80. Mostofi FK (1975) Grading of prostate carcinoma. Cancer Chemother Rep 59:111
81. Moul JW (1997) Increased risk of prostate cancer in African American men. Mol Urol 1:119–127
82. Moul JW, Gaddipati J, Srivastava S (1994) Molecular biology of prostate cancer. Oncogenes and tumor suppressor genes. In: Dawson NA, Vogelzang NJ (eds) Current clinical oncology: prostate cancer. Wiley-Liss, pp 19–46
83. Moul JW, Bettencourt M-C, Sesterhenn IA, Mostofi FK, McLeod DG, Srivastava S, Bauer JJ (1996) Protein expression of p53, bcl-2 and KI-67 (MIB-1) as prognostic biomarkers in patients with surgically treated, clinically localized prostate cancer. Surgery 120:159–167
84. Murphy GP, Tjoa BA, Simmons SJ, Jarisch J, Bowes VA, Ragde H, Rogers M, Elgamal A, Kenny GM, Cobb OE, Ireton RC, Troychak MJ, Salgaller ML, Boynton AL (1999) Infusion of endritic cells pulsed with HLA-A2- specific prostate specific membrane antigen peptides: a phase 11 prostate cancer vaccine trail involving patients with hormone-refractory metastatic disease. Prostate 38:73–88
85. Myers RB, Brown D, Oelschlager DK, Waterbor JW, Marshall ME, Srivastava S, Stockard CR, Urban DA, Grizzle WE (1996) Elevated serum levels of p105 *(c-erbB-2* in patients with advanced-stage prostatic adenocarcinoma. Int J Cancer 69:398–402
86. Newsham IF, Hadjistilianou T, Cavenee WK (1998) Retinoblastoma. In: Vogelstein B, Kinzler K (eds) The genetic basis of human cancer. McGraw-Hill, New York, pp 363–392
87. Park M (1998) Oncogenes. In: Vogelstein B, Kinzler K (eds) The genetic basis of human cancer. McGraw-Hill, pp 205–228
88. Parker SL, Tong T, Bolden S, Wingo PA (1996) Cancer statistics. CA Cancer J Clin 46:5–27
89. Partin AW, Oesterling JE (1994) The clinical usefulness of prostate-specific antigen: update 1994. J Urol 152:1358–1368
90. Phillips SM, Barton CM, Lee SJ, Morton DG, Wallace DM, Lemoine NR, Neoptolemos JP (1994) Loss of the retinoblastoma susceptibility gene (RB1) is a frequent and early event in prostate tumorigenesis. Br J Cancer 70:1252–1257

91. Raffo AJ, Perlman H, Chen MW, Day ML, Streitman JS, Buttyan R (1995) Overexpression of bcl-2 protects prostate cancer cells from apoptosis *in vitro* and confers resistance to androgen ablation in vivo. Cancer Res 55:4438–4445
92. Reiter ER, Gu Z, Watabe T, Thomas G, Szigeti K, Davis E, Wahl M, Nisitani S, Yamashiro J, LeBeau MM, Loda M (1998) Prostate stem cell antigen: a cell surface marker overexpressed in prostate cancer. Proc Natl Acad Sci USA 95:1735–1740
93. Ross JS, Sheehan CE, Haynor-Buchan AM, Ambros RA, Kallakury BV, Kauffman RP, Fisher HA, Muraca PJ (1997) HER-2/*neu* gene amplification status in prostate cancer by fluorescence *in situ* hybridization. Human Pathol 28:827–833
94. Ross JS, Sheehan CE, Haynor-Buchan AM, Ambros RA, Kallakury BV, Kauffman RP, Fisher HA, Rifkin, MD, Muraca PJ (1997) Prognostic significance of HER-2/*neu* gene amplification status by fluorescence *in situ* hybridization of prostate carcinoma. Cancer 79:162–170
95. Sadasivan R, Morgan R, Jennings S, Austenfeld M, Van Veldhuizen P, Stephens R, Noble M (1993) Overexpression of HER-2/*neu* may be an indicator of poor prognosis in prostate cancer. J Urol 150:126–131
96. Schoenberg MP, Hakimi JM, Wang S, Bova GS, Epstein JI, Fischbeck KH, Isaacs WB, Walsh PC, Barrack ER (1994) Microsatellite mutation (CAG_{24-18}) in the androgen receptor gene in human prostate cancer. Biochem Biophys Res Commun 198:74–80
97. Semba K, Kamata N, Toyoshima K, et al (1985) A *V-erb* related proto-oncogene, *c-erbB-2* is distinct from the *c-erbB-1* epidermal growth factor receptor gene and is amplified in a human salivary gland adenocarcinoma. Proc Natl Acad Sci 82:6497
98. Shi XB, Gumerlock PH, deVere White RW (1996) Molecular biology of prostate cancer. World J Urol 14:318–328
99. Smith JR, Freije D, Carpten JD, Gronberg H, et al (1996) Major susceptibility locus for prostate cancer on chromosome 1 suggested by a genome-wide search. Science 276:1371–1374
100. Srikantan V, Sesterhenn IA, Davis L, Hankins GR, Avellone FA, Livezey JR, Connelly R, Mostofi FK, McLeod DG, Moul JW, Chandrasekha rappa S, Srivastava S (1999) Allelic loss on chromosome 6q in primary prostate cancer. Int J Cancer 84:331–335
101. Srikantan V, Zou Z, Petrovics G, Xu LL, Augustus M, Davis L, Livezey JR, Connell T, Sesterhenn IA, Yoshino K, Buzard GS, Mostofi FK, McLeod DG, Moul JW, Srivastava S (2000) PCGEM1, a prostate-specific gene, is overexpressed in prostate cancer. Proc Natl Acad Sci 97:12216–12221
102. Srivastava S, Katayose D, Tong YA, Craig CR, McLeod DG, Moul JW, Cowan K, Seth P (1995) Recombinant adenovirus vector expressing wild-type p53 is a potent inhibitor of prostate cancer cell proliferation. Urology 46:843–848
103. Stapleton AMF, Timme TL, Gousse AE, Li Q-F, Tobon AA, Kattan MW, Slawin KM, Wheeler TM, Scardino PT, Thompson TC (1997) Primary prostate cancer cells harboring p53 mutations are clonally expanded in metastases. Clin Cancer Res 3:1389–1397
104. Steck PA, Pershouse MA, Jasser SA, Yung WAK, Lin H, Ligon AH, Langford LA, Baumgard ML, Hattier T, Davis T, Frye C, Hu R, Swedlund B, Teng DHF, Tavtigian SV (1997) Identification of a candidate tumor suppressor gene, *MMAC1*, at chromosome 10q23.3 that is mutated in multiple advanced cancers. Nat Genet 15:356–362
105. Stricker HJ, Jay JK, Linder MD, Tamboli P, Amin MB (1996) Determining prognosis of clinically localized prostate cancer by immunohistochemical detection of mutant p53. Urology 47:366–369
106. Suzuki H, Sato N, Watabe Y, Msai M, Seino S, Shimazaki J (1993) Androgen receptor gene mutations in human prostate cancer. J Steroid Biochem Mol Biol 46:759–765
107. Suzuki H, Koichiro A, Komiya A, Aida S, Akimoato S, Shimazaki J (1996) Codon 877 mutation in the androgen receptor gene in advanced prostate cancer: relation to antiandrogen withdrawal syndrome. Prostate 29:153–158
108. Suzuki H, Freije D, Nusskern DR, Okami K, Cairns P, Sidransky D, Isaacs WB, Bova GS (1998) Interfocal heterogeneity of PTEN/MMAC1 gene alterations in multiple metastatic prostate cancer tissues. Cancer Res 58:204–209
109. Taiguchi J, Moriyama N, Kasimoto S, Kameyama S, Kawabe K (1996) Histochemical detection of intranuclear DNA fragmentation and its relation to the expression of bcl-2 oncoprotein in human prostate cancer. Br J Urol 74:719–723
110. Tavtigian SV, Simard J, Teng DHF, Abtin V, Baumgard M, et al (2001) A candidate prostate cancer susceptibility gene at chromosome 17p. Nat Genet 27:172–180
111. Tilley WD, Buchanan G, Hickey TE, Bentel JM (1996) Mutations in the androgen receptor gene are associated with progression of human prostate cancer to androgen independence. Clin Cancer Res 2:277–285
112. Trapman J, Sleddens HF, van der Weiden MM, Dinjens WN, Koing JJ, Schroder FH, Faber PW, Bosman FT (1994) Loss of heterozygosity of chromosome 8 microsatellite loci implicates a candidate tumor suppressor gene between the loci D8S87 and D8S133 in human prostate cancer. Cancer Res 54:6061–6064
113. Van Veldhuizen PJ, Sadasivan R, Garcia F, Austenfield MD, Stephens RL (1993) Mutant p53 expression in prostate carcinoma. Prostate 22:23–30

114. Visakorpi T, Kallioniemi OP, Koivula T, Harvey J, Isola J (1992) Expression of epidermal growth factor receptor and ERBB2 (HER-2/*neu*) oncoprotein in prostatic carcinomas. Mod Pathol 5:643–648
115. Visakorpi T, Kallioniemi OP, Heikinen A, Koivula T, Isola J (1992) Small subgroup of aggressive, highly proliferative prostatic carcinomas defined by p53 accumulation. J Natl Cancer Inst 84:883–887
116. Visakorpi T, Kallioniemi OP, Koivula T, Isola J (1993) New prognostic factors in prostate carcinoma. Eur Urol 24:438–449
117. Vocke CD, Pozzatti RO, Bostwick DG, Florence CD, Jennings SB, Strup SE, Duray PH, Liotta LA, Emmert-Buck MR, Linehan WM (1996) Analysis of 99 microdissected prostate carcinomas reveals a high frequency of allelic loss on chromosome 8p21–22. Cancer Res 56:2411–2416
118. Ware JL, Maygarden SJ, Koontz WW, Strom SC (1991) Immunohistochemical detection of *c-erbB-2* protein in human benign and neoplastic prostate. Hum Pathol 22:254
119. Wasson JH, Cushman CC, Bruskewit RC, Littenberg B, Mulley AG, Wennberg JE (1993) A structured literature review of treatment for localized prostate cancer. Arch Fam Med 2:487–493
120. Weinberg RA (1996) How cancer arises. Sci Am 9:62–70
121. Wen Y, Hu MC, Makino K, Spohn B, Bartholomeusz G, Yan DH, Hung MC (2000) Her-2/neo promotes androgen-independent survival and growth of prostate cancer cells through the Akt pathway. Cancer Res 60:6841–6845
122. Xu J, Meyers DA, Freije D, Issacs S, Wiley K, Nusskern D, Ewing C, et al (1998) Evidence for a prostate cancer susceptibility focus on the X chromosome. Nat Genet 20:175–179
123. Xu LL, Srikantan V, Sesterhenn IA, Augustus M, Dean R, Moul JW, Carter KC, Srivastava S (2000) Expression profile of an androgen-regulated prostate specific homeobox gene *NKX3.1* in primary prostate cancer. J Urol 163:972–979
124. Xu LL, Stackhouse BG, Florence K, Zhang W, Shanmugam N, Sesterhenn IA, Zou Z, Srikantan V, Augustus M, Roschke V, Carter K, McLeod DG, Moul JW, Soppett D, Srivastava S (2000) PSGR, a novel prostate-specific gene with homology to a G-protein-coupled receptor, is overexpressed in prostate cancer. Cancer Res 60:6568–6572
125. Yang G, Stapleton AMF, Wheeler TM, Truong LD, Timme TL, Scardino PT, Thompson TC (1996) Clustered p53 immunostaining: a novel pattern associated with prostate cancer progression. Clin Cancer Res 2:399–401
126. Zhau HE, Wan DS, Zhou J, Miller GJ, Von Eschenbach AC (1992) Expression of *c-erbB-2/neu* proto-oncogene in human prostatic cancer tissues and cell lines. Mol Carcinog 5:320–327
127. Zhau HY, Zhou J, Symmans WF, Chen BQ, Chang SM, Sikes RA, Chung LW (1996) Transfected *neu* oncogene induces human prostate cancer metastasis. Prostate 28:73–83
128. Zhau HY, Chang SM, Chen BQ, Wang Y, Zhang H, Kao C, Sang QA, Chung LW (1996) Androgen repressed phenotype in human prostate cancer. Proc Natl Acad Sci USA 93:15152–15157

4 Diagnosis and Clinical Significance of Prostatic Intraepithelial Neoplasia

V. Ravery, L. Boccon-Gibod

4.1 Definition

The term prostatic intraepithelial neoplasia (PIN) was endorsed by consensus to replace other synonymous terms used in the literature, including intraductal dysplasia, large acinar atypical hyperplasia, atypical primary hyperplasia, hyperplasia with malignant change, marked atypia, and duct-acinar dysplasia. Further, PIN divided into two categories, low grade and high grade, replacing the previous three-grade system initially described by McNeal and Bostwick [5]. PIN grade 1 is now considered low grade and grade 2 and 3 are high grade.

PIN affects ducts and acini and is defined as abnormal proliferation with nuclear and nucleolar changes. In low-grade PIN (formerly type 1), general architecture shows stratification with irregular spacing and crowding of epithelial cells. Nuclei are enlarged with marked size variation, chromatin is normal, and nucleoli are rarely prominent. The basal cell layer and basement membrane are intact [11].

In high-grade PIN (formerly types 2 and 3), four patterns of cell stratification are described: tufting, micropapillary, cribriform, and flat. Nuclei are enlarged with some size and shape variations. Chromatin is clumped and is dense. Nucleoli are occasionally to frequently large and prominent, sometimes multiple. Basal cells are large and the basement membrane may show up to 50% disruption. Most pathologists currently use the term PIN to indicate high-grade PIN because low-grade PIN is difficult to recognize; several authors think that the distinction between low-grade PIN and normal epithelium is somewhat subjective [1].

4.2 Is PIN a Premalignant Lesion?

If PIN represents a premalignant lesion, one would expect it to be more common in younger men and to decrease in incidence with age in glands without cancer [5]. Lee et al. [15] reported that patients with cancer were younger than those with PIN alone. Recently, Sakr et al. [24] explored 152 prostate glands removed at autopsy from young men and found the incidence of PIN in those in the fourth and fifth decades to exceed the incidence of carcinoma. However, it is still difficult to state whether PIN is a true premalignant lesion or only a tumor-associated condition.

What may be emphasized is that PIN and prostatic cancer have similar architectural and cytological features. Both are commonly located in the peripheral zone and in the apical portion. Twenty-one percent are located in the central zone and 18%–31% in the transitional zone. PIN and malignant tumor have at least three times the proliferative rate of benign glands.

Moreover, PIN occurs more commonly in prostates with invasive carcinoma than in those without it. Many studies based on glands removed at autopsy, radical prostatectomy, and cystoprostatectomy have shown a strong association between PIN, especially high-grade PIN, and invasive cancer. PIN (high and low grades) was present in 59%–100% of glands with concomitant prostate cancer compared with 32% of those with no carcinoma [27].

4.3 Incidence and Prevalence of PIN

- Autopsy series : autopsy series show that the prevalence of PIN increases with age and that 70% of high-grade PIN is associated with cancer. These findings suggest that PIN lesions observed as early as the 30s precede cancer by at least 10 years [24].
- Biopsy series : the incidence of PIN within prostate biopsy tissue ranges from 0.7 to 19%, depending on the population studied and grade being considered [7].

In a series of 330 biopsies reported by the American Cancer Society National Prostate Cancer Detection Project, the rate of PIN was 5.2% versus 15.8% for cancer [16].

In 256 biopsies directed toward hypoechoic lesions Lee found 27 cases of PIN (10.5%) and 103 cancers (40.2%). In the same study the authors showed that the mean age at diagnosis was 65 years versus 70 years for cancer [15].

In a biopsy series from Mayo Clinic, the rate of high-grade PIN was 16.5%. [4, 10] while for Wills et al. [26] this rate was 5.5% in a series of 439 biopsies.

In a more recent study (European Randomized Study of Screening for Prostate Cancer) of biopsies performed on 1824 men for screening purposes, 2.7% and 3.4% of low-grade and high-grade PIN were detected, respectively – in 0.7% of these men, high-grade PIN was present with no concomitant cancer [13].

- Since PIN occurs more frequently in peripheral zones, in a series of transurethral resections of the prostate (TURPs), the incidence of isolated PIN lesions within the resected chips ranged only from 2.3% to 4.2% [6].

A finding of PIN within TURP material has should be reported, and all the TURP chips should then be subjected to complete pathological analysis in order to rule out concomitant prostate cancer.

4.4 Genetic and Molecular Changes

Fluorescence in situ hybridization (FISH) is a useful technique for determining genetic relationships between cancer and its precursors. PIN and prostatic carcinoma foci have a similar proportion of genetic changes, but cancer usually has more alterations, for instance, densification of chromatin and loss of basal cell layer [21]. The most common genetic alterations in PIN are:

1. Gain of chromosome 7, particularly 7q3 l (30% in prostate cancer versus 17% in PIN) [5].
2. Loss of 8p and gain of 8q. The rate of 8p22 loss, for example, ranges from 29% to 50% in PIN and from 32% to 69% in primary malignancies [8].
3. Loss of 10q, 16q, and 18q – inactivation of tumor suppressor genes and/ or overexpression of oncogenes at these regions may be important for the initiation and progression of prostate cancer.

As previously mentioned, numeric chromosomal anomalies in PIN and carcinoma are remarkably similar, suggesting that they share a similar underlying pathogenesis. Moreover, in some prostates, one or more foci of PIN contains more anomalies than carcinoma foci [20]. This indicates that either PIN foci may have some divergence in pathogenetic pathways, that some PIN foci may morphologically progress to cancer more slowly than others, or that foci of carcinoma may occasionally be derived from other precursor lesions such as atypical adenomatous hyperplasia [8].

It has been shown that the nuclear chromatin in secretory cells in prostates with either PIN or cancer undergoes distinct changes in texture and spatial distribution.

Recent studies have pointed out that expression of gluthathione S-transferase (GST) in PIN lesions may be altered. GST may prevent carcinogenesis through its role in cellular detoxification. It has been reported that GST staining in PIN foci may deviate from the normal in terms of extension and intensity in that the gaps in the stained basal cell layer are wider and the cells themselves appear paler than normal ones.

Telomerase activity is considered to be a useful diagnostic marker of prostate cancer [17]. Its expression is occasionally detected in benign prostatic tissue bordering prostate cancer and may result from either the presence of a primary undetected preneoplastic lesion or a secondary response to adjacent neoplasic tissue. The finding of telomerase activity has been therefore indicated as an early change in prostate carcinogenesis and as a putative biomarker of unfavorable outcome in benign prostatic hyperplasia (BPH) patients.

Substantial changes, including angiogenesis, occur in the stroma surrounding ducts, and acini in PIN tissue[18]. It has been shown that, going from normal prostate through PIN to cancer, an increasing proportion of capillaries become shorter, have an open lumen, an undulated external contour, and contain a greater number of endothelial cells. The highest proportion of touching capillaries has been seen in normal prostate, the lowest in cancer, while PIN is intermediate. With regard to this feature, values in low grade PIN approach those in normal prostate whereas in the high grade variety they are close to cancer [18].

4.5 PIN and Prostate-Specific Antigen

Conflicting results have been reported regarding the relationship between PIN and prostate-specific antigen (PSA).

Brawer et al. [6] studied 65 men undergoing transurethral or open simple prostatectomy to evaluate the contribution of PIN to serum PSA concentration. Mean serum PSA concentration in patients with PIN alone (5.6 ng/ml) was intermediate between that of benign tissue (2.1 ng/ml) and carcinoma (35.1 ng/ml).

Lee et al. [15] evaluated 248 consecutive needle biopsy specimens. Mean log serum concentration of PSA in patients with high-grade PIN (1.85) was intermediate between patients with BPH (1.09) and those with carcinoma (2.79); these studies suggest that PIN contributes to serum PSA concentration.

Conversely, Ronet et al. [22] studied 65 patients with prostate cancer who underwent radical prostatectomy; they found that high-grade PIN did not correlate with serum PSA concentration and PSA density. Immunohistochemical studies have demonstrated that expression of PSA in PIN is weaker than that observed in benign epithelium and cancer [26].

Alexander et al. [2] suggested that the elevated serum PSA concentrations found in patients on transrectal biopsy were not attributable to high-grade PIN that was discovered concurrently.

Only few data are available regarding PIN and the ratio of free to total PSA. Kilic et al. [14] found in a 46-patient study that free PSA values from BPH to high-grade PIN were increased, whereas a decrease was observed from high-grade PIN to prostate cancer. In this series, although free to total PSA ratio was lower in patients with cancer than in those with high-grade PIN, the difference was not statistically significant.

4.6 PIN and Repeat Biopsy

Thorough biopsy should be performed if PIN is discovered at initial biopsy. Indeed, the literature reveals that the rates of cancer found upon repeat biopsy were 13%–20% in cases of low-grade PIN at initial biopsy and 35%–100% when high-grade PIN was found initially [7, 9, 25].

From proportional hazards models, we know that there is a 15-fold relative risk of prostate cancer on repeat biopsy if high-grade PIN appears in the initial series [25]. Moreover, autopsy series show that there is a high association rate between prostate cancer and high-grade PIN [24].

Since high-grade PIN is considered as a strong indicator of prostate cancer [9, 25], one may therefore be justified in performing a third series of biopsies if rebiopsy was negative for cancer although high-grade PIN was found on initial biopsy.

Extensive biopsy protocols, including additional biopsies of the peripheral zone, have significantly increased the discovery of prostate cancer in patients with an elevated PSA or an abnormal digital rectal examination. We believe also that both the increased number of biopsies and the strategic acquisition of biopsies from the far lateral area of the gland (where the peripheral zone is more prominent) increases the possibility of detecting PIN and prostate cancer [23].

Finally, it is known that prostate cancer in rebiopsy is not necessarily found in the same area as was PIN in the first series; it is thus important to rebiopsy PIN patients using extensive systematic biopsy protocols and not only to biopsy in and near the initial PIN area.

4.7 Chemoprevention

The chemoprevention of cancer may be described as the application of natural or synthetic compounds to prevent or reverse carcinogenesis.

The epidemiological, anatomical, histological, and molecular data present a clear endorsement of PIN as a precursor to carcinoma. The available data support this role only for PIN characterized as high grade, which becomes therefore a logical target for chemoprevention [19]. Several chemopreventive agents have been studied and some of them are still under investigation.

The retinoid compounds may be especially attractive in the chemoprevention of PIN via the induction of differentiation and inhibition of growth. A major drawback to the use of these agents is the spectrum of dose-related side effects, including liver damage and central nervous system changes.

α-Tocopherol, β-carotene, or both, were provided in a randomized, double-blind, placebo-controlled prevention study to determine whether a reduction in lung and others cancers could be achieved. Although neither compound diminished lung cancer incidence α-tocopherol unexpectedly reduced prostate cancer incidence [3].

The homeostasis of normal and neoplastic prostate epithelium is dependent upon circulating and intraprostatic androgens which regulate the balance between prostatic cell death and proliferation. Having been shown to reduce serum and intraprostatic 5 α-dihydrotestosterone, finasteride is the first 5α-reductase inhibitor to undergo clinical evaluation. A rationale is that anticancer activity is not required for a drug to exert a chemopreventive effect. Since the process of carcinogenesis can be regarded as a continuum, the reduction of androgen-stimulated proliferation may, over time, reduce the incidence of neoplastic transformation or progression.

The incidence supporting a potential chemopreventive role for finasteride, coupled with an extremely low side effect profile, prompted the initiation of the Prostate Cancer Prevention Trial (PC PT). This study, begun in the mid-1990s, randomizes a total of 18,000 healthy men aged 55 years and older to receive either finasteride (5 mg/day) or placebo for a duration of 7 years [12]. Prostate biopsies will be obtained on all patients at the completion of the study and thus an assessment of PIN may further delineate the relationship between PIN and invasive cancer and provide valuable prognostic information.

In addition to the agents mentioned already, there are numerous other compounds which have the potential to exert a chemopreventive effect on prostate carcinogenesis. These agents include vitamin D and selenium. Their utility in modulating the development and progression of premalignant prostate changes has yet to be determined, and the major obstacle in the evaluation of agents designed to modify these mechanisms is the great amount of time needed for trials due to the protracted developmental period of prostate cancer.

4.8 Conclusions

The clinical importance of recognizing prostatic intraepithelial neoplasia is based on its strong association with prostatic carcinoma.

High-grade PIN also offers promise as an intermediate point in studies of chemoprevention of prostatic carcinoma. Furthermore, high-grade PIN does not significantly contribute to serum PSA concentration. Patients with high-grade PIN on prostatic biopsy should be rebiopsied regardless of their PSA levels.

References

1. Aboseif S, Shinohara K, Weidner N, Narayan P, Carroll PR (1995) The significance of prostatic intraepithelial neoplasia. Br J Urol 76:355–359
2. Alexander EE, Qian J, Wollan PC, Myers RP, Bostwick D (1996) Prostatic intraepithelial neoplasia does not appear to raise serum prostate-speficic antigen concentration. Urology 47: 693–698
3. Alpha-tocopherol BCCPSG (1994) The effect of vitamin E and beta carotene on the incidence of lung cancer and other cancers in male smokers. N Engl J Med 330:1029–1035
4. Bostwick DG, Qian J, Frankel K (1995) The incidence of high grade prostatic intraepithelial neoplasia in needle biopsies. J Urol 154:1791–1794
5. Bostwick FG, Qian J, Shan A, Borell TJ, Darson M, Maihle NJ, Jenkins RB, Cheng L (1998) Independent origin of multiple foci of prostatic intraepithelial neoplasia. Cancer 83:1995–2002
6. Brawer MK, Rennels MA, Nagle RB, Schifman R, Gaines JA (1989) Serum prostate-specific antigen and prostate pathology in men having simple prostatectomy. Am J Clin Pathol 92:760–764

7. Brawer MK, Bigler SA, Sohlbert OE, Nagle RB, Lange PH (1991) Significance of prostatic intraepithelial neoplasia on prostate needle biopsy. Urology 38:103–107
8. Cheng L, Shan A, Cheville JC, Qian J, Bostwick FG (1998) Atypical adenomatous hyperplasia of the prostate: a premalignant lesion? Cancer Res 58:389–391
9. Davidson D, Bostwick DG, Qian J, Wollan PC, Oesterling JE, Rudders RA, Siroky M, Stilmant M (1995) Prostatic intraepithelial neoplasia is a risk factor for adenocarcinoma: predictive accuracy in needle biopsies. J Urol 154:1295–1299
10. Davidson D, Bostwick DG, Qian J, Wollan P, Oestrerling JE, Rudders RA, et al (1995) Prostatic intraepithelial neoplasia is a risk factor for adenocarcinoma: predictive accuracy in needle biopsies. J Urol 154:1295–1299
11. Drago JR, Mostofi FK, Lee F (1989) Introductory remarks and workshop summary. Urology 34 [Suppl]:2
12. Feigl P, Blumenstein B, Thompson I, Crowley J, Wolf M, Kramer BS, Coltman CA, Brawley OW, Ford LG (1995) Design of the Prostate Cancer Prevention Trial (PCPT). Control Clin Trials 16: 150–163
13. Hoedemaeker R, Kranse R, Rietbergen J, Boeken Kruger A, Schoder F, Van Der Kwast T, et al (1999) Evaluation of prostate needle biopsy in a population-based screening study. The impact of borderline lesions. Cancer 85:145–152
14. Kilic S, Kukul E, Danisman A, Güntekin E, Sevük M (1998) Ratio of free to total prostate-specific antigen in patients with prostatic intraepithelial neoplasia. Eur Urol 34:176–180
15. Lee F, Torp-Pedersen ST, Carroll JT, Siders DB, Christenesen-Day C, Mitchell AE (1989) Use of transrectal ultrasound and prostate-specific antigen in diagnosis of prostatic intraepithelial neoplasia. Urology 34 [Suppl 6]:4–8
16. Metlin C, Lee F, Drago J, Murphy JP (1991) The American Cancer Society National Prostate Cancer detection of early prostate cancer in 2425 men. Cancer 67:2949–2958
17. Colanzi P, Satinelli A, Mazzucchelli R, Pomante R, Montironi E (1998) Prostatic intraepithelial neoplasia and prostate cancer: analytical evaluation. Adv Clin Pathol 2:271–284
18. Montironi RW, Hamilton P, Scarpelli M, Thompson D, Bartels PH (1999) Subtle morphological and molecular changes in normal-looking epithelium in prostates with prostatic intraepithelial neoplasia or cancer. Eur Urol 35:468–473
19. Nelson PS, Gleason TP, Brawer MK (1996) Chemoprevention for prostatic intraepithelial neoplasia. Eur Urol 30:269–278
20. Qian J, Bostwick FG, Takahashi S, Borell TJ, Herath JF, Lieber MM, Jenkins RB (1995) Chromosomal anomalies in prostatic intraepithelial neoplasia and carcinoma detected by fluorescence in situ hybridization. Cancer Res 55:5408–5414
21. Qian J, Jenkins RB, Bostwick DG (1999) Genetic and chromosomal alterations in prostatic intraepithelial neoplasia and carcinoma detected by fluorescence in situ hybridization. Eur Urol 356:479–483
22. Ronnet BM, Carmichael MJ, Carter HB, Epstein JI (1993) Does high grade prostatic intraepithelial neoplasia result in elevated serum prostate specific antigen levels. J Urol 150:386–389
23. Rosser CJ, Broberg J, Case D, Eskew LA, McCullough D (1999) Detection of high-grade prostatic intraepithelial neoplasia with the five-region biopsy technique. Urology 54:853–856
24. Sakr WA, Haas GP, Cassin BF, Pontes JE, Crissman JD (1993) The frequency of carcinoma and intraepithelial neoplasia of the prostate in young male patients. J Urol 150:379–385
25. Villers A, Molinie V (2000) Indication et stratégie de nouvelles biopsies après diagnostic de néoplasie intra-épithéliale prostatique. Prog Urol 10:1267–1270
26. Wills ML, Hamper UM, Partin AW, Epstein JI (1997) Incidence of high-grade prostatic intraepithelial neoplasia in sextant needle biopsy specimens. Urology 49:367–373
27. Zlotta AR, Schulman CC (1999) Clinical evolution of prostatic intraepithelial neoplasia. Eur Urol 35:498–503

Diagnosis and Staging of Prostate Cancer

5 Prostate Biopsy – When, How, and When to Repeat?

W. Höltl

5.1 Introduction

Transrectal prostate biopsy (PB) is the standard procedure for diagnosing prostate cancer. Up to 1989 it was done with digital image guidance or transperineally (usually under general anesthesia). These techniques were replaced by transrectal sextant biopsy, which was introduced by Hodge, and has since been the standard procedure [11]. It is routinely performed with ultrasound guidance. However, experience in the past few years has shown that the six biopsy specimens taken on initial biopsy according to that protocol are not sufficient for detecting all clinically relevant cancers (>0.5 cm³). This is why altered sampling schemes have been described (Table 5.1). Basically, the trend is to take as many samples during initial biopsy as needed for detecting cancer with a high probability and to keep the repeat biopsy rate low. The eight-core scheme recommended by Presti is currently considered to be most useful [20]. The pattern proposed by Karakiewicz, to take one core for every 5 cm³ prostate volume, is an alternative [13].

5.2 Indications for Initial Biopsy

Indications for initial biopsy mainly depend on the patient's age and his general condition. At an age from 45 to 50 and 75 years PB is invariably indicated in patients with elevated prostate-specific antigen (PSA) levels (corrected for age) and/or suspicious digital rectal examination (DRE) findings who are candidates for curative treatment. In patients with other morbid conditions and a substantially reduced life expectancy the usefulness of both prostate biopsies and PSA assays is questionable. This applies to men with prostates found

Table 5.1. Biopsy schemes (initial prostate biopsy)

	Biopsies (*n*)	Source
Hodge (1989)	6	[11]
Presti (2000)	8	[20]
Babaian (2000)	6 vs. 11	[1]
Naughton (2000)	6 vs. 12	[18]
Ravery (2000)	12	[22]
Norberg (1997)	8 vs. 10	[19]
Eskew (1997)	at least 13 (mean, 18)	[9]

to be normal on DRE. In those with suspect DRE findings, PB only has a place when the underlying histology can be expected to be relevant for treatment. If this is not so, patients should be spared the emotional stress of a potential prostate cancer diagnosis, and at best be subjected to biopsy when they develop symptoms and PB is likely to give guidance for treatment. After all, immediate androgen deprivation has still not been shown to provide a survival benefit versus delayed treatment, but is known to substantially reduce the patient's quality of life.

5.3 Interpretation of Negative Initial Biopsies

On classical sextant biopsy as described by Hodge, the rate of false-negative findings is 12%–30% [25]. Closer tolerances cannot be given because the intervals reported in the literature between initial and repeat biopsies vary from 6 weeks to 1 year. During long intervals the tumor volume may increase and thus make the data incomparable [21].

Inconclusive findings on initial biopsy should be interpreted with particular caution. Increasingly thin biopsy needles and earlier PBs prompted by PSA screening at a time at which the tumor volume is still small provide the pathologist with specimens that often all but defy analysis. The detection of so-called ASAPs (atypical small acinar proliferations) should always raise suspicion of prostate cancer. ASAPs are found in 1.5%–9% of all PBs. High-grade prostatic intraepithelial neoplasia (PIN – previously known as PIN 2 and PIN 3) is another high-risk factor for concomitant prostate cancer. Its reported incidence varies between 1.5% and 16.5% [3, 5].

5.4 Indications for Repeat Biopsies

Repeat biopsies should be performed whenever initial biopsies were found to be negative although prompted by suspect DRE findings and/or elevated PSA levels with a tendency to rise. Increasing PSA levels (PSA slope >0.75 ng/ml per year) and a ratio <0.18–0.20 between free and total PSA mandate repeat biopsy. Histologic details seen on initial biopsy may also dictate repeat biopsy. These include high-grade PIN and ASAP. Sixty percent of the glands with ASAP on initial biopsy are found to contain prostate cancer on repeat biopsy [5]. Of the patients presenting with high-grade PIN on initial biopsy, 30%–50% can be expected to show prostate cancer on repeat PB [6, 23] versus only 10%–20% of those who initially underwent standard sextant biopsy without PIN or ASAP by histologic evidence. What the optimal timing of repeat PB is has not yet been defined. An interval of 3–6 months is a useful guideline (Table 5.2) [14].

Table 5.2. The author's scheme

First PB:	<30 g – sextant + 2 lateral + areas suspect on TRUS±DRE >30 g – sextant + 4 lateral + suspect areas
Second PB:	As first PB + high-grade PIN areas + 2 transitional zone (about 3 months following first PB)

PB, prostate biopsy; TRUS, transrectal ultrasound; DRE, digital rectal excamination; PIN, prostatic intraepithelial neoplasia.

5.5 Evaluation and Reporting by the Pathologist

Reliable generally valid guidelines for evaluating the biopsy material by the pathologist are not available [4]. Recommendations vary from three sections to a complete analysis of the entire specimen [25]. Whether one or several cores per tissue block are processed makes a difference in qualitative terms. For optimal evaluation at least six sections should obtained from each core. Evaluation depends critically on the quality with which the cores are processed, from retrieval to being embedded in paraffin. Neatly keeping the specimens in separate containers is important for assigning the histologic findings to the correct site (e.g., capsular perforation; suspect areas to be considered in future repeat PBs). For reporting, the guidelines of the Cancer Committee of the College of American Pathologists are helpful [10].

5.6 Biopsy Technique

Ultrasound-guided transrectal biopsy is the contemporary method of choice. It is usually performed with an 18-gauge needle. With the use of thinner needles the complication rate has dropped despite the larger number of samples taken. Both infections and hemorrhages are clearly less common than with 14-gauge needles (7%–39% versus 0.8% infections, and 3.2% versus 1% hemorrhages in need of treatment) [2]. One drawback associated with thinner needles is that the specimens are substantially smaller (less than half the core volume obtained with a 14-gauge needle). The core length is another problem. It depends on the needle used and the penetration depth in the prostate tissue. Commercial PB needles have a core length of 17 or 19 mm. This is inadequate for large glands. Needles designed for a greater penetration depth are a problem technically. They tend to be unstable on insertion and break easily, so that they are rarely used. As a consequence, more cores must inevitably be taken to cover all areas of interest.

Ideally assuming a full core (which, in reality, is no more than half a core, because the other half of the volume is occupied by the needle), the tissue volume of a 17-mm core taken with an 18-gauge needle is 8.3 mm^3, that of a 19-mm core taken with an 18-gauge needle 9.31 mm^3. As at least eight cores are standard today, the total tissue volume available will be 66.64 mm^3 versus 74.48 mm^3 using the longer core.

What does this mean for a 30-cm^3 prostate? Assuming, like McNeal [17], that the mean volume of the peripheral zone is 25% of the total volume, eight cores will contain about 1% of the peripheral zone volume in the ideal case (all cores are targeted to the peripheral zone and contain as much tissue as possible).

Classical sextant biopsy is no longer thought to be adequate today, because it misses about one fifth of what are deemed clinically relevant prostate cancers (tumor volume >0.5 cm^3) on initial examination. Numerous improvements to enhance its diagnostic accuracy were proposed in the past few years. The cancer detection rate depends on various factors. Among these, the distribution of sampling sites in the prostate (Table 5.1), the number of cores taken, and the volume of the gland (particularly of its peripheral zone) are most important. In glands <50 cm^3 significantly more lesions are detected than in those with a volume >50 cm^3. This would logically imply that more cores should be taken from large glands in order to match the detection rate known from smaller glands.

But the percentage of discovery of clinically relevant prostate cancers decreases as the number of samples increases. Consequently, clinically practicable PB techniques are needed. These should account for the size of the prostate, the patient's age, the DRE findings (suspect or not suspect), suspicious areas seen on transrectal ultrasound (TRUS) and the outcome of prior initial PB, if any. Rigid schemes offer, at best, some orientation in the decision-making process. The number of cores to be taken are best decided on an individualized basis, taking into consideration the above criteria.

Pain tolerance also decreases as the number of samples increases. This is why several authors recommended a local anesthetic to be injected in the neurovascular bundle or to be applied by enema prior to PB. In our experience this is, however, rarely necessary.

5.7 Nomograms

Based on various criteria, nomograms are calculatory models that are intended to increase the probability of obtaining meaningful results from an examination. They are also available for PB to improve its diagnostic accuracy. Among them, the nomogram by Vashi et al. is most helpful. It correlates the number of cores required with the patient's age and the gland volume [29]. Eastham et al. developed a nomogram for predicting prostate cancer in patients with a PSA of 0 to 4 ng/ml and suspect DRE. The variables considered for it included patient age, race, and PSA levels. Of these, only PSA levels were statistically significant predictors of a positive PB [8]. Djavan et al. introduced a nomogram for improving the diagnostic accuracy of repeat PB in patients with PSA levels between 4 and 10 ng (Vienna Nomogram). This nomogram is based on total PSA, f-PSA, PSA density, and PSA-TZ [7].

5.8 Transitional Zone and Seminal Vesicle Biopsy

Transitional zone biopsies have no place in the initial examination. They should, however, be obtained during repeat PB, even though the likelihood of a positive outcome is low when cores are taken only from the transitional zone (0.6%–1%) [27]. Seminal vesicle biopsy is useful in patients with a PSA level >15 to 20 ng/ml. In these, the likelihood of seminal vesicle invasion is increased to about 20%–25%. On account of their poor prognosis in terms of systemic progression they are no longer thought to qualify for (RPE) by some authors [15].

5.9 PB Volume Versus Total Tumor Volume

The amount of tumor present in the cores is not a reliable predictor of the total tumor volume. Only a large number of positive cores predicts a large tumor volume in the entire gland. A small number of positive cores, by contrast, does not correlate with a small tumor volume. This means that a small tumor volume found on PB does not conclusively predict the tumor volume present in the entire gland [2, 27]. Terris et al. showed that, if 1/6 cores is positive, the tumor volume is >0.5 cm^3 in 70% of cases [26].

References

1. Babaian RJ, Toi A, Kamoi K, et al (2000) A comparative analysis of sextant and an extended 11-core multisite directed biopsy strategy. J Urol 163:152–157
2. Bostwick DG (1997) Evaluating prostate needle biopsy: therapeutic and prognostic importance. CA Cancer J Clin 47:297–319
3. Bostwick DG, Qian J, Frankel K (1995) The incidence of high grade prostatic intraepithelial neoplasia in needle biopsies. J Urol 154:1791–1794
4. Brat DJ, Wills ML, Lecksell KL, et al (1999) How often are diagnostic features missed with less extensive histologic sampling of prostate needle biopsy specimens? Am J Surg Pathol 23:257–262
5. Cheville JC, Reznicek MJ, Bostwich DG (1997) The focus of "atypical glands, suspicious for malignancy" in prostatic needle biopsy specimens. Am J Clin Pathol 108:633–640
6. Davidson D, Bostwick DG, Qian J, et al (1996) Prostatic intraepithelial neoplasia is a risk factor for adenocarcinoma: predictive accuracy in needle biopsies. J Urol 154:1295–1299
7. Djavan B, Zlotta A, Remzi M, et al (2000) Optimal predictors of prostate cancer on repeat biopsy: a prospective study of 1051 men. J Urol 1144–1149
8. Eastham JA, May R, Robertson JL, et al (1999) Development of a nomogram that predicts the probability of a positive biopsy in men with an abnormal digital rectal examination and a prostate-specific antigen between 0 and 4 ng/ml. Urology 54:709–713
9. Eskew LA, Bare RL, McCullogh DL (1997) Systematic 5-region biopsy is superior to sextant method for diagnosing carcinoma of the prostate. J Urol 157:199–203
10. Henson DE, Hutter RVP, Farrow G (1994) Practice protocol for the examination of specimens removed from patients with adenocarcinoma of the prostate gland. A publication of the cancer committee, College of American Pathologists. Arch Pathol Lab Med 118:779–783
11. Hodge KK, McNeal JE, Terris MK (1989) Random systematic versus directed ultrasound guided transrectal core biopsies of the prostate. J Urol 142:66–70
12. Karakiewicz PI, Bazinet M, Aprikian AG (1997) Outcome of sextant biopsy according to gland volume. Urology 49:55–59
13. Karakiewicz PI, Hanley JA, Bazinet M (1998) Three-dimensional computer assisted analysis of sector biopsy of the prostate. Urology 52:208–212
14. Karakiewicz PI, Aprikian AG (1998) Prostate cancer. V. Diagnostic tools for early detection. CMAJ 159:1139–1146
15. Linzer DG, Stock RG, Stone NN, et al (1996) Seminal vesical biopsy: accuracy and implications for staging of prostate cancer. Urology 48:757–761
16. Manivel CJ (1997) Inconclusive results of needle biopsies of the prostate gland. What they mean and what to do [editorial]. Am J Clin Pathol 108:611–615
17. McNeal JE (1967) Regional morphology and pathology of the prostate. Am J Clin Pathol 49: 347–357
18. Naughton CK, Miller DC, Mager DE, et al (2000) A prospective randomized trial comparing 6 versus 12 prostate biopsy cores: impact on cancer detection. J Urol 164:388–392
19. Norberg M, Egevad L, Holmberg L, et al (1997) The sextant protocol for ultrasound guided biopsies of the prostate underestimates the presence of cancer. Urology 50:562–566
20. Presti JC, Chang JJ, Bhargava V, Shinohara K (2000) Optimal systematic prostate biopsy scheme should include 8 rather than 6 biopsies: results of a prospective clinical trial. J Urol 163: 163–167
21. Rabbani F, Stroumbakis N, Kava BR, et al (1998) Incidence and clinical significance of false-negative sextant prostate biopsies. J Urol 159:1247–1250
22. Ravery V, Goldblatt L, Royre B, et al (2000) Extensive biopsy protocol improves the detection rate of prostate cancer. J Urol 164:393–396
23. Raviv G, Zlotta AR, Janssen TH, et al (1996) Do prostate specific antigen and prostate specific antigen density enhance the detection of prostate carcinoma after initial diagnosis of prostatic intraepithelial neoplasia without concurrent carcinoma? Cancer 77:2103–2108
24. Reyes AO, Humphrey PA (1998) Diagnostic effect of complete histologic sampling of prostate needle biopsiy specimens. Am J Clin Pathol 109:416–422
25. Stroumbakis N, Cookson MS, Reuter VE, et al (1997) Clinical significance of repeat sextant biopsies in prostate cancer patients. Urology 49 [Suppl 3A]:113–118
26. Terris MK, McNeal JE, Stamey TA (1992) Detection of clinically significant prostate cancer by transrectal ultrasound guided systematic biopsies. J Urol 148:829–832
27. Terris MK, Pham TQ, Issa MM, et al (1997) Routine transition zone and seminal vesical biopsies in all patients undergoing transrectal ultrasound guided biopsies are not indicated. J Urol 157:204–206
28. Uzzo RG, Wie JT (1995) The influence of prostate size on cancer detection. Urology 46:831–836
29. Vashi AR, Wojno KJ, Gillespie B, et al (1998) A model for the number of cores per prostate biopsy based on patient age and prostate gland volume. J Urol 159:920–924

6 Molecular Forms of Prostate-Specific Antigen for Prostate Cancer Detection

B. Djavan, M.K. Brawer, M. Marberger

6.1 Introduction

Prostate cancer has become the most common neoplasm in men and the second leading cause of cancer death [28, 29, 67]. Attempts to reduce the mortality have mainly focused on early detection of this disease. Since its discovery in 1979, prostate-specific antigen (PSA) has unequivocally proved its usefulness as a serum marker for prostate cancer. However, in patients with a PSA below 10 ng/ml an important overlap exists between benign prostatic hyperplasia (BPH) and prostate cancer. Indeed, PSA is not prostate cancer specific and develops at an age when the prevalence of BPH is high. Previous reports indicate that two-thirds of the patients who undergo biopsies based on a PSA of 4–10 ng/ml have no histological evidence of prostate cancer [10]. Largely because of this large number of false positives, several concepts have been introduced, all aiming to optimize the clinical use of PSA by improving its sensitivity and specificity and trying to decrease the number of unnecessary biopsies in men with benign disease. These concepts include PSA density (relating the serum PSA to the volume of the prostate), PSA velocity (evaluating the rate of change of PSA values with time), age-adjusted PSA reference ranges (adjusting the PSA level with patient age), and determination of PSA molecular forms (free versus protein-bound forms of PSA).

Undoubtedly the most exciting advance in PSA testing has been the recognition that PSA circulates not in one form, but in a complex to protease inhibitors [20, 77]. This is because PSA, like other serine proteases, does not occur in an enzymatically active form in blood. Hence, regulation of enzymatic action of PSA is controlled by different means. First, PSA is produced as an inactive protease which is converted to the active enzyme by release of a small propeptide [56]. This activation is suggested to be dependent on the action of human glandular kallikrein (hK2) [42, 53, 56, 79], a closely homologous protein which, like PSA, is exclusively expressed by the prostate [16]. Second, although no candidate enzyme has been identified yet to be responsible, internal peptide bonds are cleaved at, e.g.,Lys145-Lys146 and Lys182-Ser183, which results in loss of enzymatic activity and the production of a PSA form often referred to as "nicked PSA" [20, 86]. The enzymatic action may also be inactivated by the reaction of PSA with several abundant extracellular protease inhibitors, such as α-2-macroglobulin (AMG), the AMG homologous inhibitor called pregnancy zone protein, α-1-antichymotrypsin (ACT), α-1-antitrypsin (API), or protein C inhibitor (PCI) [19, 20, 34, 77].

6.2 PSA, Free PSA, and Free to Total PSA Ratio

Most of the PSA that is in circulation is complexed to α-1-antichymotrypsin and other inhibitor complexes, including the PSA–AMG complex, which is complicated to measure, only occuring at low or very low levels in blood [19, 49, 50, 77, 87]. Free or noncomplexed PSA comprises a much smaller amount in the circulation, although this is the major form found in the ejaculate. Free PSA in blood differs from enzymatically active PSA in the ejaculate, being enzymatically inactive, hence unreactive with the large excess of inhibitors in blood [20, 49, 50, 71]. PSA is also bound to the α-2 macroglobulin, but this fraction is present at very low blood levels in blood in vivo [50, 87]. It forms, however, during imperfect storage of samples in vitro, is not detected by commercial immunoassays, and can only be measured by complicated relatively insensitive assays used for research purposes [50, 87].

Little is known about the site of formation of the complex of PSA with the protease inhibitors. This knowledge appears essential for understanding such basic apparent dilemmas as the fact that much more of the PSA–ACT complex is found in blood than is the PSA-AMG complex, when in fact enzymatically active PSA reacts much faster with AMG than with ACT in vitro [45, 50, 87]. It has been suggested that α-1-anti-chymotrypsin may be present to a greater degree in normal and transformed prostatic epithelium as compared to that represented by benign prostatic hyperplasia [7]. Thus the PSA–ACT complex formation could conceivably occur within the prostate itself as opposed the systemic blood circulation. We know that the free form of PSA occurs to a greater proportion in men without carcinoma, and by contrast the α-1-anti-chymotrypsin complex with PSA comprises a greater proportion of the total PSA in men with malignancy. Still, we do not know why the proportion of PSA–ACT complex is greater in blood from cancer patients than those with BPH.

In 1991 Stenman and associates demonstrated a correlation between the level of a PSA complex and prostate cancer [77]. Subsequently, Christensson et al. demonstrated the ratio of free to total PSA was lower in men with cancer [21]. Luderer et al. [55] demonstrated that over the truncated range of total PSA between 4.0 and 10.0 ng/ml the total PSA did not differ between men with and without carcinoma. However, free PSA was significantly lower in men with cancer. Other results have also been reported by Higashihara et al. [40], Chen et al. [18], and Djavan et al. [29] (Table 6.1).

Perhaps the most definitive trial of free to total PSA measurement was recently reported by Catalona and colleagues [15]. This seven-institution

Table 6.1. Sensitivity, specificity and positive predictive and negative values at different cutoff values. Free-to-total prostate-specific antigen (PSA) and PSA 4.0–10 ng/ml (521 patients)

% Free-to-total PSA cut-off	% Sensitivity	% Specificity	Positive predictive value	Negative predictive value
10	33.690	92.308	0.74118	0.68041
15	54.545	79.021	0.62963	0.72669
20	68.984	69.930	0.60000	0.77519
30	87.701	54.196	0.55593	0.87079
40	96.257	32.168	0.48128	0.92929

Djavan et al. [29].

Table 6.2. Specificity of free-to-total prostate-specific antigen level at various sensitivity levels

Sensitivity (%)	Cut-off	Specificity (%)
90	22	29
95	25	20
98	32	6

Catalona et al. [15].

study evaluated men with a total PSA between 4.0 and 10.0 ng/ml with no evidence of cancer at digital rectal examination. Utilizing the Hybritech method, these authors observed that when the free to total PSA ratio was less than 25%, the sensitivity of the test was 95% and the specificity enhanced by 20%. These results indicate that if a clinician is willing to miss 5% of cancers, one out of five negative biopsies can be avoided (Table 6.2). Another trial performed by Hugosson et al. in 1995–1996 [41] in Sweden included 5853 of almost 10,000 (about 60%) invited, randomly selected men, aged 50–66 years, who were tested for free and total PSA levels in blood [41]. There were 145 men diagnosed with cancer among 612 biopsied men with total PSA >3.0 ng/ml. Twenty-four percent of the men diagnosed with cancer (i.e., 36/145 men) had total PSA levels from 3.0–4.0 ng/ml using the EG&G Wallace Dual Prostatus assay. Only 5/36 of these men had abnormal digital rectal examination (DRE) findings [51].

The large number of men with benign biopsy findings (466/611 biopsied men) were reduced by 44% using a cut-off ≤18% free PSA. This occurred at the expense of not detecting 11% (16/145) of men with cancer, who had >18% free PSA mainly resulting from an enlarged prostate gland [41]. Analysis of percent free PSA may also be useful in men with total PSA levels <3.0 ng/ml, as shown by another trial undertaken in 1988–1989 of 1748 of 2400 invited men aged 55–70 years who were examined by DRE, transrectal ultrasound (TRUS) and PSA. The carefully stored samples (–70 C) were analyzed for percentage of free PSA in 1995 [80]. In total, 367 of the 1748 examined men were biopsied and 64 men diagnosed with cancer. In 9/9 cancer patients with total PSA levels below 3.0 ng/ml, ≤18% free PSA was indicative of cancer as opposed to no cancer detected in 159 biopsied men with >18% free PSA [80].

While it is apparent that the measurement of free to total PSA ratio is a significant advance in cancer detection several concerns exist. First of all, the detailed molecular nature of the free form has yet to be clarified. Further, it is essential that the vital importance of introducing pre-analytical handling instructions be stressed as the levels and percentage of free PSA may decrease during sample storage in vitro [71]. This loss may, at least in part, be due to protease activity in the sample released by blood clotting and/or granulocytes. This might account for inferior stability of free PSA in serum compared to samples collected as EDTA- or heparin-anticoagulated plasma [71, 83]. Further the PSA–ACT complex may also decompose and increase the free PSA levels in serum [78], although the dissociation rate of the complex is insignificant under optimal storage conditions [69]. For further details, the reader is referred to the excellent summary by Woodrum and associates [84]. Perhaps of greatest concern is the fact that different manufacturer assays may give different results on the same sera with respect to the free to total PSA ratio. Measurement of two analytes potentially compounds the bias between different manufacturer assays. We have observed

Table 6.3

Assay	Cut-off for 95% sensitivity	Specificity
Hyb. F / Hyb. T	22%	38%
Dia. F / Hyb. T	35%	19%
Chi. F / Hyb. T	35%	33%
DELFIA/ WALLAC	37%	36%

Djavan et al. [29], Nixon et al. [63].
Hyb., Hybritech; Dia., Dianon; Chi., Chiron; F, free prostate-specific antigen; T, total prostate-specific antigen.

considerable bias in total PSA [63, 74] and also free PSA [63]. More recently, we have demonstrated significant bias when the free assays of different manufacturers are compared and when the free and total PSA assays from the same manufacturers are contrasted [74]. In this latter investigation, 240 sera referred for routine PSA testing were compared utilizing three different manufacturers' free assays and their corresponding total assays. Tables 6.3 and 6.4 demonstrate the significant findings. We observed similarity between the Chiron ACS-180 and Tandem R assays but different results with the Enzymum assay.

These data show marked variability when different manufacturer assays are employed. Clinicians should be aware of the assays used in their institutions, and laboratory staff should define the performance of each free to total PSA assay in their patient setting prior to utilizing this test clinically.

A number of issues remain with respect to understanding the proper utilization of the free to total PSA ratio. Of course one of the most important is: Who should this test be used on? All men, or only those within a more restricted PSA range, say 4.0–10.0 ng/ml? Another possible cohort would be those men with a PSA of less than 4.0 ng/ml, where approximately 25% of carcinomas are detected. Finally, an ideal situation may be the use in those patients who have undergone a previously negative prostate needle biopsy. It is widely recognized that 20%–30% of such men harbor malignancy, which is detected on repeat biopsy. Recently we have demonstrated that free to total PSA may help to stratify those men who have carcinoma despite an initial negative biopsy [46].

Table 6.4. Sensitivity and specificity of total prostate specific antigen (PSA) and the free-to-total (FT) prostate-specific antigen ratio

Assay	Sensitivity (%)	Specificity (%) Total PSA	Specificity (%) F/T PSA	Cut-point Total PSA (ng/ml)	Cut-point F/T PSA (%)
ACS:180 PSA2 and free PSA	100	0	0	0.02	90
	95	10	17	1.7	25
	90	25	54	3.3	15
Enzymun PSA and free PSA	100	0	0	0.02	100
	95	5	7	1.1	43
	90	24	32	3.0	23
Tandem-R PSA and free PSA	100	1	1	0.4	52
	95	7	22	2.1	25
	90	17	31	3.4	21

Data from Roth et al. [74].

6.3 Complexed PSA

Although utilization of serum PSA testing for early detection of prostate cancer is generally accepted, the specifity of PSA assays is low. Studies have demonstrated that 70%–80% of men on whom biopsies were performed did not have prostate cancer [11, 14]. Thus, improvement of specificity in early detection of prostate carcinoma is needed to avoid costly and unnecessary biopsies. It has been recognized that the majority of PSA found in men with cancer is complexed to α-1-antichymotrypsin as opposed to PSA found in healthy men [21, 77]. However, early work to measure PSA–ACT complexes encountered difficulties demonstrating nonspecific binding or over-recovery due to technical problems in accurate measurement of complexed PSA [21, 82]. Indeed, the reason we used free to total PSA is because complexed PSA assays were not available despite recognition that it was the most important moiety to measure. This statement derives from the fact that this form is found in greater proportion in men with carcinoma. The previous technical problems in designing specific PSA–ACT complex assay procedures have largely been overcome [69]. However, decomposition of the PSA–ACT complex during storage under suboptimal conditions may release enzymatically active PSA in vitro [69]. In vitro this may result in formation of either AMG-PSA complexes, or, if the AMG fraction in blood has become inactivated, false elevatation of free PSA. These factors could explain some of the data reported on samples stored at –20°C for more than 20 years [78].

Recently the Bayer Corporation (Tarrytown, NY) has developed a PSA assay, Immuno 1 cPSA, specific for complexed PSA. The design of this assay reflects the level of PSA complexed to different serpin-inhibitor ligands, such ACT, API, and PCI: The PSA–ACT complex fraction is by far the predominant complex PSA form [49, 77] measured by this assay. A multicenter evaluation established the analytical performance and clinical effectiveness of this Bayer assay in monitoring of prostate cancer patients during the course disease and therapy. The cPSA assay demonstrated an increased trend in clinical sensitivity (71%–86%) for prostate carcinoma with increasing stage of disease. Clinical specificity for patients with benign urogenital disease was 74.8%. For other nonprostate diseases specificity ranged from 91.1% to 100%. Retrospective serial monitoring of 155 patients with prostate carcinoma showed concordance of the PSA complex measurements to clinical status for 97% of the patients analyzed. The results from the multicenter clinical evaluation using the Bayer Immuno 1 cPSA assay were comparable to the results obtained with the Bayer Immuno 1 PSA assay.

We performed an initial evaluation of this assay utilizing a series of men who previously underwent ultrasound-guided needle biopsy of whom archival serum was available [12]. We compared the results of the Bayer Immuno-1 cPSA assay and the Hybritech Tandem R free and total assays (Hybritech, Incorporated, San Diego, CA). As expected the mean-to-total PSA and PSA complex were higher in those men with carcinoma and the free-to-total PSA was lower. A good correlation between total PSA and the sum of free PSA and PSA complex was observed. Performance characteristics for total PSA, PSA complex, and free to total PSA are shown in Table 6.5. At 95% sensitivity specificity for total PSA was 22%. A complexed PSA cut-off of 2.52 demonstrated an enhanced specificity of 26.7%. The free to total PSA ratio at 28% resulted in a specificity of only 15.6%. Moreover, similar findings have recently been reported in a multicenter investigations with a Bayer PSA complex [8] (Table 6.6).

Table 6.5. Specificity of the cut-off values of the different prostate-specific antigen (PSA) assays at selected sensitivities

% Sensitivity	Total PSA		PSA complex		Free/total PSA	
	Cut-off (ng/ml)	% Specificity	Cut-off (ng/ml)	% Specificity	Cut-off (%)	% Specificity
80	4.11	35.6	3.98	51.6	19	46.2
85	3.86	31.1	3.34	38.7	22	32.4
90	3.4	25.3	2.94	33.8	24	26.2
95	3.06	21.8	2.52	26.7	28	15.6
97.5	2.28	12.9	1.67	14.7	32	8.9
100	1.0	3.1	0.89	6.2	67	0

Data from Brawer et al. [12].

Table 6.6. Performance of total prostate-specific antigen (tPSA), PSA in complex (cPSA) and free-to-total PSA (F/T PSA) in multiple study centers

Entire tPSA range	Sensitivity				Specificity			
Study center	*n*	tPSA[a]	cPSA[b]	f/t PSA[c]	n	tPSA[a]	cPSA[b]	f/t PSA[c]
Vienna	52	82	–	87	52	33	–	54
Seattle	75	85	83	77	225	37	48	48
Johns Hopkins	167	90	85	87	128	20	29	27

[a] Cutoff = 4.0 ng/ml.
[b] Cutoff = 3.75 ng/ml.
[c] Cutoff = 25% when total PSA >4.0 ng/ml.

6.4 PSA Complex in Screening

Currently, we are carrying out a prospective screening study with this assay and have shown that cPSA identifies all men with prostate cancer who would be found with a total PSA of greater than 4.0 ng/ml, and does so with a significant reduction in the negative biopsy rate (unpublished observation). Assuming that similar results are found in other investigations, it would appear that the PSA complex offers a significant advance over total PSA for early detection and screening due to specificity enhancement. Recently cPSA has been approved for monitoring men with prostate cancer. In this application, for staging, and for other applications this assay should provide the same information as afforded by total PSA.

6.5 Combination of PSA and PSA Derivatives

PSA based parameters can be combined to improve CaP detection. In a recent study by Djavan et al. [30], the ability of PSAD, PSA-TZ, PSA velocity, percent free PSA, and their combination to improve the detection of CaP, was evaluated with univariate and multivariate analyses as well as receiver operating characteristic (ROC) curves. The combination of PSA-TZ and free-to-total (f/t) PSA

Table 6.7. Area under the curve in the receiver operating charactristic curves for each of the different parameters used, separately or in combination

	PSA 4.0–10 ng/ml
1. PSA	61.2%
2. PSA velocity	58.0%
3. f/t PSA	77.8%
4. PSAD	76.2%
5. PSA-TZ	82.7%
6. Combination PSA-TZ and f/t PSA	88.1%
7. Combination PSA-TZ and PSAD	82.9%
8. Combination PSA-TZ and PSA	82.4%
9. Combination f/t PSA and PSA	78.9%
10. Combination f/t PSA and PSAD	73.4%
11. Combination PSAD and PSA	78.4%

Areas are given in percentage.
Djavan et al. [30].
tPSA, total prostate-specific antigen; cPSA, PSA in complex; f/t PSA, free-to-total PSA; PSA-TZ.

significantly increased the area under the curve (AUC) as compared to the use of any other combination ($P = 0.020$, Mc Nemar test). In fact, PSA-TZ + f/t PSA showed an AUC of 88.1% followed by PSA-TZ + PSAD (82.9%), PSA-TZ + PSA (82.4%), PSAD + PSA (78.4%) and f/t PSA + PSAD (73.4%). Obviously, volume-dependent PSA parameters such as PSAD and PSA-TZ were crucial when PSA parameters were combined. However, if volume independent PSA combinations are to be considered, f/t PSA + PSA clearly outperformed all other possible combinations.

6.6 Human Glandular Kallikrein 2

PSA and human glandular kallikrein 2 (hK2) are proteases that, along with human kallikrein 1 (hK1), comprise the kallikrein family, a subgroup of a large family of serine proteases [2, 5, 47, 48, 81]. Numerous review articles on kallikreins, PSA, and, more recently, hK2, are available [1, 5, 6, 9, 13, 22, 23, 24, 25, 31, 32, 33, 37, 39, 44, 48, 57, 58, 59, 62, 64, 65, 66, 68, 73, 76, 85].

There are structural similarities between hK1, hK2, and PSA [13, 72, 75]. The first known protein in this family is a true kallikrein, termed tissue kallikrein or hK1. That was discovered over 60 years ago [6, 36, 60]. The kallikrein function of hK1 is to cleave polypeptide substrates from low-molecular-weight (l) kininogen to release a vasoactive decapeptide Lys-bradykinin (kallidin) [6]. Initial studies indicated that PSA was capable of generating small amounts of kinin-like substances when incubated with seminal vesicle fluid [35]. However, recent studies with PSA preparations, free of trypsin-like activity, demonstrated that PSA does not appear to act as a true kallikrein despite its structural similarity to hK1 [27]. A small amount of kininogenase activity has been observed with hK2 on high-molecular-weight kininogen, although this activity is 1000-fold lower than that of hK1 [27].

The hK2 protein has an appoximately 79% identity in primary structure to PSA [75] and shares several important properties with PSA, such as tissue-restricted expression pattern; however, hK2 has markedly different enzymatic properties [26, 54, 61]. Several of these properties suggest that hK2 may also be useful in diagnosis of prostate cancer. Several immunoassays specific for hK2 have now been developed [17, 70], which have demonstrated that the hK2 levels are in the picograms per milliliter range and therefore only 1%–2% of the total PSA concentration [43, 70], though not directly proportional to PSA, and may hence provide additional clinical information. Low analyte concentration and immunological cross-reactivity relating to similarity [52, 70] with PSA initially hampered progress in this field, but can now be overcome in as much as hK2 assays have now been reported which detect 0.03 ng/ml of hK2, cross-react insignificantly with PSA (<0.01%), and provide equimolar detection of free and forms of hK2 in complex [4]. The majority of hK2 in serum is free, only about 5%–20% of hK2 is believed to be present in a complex form, mainly with ACT [4, 38, 70]. The serum levels of hK2 are very low in females and in prostate cancer patients following radical prostatectomy. These levels are significantly higher in men with benign prostatic disease than in young healthy men. Further, hK2 levels are significantly elevated in the men with localized prostate cancer compared to to those with BPH [3, 17]. Recently, it has been proposed that hK2 measurements in combination with free and total PSA can improve the sensitivity and specificity of cancer detection and avoid unnecessary biopsies, also in total PSA levels from 2.5 to 4.0 ng/ml. Certainly, more comprehensive studies are needed to confirm the utility of the hK2 measurements in serum. The interrelationships of hK2 with free and total PSA may require appropriate algorithms, such as logistic regression or artificial neural networks. Overall, hK2 seems to offer complementary information to that of PSA. Its potential for replacing the latter, however, is doubtful.

In summary, PSA, free PSA and lately complex PSA have revolutionized our management of men with prostate cancer. They offer the best means of detecting early stage disease. Significant advances particularly in the realm of increased specificity will undoubtedly continue to unfold. Novel markers such as human kallikrein type 2, prostate specific membrane antigen, and other tests will surely aid clinicians and their patients.

References

1. Armbruster DA (1993) Prostate-specific antigen: biochemistry, analytical methods and clinical application. Clin Chem 39: 181–195
2. Ban Y, Wang MC, Watt KW, et al (1984) The proteolytic activity of human prostate-specific antigen. Biochem Biophys Res Commun 123: 482–488
3. Becker C, Piironen T, Pettersson K, et al. (2000) Discrimination of men with prostate cancer from those with benign disease by measurements of human glandular kallikrein (hK2) in serum. J Urol 163: 311–316
4. Becker C, Piironen T, Kiviniemi J, Lilja H, Petersson K (2000) Sensitive and specific immunodetection of human glandular kallikrein 2 (hK2) in serum. Clin Chem 46: 198–206
5. Berg T, Bratshaw RA, Carretero OA, et al (1996) A common nomenclature for members of the tissue (glandular) kallikrein gene families. Agents Actions Suppl 38: 19–25
6. Bhoola KD, Figueroa CD, Worthy K (1992) Bioregulation of kinins: kallikreins, kininogens, and kininases. Pharmacol Rev 44: 1–80
7. Bjork T, Bjartell A, Abrahamsson PA, Hulkko S, diSant'Agnese A, Lilja H (1994) Alpha-1-antichymotrypsin production in PSA producing cells is common in prostate cancer but rare in benign prostatic hyperplasia. Urology 43: 427–434
8. Brawer M, Partin A (1999) The promise of new serum markers for prostate cancer. Contemp Urol 11: 44–75
9. Brawer MK (1991) Prostate-specific antigen: a review. Acta Oncol 30: 161–168
10. Brawer MK (1994) Prosate-specific antigen: critical issues. Urology 44: 9

11. Brawer MK, Chetner MP, Beati J, Buchner MD, Vessela RL, Lange PH (1994) Screening for prostatic carcinoma with PSA. J Urol 147: 841–845
12. Brawer MK, Meyer GE, Letran JL, et al. (1998) Measurement of complexed PSA improves specificity for early detection of prostate cancer. Urology 52: 372–378
13. Carbini LA, Scicli GA, Carretero OA (1993) The molecular biology of the kallikrein-chinin system. III. The human kallikrein gene family and kallikrein substrate. J Hypertens 11: 893–898
14. Catalona WJ, Hudson MA, Scardino PT, et al. (1994) Selection of optimal PSA cutoffs for early detection of prostate cancer: receiver operating characteristic curves. J Urol 152: 2037–2042
15. Catalona WJ, Partin AW, Slawin KM, et al. (1998) Use of the percentage of free prostate-specific antigen to enhance differentiation of prostate cancer from benign prostatic disease: a prospective multicenter clinical trial. JAMA 279: 1542–1547
16. Chapdelaine P, Paradis G, Temblay RR, Dube JY (1988) High level of expression in the prostate of a human glandular kallikrein mRNA related to prostate-specific antigen. FEBS Lett 236: 205– 208
17. Charlesworth MC, Young Cyf, Klee GG, et al. (1997) Detection of a prostate-specific protein, hK2, in sera of patients with elevated prostate-specific antigen levels. Urology 49: 487–493
18. Chen Y, Luderer AA, Thiel RP, Carlson G, Cuny CL, Soriano TF (1996) Using proportions of free to total prostate-specific antigen, age, and total prostate-specific antigen to predict the probability of prostate cancer. Urology 47: 518–524
19. Christensson A, Lilja H (1994) Complex formation between protein C inhibitor and prostate-specific antigen in vitro and in human semen. Eur J Biochem 220: 45–53
20. Christensson A, Laurell CB, Lilja H (1990) Enzymatic activity of prostate-specific antigen and its reaction with extracellular serine proteinase inhibitors. Eur J Biochem 194: 755
21. Christensson A, Bjork T, Nilsson O, et al (1993) Serum prostate-specific antigen complexed to alpha 1-antichymotrypsin as an indicator of prostate cancer. J Urol 150: 100–105
22. Chu TM (1990) Prostate cancer-associated markers. In: Herbermann RB, Mercer GW (eds) Immunodiagnosis of cancer. Immunology series. Marcel Deker, New York, pp 339–356
23. Chu TM (1992) Prostate-specific antigen. In: Sell S (ed) Serological cancer markers. Humana Press, Totowa, pp 99–115
24. Chu TM (1994) Prostate-specific antigen in screening of prostate cancer. J Clin Lab Anal 8: 323–326
25. Clements JA (1994) The human kallikrein family: a diversity of expression and function. Mol Cell Endocrinol 99: 1–6
26. Denmeade SR, Lou W, Lovgren J, Malm J, Lilja H, Issacs JT (1997) Specific and efficient peptide substrates for assaying the proteolytic activity of prostate-specific antigen. Cancer Res 57: 4924–4930
27. Deperthes D, Marceau S, Frenette G, et al (1997) Human kallikrein hK2 has low kininogenase activity while prostate-specific antigen (hK3) has none. Biochem Biophys Acta 1343: 102–106
28. Dijkman GA, Debruyne FM (1996) Epidemiology of prostate cancer. Eur Urol 30: 281–295
29. Djavan B, Zlotta AR, Byttebier G, Shariat S, Omar M, Schulman CC, Marberger M (1998) Prostate specific antigen density of the transitional zone for early detection of prostate cancer. J Urol 160: 411–419
30. Djavan B, Remzi M, Zlotta AR, et al (1999) Combination and multivariate analysis of PSA-based parameters for prostate cancer. Tech Urol 5: 71–76
31. Dube JY (1992) Tissue kallikreins and prostatic diseases in men: new questions. Biochem Cell Biol 70: 177–178
32. Dube JY (1994) Prostatic kallikreins: biochemistry and physiology. Comp Biochem Physiol 107: 13–20
33. Dube JY, Tremblay RR (1997) Biochemistry and potential roles of prostatic kallikrein hK2. Mol Urol 1: 279–285
34. Espana F, Sanchez CJ, Vera CD, Estelles A, Gilabert J (1993) A quantitative ELISA for a measurement of complexes of prostate-specific antigen with a protein C inhibitor when using a purified standard. J Lab Clin Med 122: 711–709
35. Fichtner J, Graves HCB, Thatcher K, et al. (1996) Prostate-specific antigen releases a kinin-like substance on proteolysis of seminal vesicle fluid that stimulates smooth muscle contraction. J Urol 155: 738–742
36. Frey EK, Kraut H, Werle E (1932) Über die blutzuckersenkende Wirkung des Kallikreins (Padutins). Klin Wochenschr 11: 846–849
37. Gittes RF (1991) Carcinoma of the prostate. N Engl J Med 324: 236–243
38. Grauer LS, Finlay JA, Mikolajczyk SD, Pusateri KD, Wolfert RL (1998) Detection of human glandular kallikrein hK2 as its precursor form, and in complex with protease inhibitors in prostate carcinoma serum. J Androl 19: 407–411
39. Henttu P, Vinko P (1994) Prostate-specific antigen and human glandular kallikrein:two kallikreins of the human prostate. Ann Med 26: 157–164
40. Higashihara E, Nutahara K, Kojima M, et al. (1996) Significance of serum free prostate-specific antigen in the screening of prostate cancer. J Urol 156: 1964–1968
41. Hugosson J, Aus G, Berdahl S, et al. (2001) Population based screening for prostate cancer by measurements of free and total concentration of prostate-specific antigen (PSA). Urology 2001 (submitted)

42. Kumar A, Mikolajczyk SD, Goel AS, Millar LS, Saedi M (1997) Expression of form of prostate-specific antigen by mammalian cells and its conversion to mature, active form by human kallikrein2. Cancer Res 57: 3111–3114
43. Kwiatkowski MK, Recker F, Piironen T, et al. (1998) In prostatism patients the ratio of human glandular kallikrein to free PSA improves the discrimination between prostate cancer and benign hyperplasia within the diagnostic grey zone of total PSA 4–10 ng/ml. Urology 52: 360–365
44. Lang RJ, Roberts KB, Wilson MJ, et al. (1997) Prostate cancer: a clinical and basic science review. J Androl 18: 15–20
45. Leinonen J, Stenman UH (1996) Complex formation between PSA isoenzymes and prostate inhibitors. J Urol 155: 1099–1103
46. Letran JL, Blase AB, Loberiza FR, Meyer GE, Ransom SD, Brawer MK (1998) Repeat ultrasound-guided prostate needle biopsy: the utility of free to total PSA ratio in predicting those men with or without prostatic carcinoma. J Urol 160: 426–429
47. Lilja H (1985) A kallikrein-like prostate protease in prostatic fluid cleaves the predominant seminal vesicle protein. J Clin Invest 76: 1899–1903
48. Lilja H (1993) Structure, function and regulation of the enzyme activity of prostate-specific antigen. World J Urol 11: 188–191
49. Lilja H, Christensson A, Dahlen U, et al. (1991) Prostate-specific antigen in human serum occurs predominantly in complex with alpha-1-antichymotrypsin. Clin Chem 37: 1618–1625
50. Lilja H, Haese A, Bjork T, et al (1999) Significance and metabolism of complexed and non-complexed prostate-specific antigen (PSA) forms and human glandular kallikrein 2 (hK2) in localized prostate cancer befor and after radical prostatectomy. J Urol 162: 2029–2034
51. Lodding P, Luderer AA, Thiel RP, Carlson G, Cuny CL, Soriano TF (1998) Characteristics of screening detected prostate cancer in men 50–65 years old with 3 to 4 ng/ml prostate-specific antigen. J Urol 159: 899–903
52. Lovgren J, Piironen T, Overmo C, et al. (1995) Production of recombinat PSA and hK2 and analysis of their immunologic cross-reactivity. Biochem Biophys Res Commun 213: 888–895
53. Lovgren J, Rajakoski K, Karp M, Lundwall A, Lilja H (1997) Activation of the zymogen form of prostate-specific-antigen by human glandular kallikrein 2. Biophys Res Comm 238: 549–555
54. Lovgren J, Airas K, Lilja H (1999) Enzymatic action of human glandular kallikrein 2 (´hK2): substrate specificity and regulation by Zn2+ and extracellular protease inhibitors. Eur J Biochem 262: 781–789
55. Luderer AA, Chen Y, Thiel R, et al. (1995) Measurement of the proportion of free to total PSA improves diagnostic performance of PSA in the diagnostic gray zone of total PSA. Urology 46: 187–194
56. Lundwall A, Lilja H (1987) Molecular cloning of human prostate-specific antigen cDNA. FEBS Lett 214: 317–322
57. Malm J, Lilja H (1995) Biochemistry of prostate-specific antigen, PSA. Scand J Clin Lab Invest Suppl 221: 15–22
58. Marinovic V, Cuperlovic M, Hajducovic-Dragojlovic L (1997) Prostate-specific antigen: biochemical characteristics, biological functions and diagnostic potential in prostate cancer screening. Yugoslav Med Biochem 16: 129–136
59. McCormack RT, Brittenhouse HG, Finlay JA, et al. (1995) Molecular forms of prostate-specific antigen and the human kallikrein gene family: a new era. Urology 45: 729–744
60. McDonald RJ, Margolius HS, Erdös EG (1988) Molecular biology of tissue kallikrein. Biochem J 253: 313–321
61. Mikolajczyk SD, Millar LS, Kumar A, Saedi MS (1998) Human glandular kallikrein 2, hK2, shows arginine-restricted specificity and forms complexes with plasma protease inhibitors. Prostate 34: 44–50
62. Murphy G (1995) Radioscintiscanning of prostate cancer. Cancer Suppl 75: 1819–1822
63. Nixon RG, Gold MH, Blase AB, Meyer GE, Brawer MK (1998) Comparison of three investigative assays for the free form of prostate-specific antigen. J Urol 160: 420–425
64. Oesterling JE (1991) Prostate-specific antigen: critical assessment of the most useful tumor marker for adenocarcinoma of the prostate. J Urol 145: 907–923
65. Oesterling JE (1993) Prostatic tumor markers. J Urol Clin North Am 20: 575–777
66. Oesterling JE (1993) PSA leads the way for detecting and following prostate cancer. Contemp Urol 5: 60–82
67. Parker SL, Tong T, Bolden S, Winog PA (1996) Cancer statistics, 1996. CA Cancer J 46: 5–27
68. Partin AW, Oesterling JE (1994) The clinical usefulness of prostate-specific antigen: update 1994. J Urol 152: 1358–1368
69. Pettersson K, Piironen T, Seppala M, et al. (1995) Free and complexed prostate-specific antigen (PSA): in vitro stability, epitope map, and development of immunofluorometric assays for specifc and sensitive detection of free PSA and PSA-alpha-1-antichymotrypsin complex. Clin Chem 41: 1480–1488
70. Piironen T, Lovgren J, Karp M, et al. (1996) Immunofluorometric assay for sensitive and specific measurement of human prostatic glandular kallikrein (hK2) in serum. Clin Chem 42: 1034–1041

71. Piironen T, Pettersson K, Suonpaa M, et al. (1996) In vitro stability of free prostate-specific antigen (PSA) and prostate-specific antigen (PSA) complexed to alpha-1-antichymotrypsin in blood samples. Urology 48: 81–87
72. Riegman PH, Vlietstra RJ, Suurmeijer L, et al. (1992) Characterization of the human kallikrein locus. Genomics 14: 6–11
73. Rittenhouse HG, Tindall DJ, Klee GG, et al. (1997) Characterisation and evaluation of hK2: a potential prostate cancer marker, closely related to PSA. In: Murphy GP, Khoury S (eds). Proceedings of the first International Consultation on prostate cancer. Scientific Communication International, Monaco, pp 133–140
74. Roth HJ, Christensen-Stewart S, Brawer MK (1998) A comparison of three free and total PSA assays. PCPD 1: 326–331
75. Schedlich LJ, Bennetts BH, Morris BJ (1987) Primary structure of human glandular kallikrein gene. DNA 6: 429–437
76. Sikes RA (1996) Prostate-specific antigen. Clin Biochem Rev 17: 50–68
77. Stenman U, Leinonen J, Alfthan H, Rannikko S, Tuhkanen K, Althan O (1991) A complex between PSA and a 1-antichymotrypsin is the major form of PSA in serum of patients with prostatic cancer: assay of the complex improves clinical sensitivity for cancer. Cancer Res 51: 222
78. Stenman UH, Hakama M, Knekt P, Aromaa A, Teppo L, Leinonen J (1994) Serum concentrations of prostate specific antigen and its complex with alpha 1-antichymotrypsin before diagnosis of prostate cancer. Lancet 344: 1594–1598
79. Takayama TK, Fujikawa K, Davie EW (1997) Characterization of the precursor of prostate-specific antigen-activation by trypsin and by human glandular kallikrein. J Biol Chem 272: 21582–21588
80. Tornblom M, Norming U, Adolfsson, et al. (1999) Diagnostic value of percent free-PSA: retrospective analysis of a population-based screening study with emphasis on men with PSA less than 3.0 ng/ml. Urology 53: 945–950
81. Watt KW, Lee PJA, Timkulu T, et al. (1986) Human prostate-specific antigen: structural and functional similarity with serine proteases. Proc Natl Acad Sci USA 83: 3166–3170
82. Wood WG, Van der sloot GE, Bohle A (1991) The establishment and evaluation of luminescent-labeled immunometric assays for PSA-alpha-1-antichymotrypsin complexes in serum. Eur J Clin Chem Biochem 29: 787–794
83. Woodrum D, French C, Shamel LB (1996) Stability of free prostate-specific antigen in serum samples under a variety of sample collection and storage conditions. Urology 33 [Suppl 6A]:9
84. Woodrum DL, Brawer MK, Partin AW, Catalona WJ, Southwick PC (1998) Interpretation of free prostate-specific antigen clinical research studies for the detection of prostate cancer. J Urol 159: 5–12
85. Young CYF, Andrews PE, Tindall DJ (1995) Expression and androgenic regulation of human prostate-specific kallikreins. J Androl 16: 97–99
86. Zhang WM, Leinonon J, Kalkkinen N, Dowell B, Stenman UH (1995) Purification and characterization of different molecular forms of prostate-specific antigen in human seminal fluid. Clin Chem 41: 1567–1573
87. Zhang WM, Finne P, Leinonen J, et al. (1998) Characterization and immunological determination of the complex between prostate-specific antigen and alpha-2-macroglobulin. Clin Chem 44: 2471–2479

7 Clinical and Pathohistological Prognosticators

H. Huland, M. Graefen, A. Haese, P.G. Hammerer, J. Palisaar, U. Pichlmeier, R.-P. Henke, A. Erbersdobler, E. Huland, H. Lilja

7.1 Synopsis

The clinical T1–T2 prostatic carcinoma is a heterogeneous tumor in respect to pathologic stage and outcome. Tumor heterogeneity can be fairly well predicted using classification and regression tree analysis (CART) with preoperative parameters, especially a quantitative analysis of Gleason grade 4–5 cancer in six systematic biopsies and a determination of preoperative prostate-specific antigen (PSA) levels, to predict lymph node status, capsular penetration, and outcome.

Several studies by other investigators and ourselves have revealed that T1–T2 prostatic carcinoma is heterogeneous with respect to pathological stage and outcome. The most important prognostic factor in prostate cancer is the quantity of Gleason grade 4–5 tumor, which can be used to predict the presence or absence of lymph node metastases and capsular penetration, respectively. Moreover, it has significant contribution to the outcome after radical prostatectomy. CART analysis that uses a panel of preoperative parameters – for example, PSA levels or a semiquantitative analysis of six systematic biopsies with respect to the percentage of Gleason 4–5 cancer – is a powerful and easy-to-use tool for predicting whether an individual patient has lymph nodes positive for cancer, and predicting the presence and side of its capsular penetration. This information can be used in making a preoperative decision of whether to perform a unilateral or bilateral nerve-sparing radical prostatectomy without compromising the completeness of cancer removal. Finally, the prognosis for cure after radical prostatectomy is also obtained.

7.2 T1–T2 Prostatic Carcinoma Is Heterogeneous

Several investigations have revealed that T1–T2 prostatic carcinoma is a heterogeneous tumor with respect to pathologic staging and outcome after radical prostatectomy. This has been shown in many studies from well-known centers throughout the world where careful work-ups of radical prostatectomy specimens were performed using the 2- or 3-mm step-section technique with an undetectable PSA level as endpoint in the follow-up of the patients [1, 6, 14, 16, 19, 23, 25, 26]. Outcome in terms of PSA-free survival is excellent for patients with a pT2 tumor; approximately 90% of tumors are cured with a follow-up of 5–10 years (Fig. 7.1). However, the outcome is less favorable for patients with pT3 tumors [24], especially for those with seminal vesicle invasion. The prognosis is poor for patients with pT4 tumors and for those with lymph nodes positive for disease. These latter groups are typically not cured by radical prostatectomy. We, like clinicians at many other centers, have observed a stage migration: the percentage of patients whose cancers were detected by elevated PSA levels has

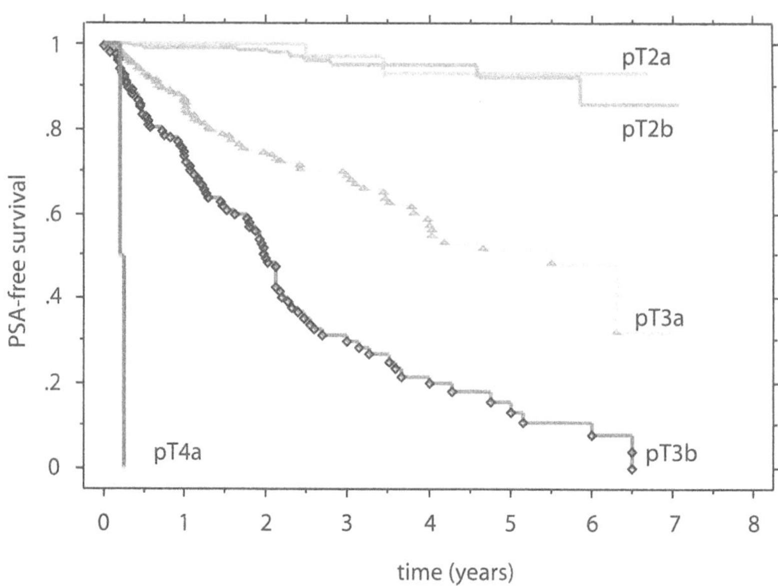

Fig. 7.1. Kaplan-Meier analysis. PSA-free survival of patients with tumors of different pT stage ($n = 789$)

Table 7.1. Stage migration of radical prostatectomy specimens 1992–1999

Variable	Year							
	1992	1993	1994	1995	1996	1997	1998	1999
No. patients	69	95	80	119	125	194	227	317
pT2 (%)	30	32	31	46	55	58	55	60
Positive margin (%)	35	27	24	22	13	14	19	19
T1c (%)	10	10	16	38	45	47	46	51
Cancer volume <0.5 cm³ (%)	7	9	4	4	2	2	2	3
Nerve sparing (%)	16	26	28	27	40	48	54	62

risen from 10% to 15% in 1992 to almost 50% in the past 5 years. As a result of increasing PSA testing, the percentage of pT2 tumors in our radical prostatectomy series has changed from 30% in 1992 to 60% in the last 5 years (Table 7.1).

No specific gene alteration has been identified as a marker for progression in prostate cancer. Although preoperative PSA levels, clinical stage, and grading of the biopsies correlate with outcome and pathologic stage, none of these alone is precise enough to enable us to advise an individual patient whether he has a good or poor prognosis. However, recently, a number of algorithms have been developed. They combine the three above-mentioned parameters to obtain a more precise prediction of patient's prognosis [4, 5, 7, 13, 15, 18, 20, 22]. Partin and colleagues [17, 18] developed the one that is most widely used. The so-called Partin table gives an estimated probability for a patient having organ-confined disease on the basis of the preoperative PSA level, clinical stage, and Gleason score in the biopsy. However, most patients fall into intermediate risk groups, and it is difficult to make treatment decisions in these patients.

7.3 Histologically Insignificant Cancer

Despite the stage migration seen in our and other centers (Table 7.1), the percentage of so-called insignificant cancers (<0.5 cm^3 in size regardless of grade) did not change during the last years, when it was observed to be in the range of 2%–4% of all patients. We recently have shown that most (91.5%) of these small, insignificant cancers are missed by the six systematic biopsies and fine-needle aspiration cytology. This was demonstrated on prostates from patients referred for bladder cancer who underwent cystoprostatectomy and who had undergone biopsy before the histologic work-up [11]. Using the definition of having less than 2 or 3 mm^3 of cancer in one or two biopsies or of having well-differentiated tumor in six systematic biopsies to identify and exclude insignificant cancer from radical prostatectomy, we could show that, indeed, all 22 of 360 cancers with a volume of less than 0.5 cm^3 fulfilled such criteria. However, another 42 of 360 patients who also fulfilled these biopsy criteria were found to have a significant cancer volume, that is, of more than 0.5 cm^3, after pathologic work-up. Because the percentage of small, insignificant cancer is so low, because there is no possibility of identifying them before treatment, and because our patients have now a mean age of 61 years when a cancer of, for example, 0.4 cm^3 might be significant, we think that this issue is not a major problem in the present treatment of T1–T2 prostatic carcinoma. However, we have to admit that our data (Table 7.1) represent prostate cancer detection characteristics in an area without any screening program where the detection is mainly based on one – seldom on two – sets of six systematic biopsies.

7.4 Gleason 4–5 Cancer: The Most Significant Predictor of Tumor Heterogeneity

The most important pieces of information required for adequate treatment of clinically localized prostatic carcinoma are the prediction of the status of the lymph nodes (to avoid unnecessary treatment), the prediction of capsular penetration (to indicate nerve-sparing or non-nerve-sparing radical prostatectomy) and an estimated prediction of the overall prognosis after therapy for each individual patient. It is our experience that the preoperative prediction of tumor heterogeneity can be improved by including a semiquantitative analysis of the six systematic biopsies with respect to the amount of Gleason grade 4–5 cancer. The basis for this rationale is the study of Stamey et al. [21], who showed in a retrospective analysis of patients with peripheral zone prostate cancer that the percentage of Gleason 4–5 grade cancer in the radical prostatectomy specimens was by far the most significant parameter for prediction of prognosis. Radical prostatectomy specimens from 379 men were retrospectively studied for the following morphologic variables: cancer volume, Gleason score, percentage of each cancer occupied by Gleason grade 4–5 tumor, vascular invasion, lymph node involvement, intraductal cancer, seminal vesicle invasion, capsular penetration, and positive surgical margin. Age, prostate weight, and preoperative PSA levels were also recorded. Multivariate analysis showed that the percentage of Gleason grade 4–5 and cancer volume were highly predictive of disease progression. Lymph node status and intraprostatic vascular invasion were the only other variables that remained significant at the 0.01 level (p).

Univariate and multivariate logistic analyses were carried out on 326 of the men with a minimum follow-up of 3 years. A cure rate of at least 80% was

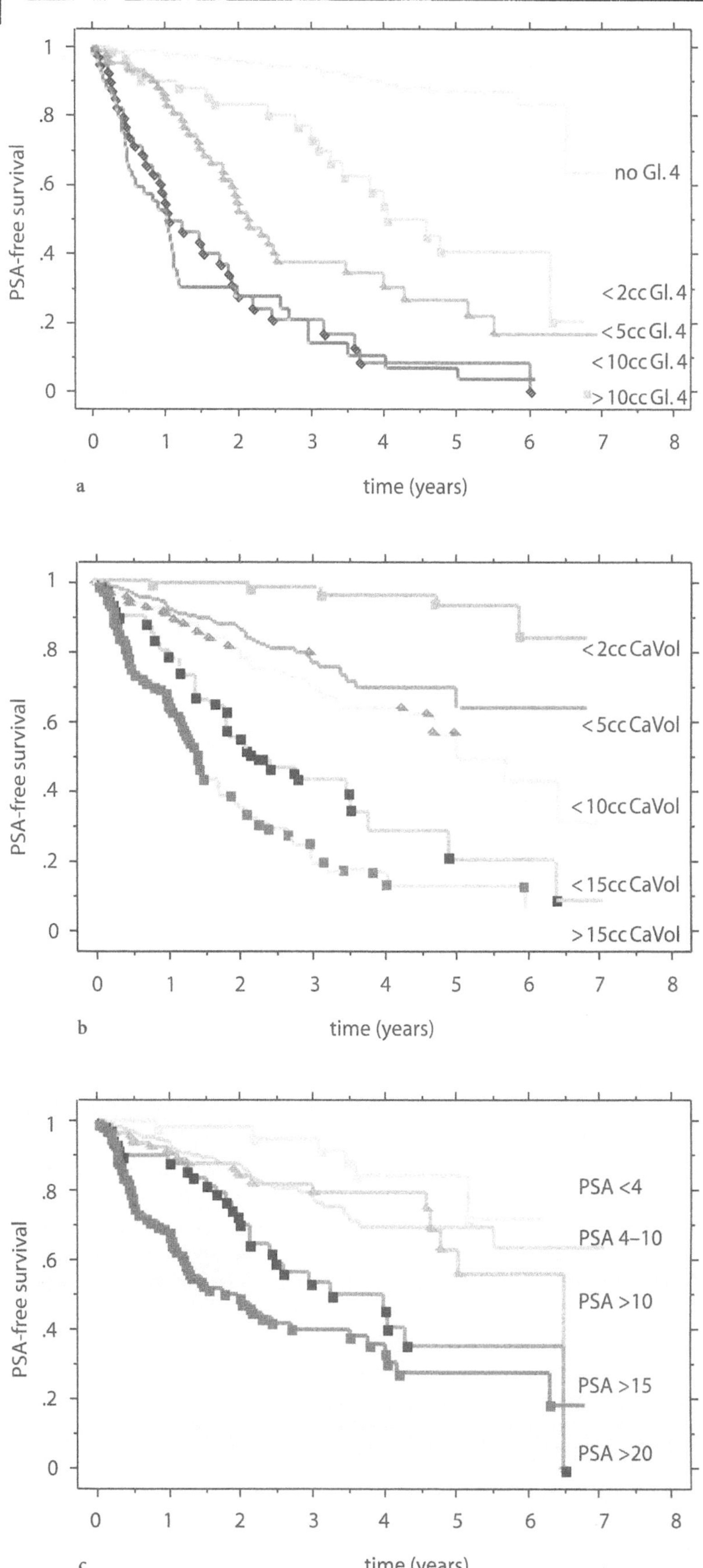

Fig. 7.2a–c. Kaplan-Meier analysis. PSA free survival (years) according to (**a**) volume of Gleason grade 4–5 cancer in the specimen ($n = 730$); (**b**) total cancer volume in the specimen ($n = 730$); and (**c**) preoperative PSA serum level ($n = 789$)

achieved for patients with up to 10% Gleason grade 4–5 disease. The cure rate decreased steadily with increasing percentage of Gleason grade 4–5, and in those patients with more than 41% Gleason grade 4–5, the cure rate was just 24%. Most patients fall within clearly defined prognostic groups: 40% have a good prognosis, and approximately 30% have a poor prognosis, leaving only 30% in the intermediate-risk group. These data show that significant information would be lost if we used the Gleason score rather than the Gleason grade to describe the tumor grade in the specimen. For a Gleason score of 7, for example, the proportion of grade 4 cancer may vary between 5% and 95% without altering the score. The prognosis of the quantity of Gleason grade 4–5 tumor in the specimen has been confirmed in our studies (Fig. 7.2a). We evaluated the absolute volume of Gleason 4–5 cancer in the specimen rather than the percentage. If the absolute volume of Gleason grade 4–5 cancer was less than 1 cm^3, then the prognosis was favorable, becoming progressively worse as the volume increased. We also confirmed the correlation between the total tumor volume in the specimen (Fig. 7.2b) and the preoperative PSA value (Fig. 7.2c) and the outcome after radical prostatectomy by use of undetectable PSA levels as an endpoint.

7.5 Gleason Grade 4–5 Tumor in Biopsies as a Predictor

We showed that the volume of the Gleason grade 4–5 cancer can be estimated by means of six high-quality (>10 mm in length) systematic biopsies. There was a weak but definite correlation with a percentage of Gleason 4–5 cancer in the specimen with the percentage of the Gleason 4–5 cancer in the biopsies, with a correlation coefficient of 0.53. The number of biopsies with any Gleason grade 4–5 cancer and the number of biopsies with dominant (>50%) Gleason grade 4–5 cancer were also found to have a good correlation with PSA-free survival (Fig. 7.3a, b). This simple semiquantitative analysis of the preoperative six systematic biopsies can be given by every pathologist as a routine evaluation; it proved to be sufficient in the CART analysis for the characterization of tumor heterogeneity, mentioned below. This means that no more sophisticated analysis of the six systematic biopsies is necessary – for example, millimeters of length of Gleason 4–5 cancer or exact percentage of Gleason 4–5 cancer in the biopsy.

7.6 CART Analysis to Predict Tumor Heterogeneity

We later included 14 preoperative parameters, as for example PSA levels, the number of positive biopsies, the number of positive biopsies with Gleason grade 4–5 disease, the percentage of Gleason grade 4–5 disease, and the percentage of volume of Gleason grade 4–5 tumor in six systematic biopsies in a CART analysis [2] to predict the lymph node status of 344 patients with clinically localized prostate cancer. This is a nonparametric modelling technique that analyzes interactions and identifies homogeneous prognostic subgroups in a data set. The algorithm starts with the set of all patients and splits them by the most predictive prognostic factor, followed by the second most predictive variable, and so on. The CART analysis demonstrated that if a patient has three or fewer biopsy cores with Gleason grade 4–5 tumor, and at least one of these cores has predominantly (>50%) Gleason grade 4–5 tumor, then he has a fairly

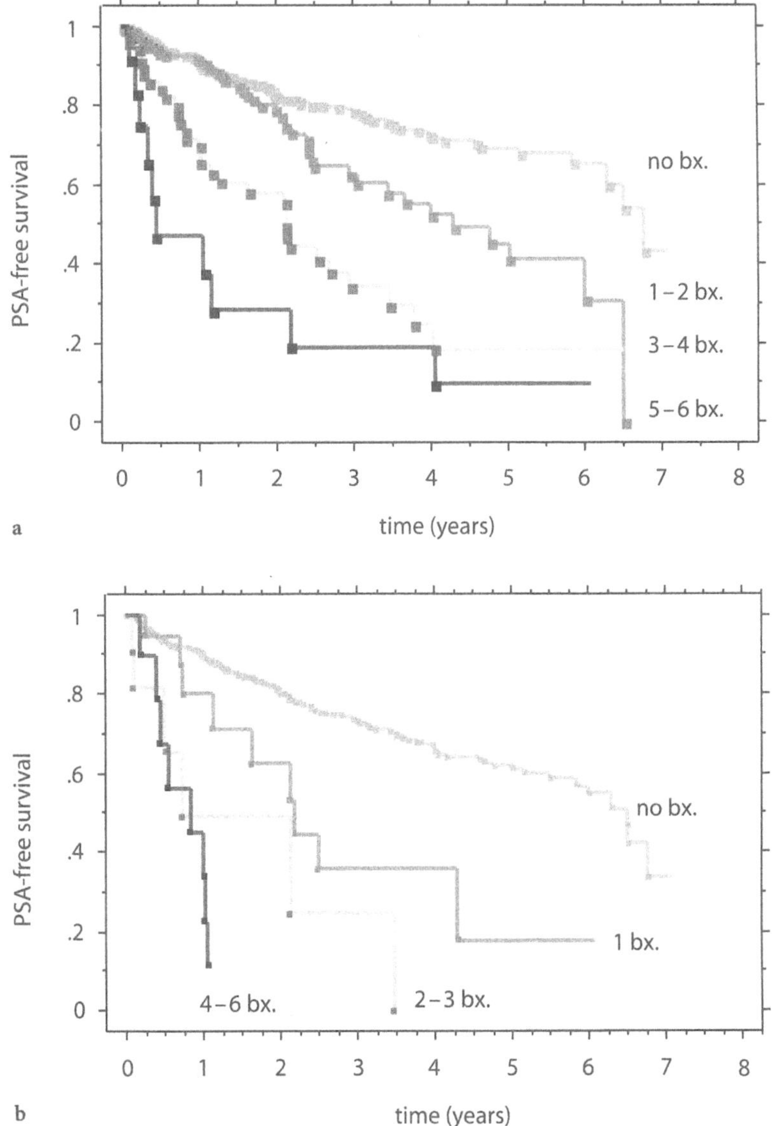

Fig. 7.3a,b. Kaplan-Meier analysis. PSA-free survival (years) according to (**a**) number of biopsy cores (bx.) with Gleason grade 4–5 cancer ($n = 642$) and (**b**) number of biopsy cores (bx.) with dominant Gleason grade 4–5 cancer ($n = 642$)

high risk (19%) of having positive lymph nodes. On the other hand, this CART analysis allowed us to identify a low-risk group, with a risk of positive lymph nodes of only 2.2% characterized by the following parameter: three or fewer biopsy cores with any Gleason grade 4 or 5 cancer, but no cores with more than 50% Gleason grade 4 or 5 cancer. A total of 79.7% of all patients belong to that low-risk group. We have validated these algorithms prospectively in 293 consecutive patients [3]: 251 of 293 in the prospective validation study belonged to the low-risk group, with a rate of positive lymph nodes of 2.8%. So the negative predictive value was 97.2% (244 of 251) with a specificity of 88.4% (244 of 276). As a result of these two studies, we do not perform lymphadenectomy in patients with prostate cancer who belong to such a well-defined low-risk group.

Similarly, we used CART analysis to predict the probability of organ-confined prostate cancer in 552 patients from our center. This is particularly important if a nerve-sparing radical prostatectomy is being considered, because such surgery can be safely done only in tumors with no capsular penetration (pT2 tumors). By use of this method, we can identify 50.8% of patients who have only a ≤13.9% probability of capsular penetration (≤1 biopsy core Gleason grade 4–5, PSA <10 ng/ml) [8]. Here, we were able to confirm the results of the retrospective CART analysis prospectively in 353 consecutive patients. In this study, we tried to identify the capsular penetration in each lobe [9]. A total of 427 (60.4%) of 706 lobes were in the low-risk group; 88.3% of those indeed had no capsular penetration (ppv). The sensitivity (the identification of those lobes without capsular penetration) was 427 of 552 (77.3%).

7.7 Human Glandular Kallikrein 2 To Improve CART Analysis

In the future, we expect to improve the CART analyses. The determination of human glandular kallikrein 2 (HK-2) showed a striking difference in the serum levels of pT2 versus pT3 tumors [10]. We have ongoing studies to include HK-2 in our CART analysis to improve the prediction of the tumor heterogeneity. Other fields of interest are promising markers or genetic alterations – for example, mutations, loss of heterozygosity, and methylation of suppressor genes. Many such markers have been implicated in the process of progression of localized prostatic carcinoma; they are correlated with pathologic grade and stage, but seldom with the outcome of radical prostatectomy.

7.8 Future Expectations for Prediction of Tumor Heterogeneity

Despite evolving literature about promising molecular biologic or genetic markers, the clinician is faced with several critical issues. First, marker information has to be available preoperatively (e.g., in the analysis of the six systematic biopsies) as well as showing a good correlation after a 5-year follow-up that used sensitive PSA determination as an end point. A multivariate analysis should compare any new marker in this setting with the classic pathologic parameters used for prediction. It must be determined whether markers complement the classic morphologic parameters, whether such markers are independent parameters, and whether the majority of the patients can be placed in clearly defined risk groups. Further, any new marker should be cheap and easy to use in daily practice. At our institution, we have been able to identify curable and incurable prostate cancer in six systematic biopsies by the use of interphase cytogenetic studies [12]. The good risk group, with almost 90% probability of cure by radical prostatectomy included – as we expected – two thirds of cancer patients with T1–T2 prostate disease. The poor risk group, with almost 0% cure rate, included one third of these patients. Only three probes for numeric aberrations in chromosome 7, chromosome 17, and chromosome X were used for interphase cytogenetic study in the biopsies. The prediction of outcome was even better than that obtained by the length or the percentage of length of Gleason 4–5 cancer in the preoperative six systematic biopsies. However, it is obvious that such an examination is not practical in daily practice.

7.9
CART Analysis for Identifying Candidates for Nerve-Sparing Radical Prostatectomy

We have used the CART analysis to identify capsular penetration on each lobe of the prostate. We have increased the nerve-sparing procedure from 10% initially to almost 62% of the radical prostatectomies we have performed in the last 5 years. The overall positive margin rate has remained stable at the 16% to 19% range over the last 4 years (Table 7.1). The positive margin rate in pT2 tumors is stable at the level of 5% to 6%. More importantly, only 2.4% of the positive margins are in the area of the nerve-sparing side of the prostate. The results of the unilateral or bilateral nerve-sparing technique were evaluated by a questionnaire. We evaluated five different periods; in the first three time periods, a nonvalidated questionnaire was used; in the last two time periods, an internationally validated questionnaire was used. The overall potency rate in these five evaluation periods was 70% to 95% after unilateral and bilateral nerve sparing, respectively. After bilateral nerve sparing, 56% of the patients were able to engage in intercourse without any additional pharmacological therapy or the use of sildenafil. After unilateral nerve sparing, this rate changed from 18% in the first evaluation period to 30% in the fifth evaluation period.

7.10
Conclusion

The clinical T1–T2 prostatic carcinoma is a heterogeneous tumor with respect to pathologic stage and outcome. We have found that 60% of the patients we treated had a pT2 prostatic carcinoma, 2%–4% with tumors less than 0.5 cm^3 in volume. The latter group cannot be predicted by the use of preoperative parameters with a sufficient sensitivity and specificity. However, "semiquantitative" analysis of six systematic biopsies, just a report of the number of biopsy cores with any Gleason grade 4–5 cancer or the number of cores with more than 50% Gleason grade 4–5 cancer, together with preoperative PSA levels, can be used to predict the different pathologic stages and risk groups of patients with T1–T2 prostatic carcinoma. CART analysis that uses these preoperative parameters is able to predict the lymph node stage and the capsular penetration on each side of the prostate with a sufficient positive and negative predictive value, and a sufficient specificity to avoid routine lymphadenectomy in about 80% of the patients who are classified as a low-risk group for having lymph nodes positive for disease. Such analysis further allows a solid identification of those in whom unilateral or bilateral nerves may be spared during surgery. The algorithms used in the analysis of the biopsies can be improved further in the future as HK-2 level in the blood are determined, and/or as other molecular biological markers are included. The clinical T1–T2 prostatic carcinoma is a heterogeneous but fairly predictable tumor.

References

1. Catalona WJ, Smith DS (1994) Five-year tumor recurrence rates after anatomical radical prostatectomy for prostate cancer. J Urol 152: 1837–1842
2. Conrad S, Graefen M, Pichlmeier U, et al (1998) Systematic sextant biopsies improve preoperative prediction of pelvic lymph node metastases in patients with clinical localized prostatic carcinoma. J Urol 159: 2023–2029
3. Conrad S, Graefen M, Pichlmeier U, et al (2002) Prospective validation of an algorithm using systematic sextant biopsies to predict pelvic lymph node metastases in patients with clinically localized prostatic carcinoma. J Urol 167:521–525
4. Epstein IJ, Pizov G, Walsh PC (1993) Correlation of pathologic findings with progression after radical retropubic prostatectomy. Cancer 71: 3582–3589
5. Epstein IJ, Partin AW, Sauvageot J, et al (1996) Prediction of progression following radical prostatectomy. A multivariate analysis of 721 men with long-term follow-up. Am J Surg Pathol 20: 286–292
6. Frohmüller H, Theiss M, Wirth MP (1991) Radical prostatectomy for carcinoma of the prostate: long-term follow-up of 115 patients. Eur Urol 19:279–284
7. Goto Y, Ohori M, Arakawa A, et al (1996) Distinguishing clinically important from unimportant prostate cancers before treatment: value of systematic biopsies. J Urol 156:1059–1066
8. Graefen M, Noldus J, Pichlmeier U, et al (1999) Early-prostate specific antigen relapse after radical retropubic prostatectomy: prediction on the basis of preoperative and postoperative tumor characteristics. Eur Urol 36: 21–30
9. Graefen M, Pichlmeier U, Hammerer PG, et al (2001) A validated strategy to select patients for nerve-sparing radical prostatectomy. J Urol 165:857–863
10. Haese A, Becker C, Noldus J, et al (2000) Human glandular kallikrein 2: a potential serum marker for predicting the organ confined versus nonorgan confined growth of prostate cancer. J Urol 163: 1491–1497
11. Hautmann S, Conrad S, Henke R-P, et al (2000) Detection rate of histologically insignificant prostate cancer with systematic sextant biopsies and fine needle aspiration cytology. J Urol 163: 1734–1738
12. Henke R-P, Hammerer P, Graefen M, et al (1998) Interphase cytogenetic study of preoperative core biopsies for the prediction of early serum prostate specific antigen recurrence after radical prostatectomy of clinically localized prostate carcinoma. Am Cancer Soc 83: 977–988
13. Huland H, Hammerer P, Henke R-P, et al (1996) Preoperative prediction of tumor heterogeneity and recurrence after radical prostatectomy for localised prostate carcinoma with digital rectal examination, PSA, and the results of six systematic biopsies. J Urol 155: 1344–1347
14. Ohori M, Wheeler TM, Dunn JK, et al (1994) The pathological features and prognosis of prostate cancer detectable with current diagnostic tests. J Urol 152: 1714–1721
15. Ohori M, Wheeler TM, Kattan MW, et al (1995) Prognostic significance of positive surgical margins in radical prostatectomy specimens. J Urol 154: 1818–1823
16. Partin AW, Pound CR, Clemens JQ, et al (1993) Serum PSA after anatomic radical prostatectomy. The Johns Hopkins' experience after 10 years. Urol Clin North Am 20: 713–719
17. Partin AW, Yoo J, Carter HB, et al (1993) The use of prostate-specific antigen, clinical stage and Gleason score to predict pathological stage in men with localized prostate cancer. J Urol 150: 110–118
18. Partin AW, Kattan MW, Subong ENP, et al (1997) Combination of prostate-specific antigen, clinical stage, and Gleason score to predict pathological stage of localized prostate cancer. A multi-institutional update. JAMA 277: 1445–1451
19. Ravery V, Boccon-Gibod LA, Meulemans A, et al (1994) Predictive value of pathologic features for progression after radical prostatectomy. Eur Urol 26: 197–201
20. Stamey TA (1995) Making the most out of six systematic sextant biopsies. Urology 45: 2–12
21. Stamey TA, McNeal JE, Yemoto CM, et al (1999) Biological determinants of cancer progression in men with prostate cancer. JAMA 281: 1395–1400
22. Stapleton AMF, Kattan MW, Eastham JA, et al (1997) Which factors best predict treatment failure after radical prostatectomy for clinically localized prostate cancer? [abstract 1533]. J Urol 157: 391
23. Trapasso JG, de Kernion JB, Smith RB, et al (1994) The incidence and significance of detectable levels of serum prostate-specific antigen after radical prostatectomy. J Urol 152: 1821–1826
24. Van den Ouden D, Davidson PJT, Hop W, et al (1994) Radical prostatectomy as a monotherapy for locally advanced (stage T3) prostate cancer. J Urol 151: 646–651
25. Walsh PC, Partin AW, Epstein IJ (1994) Cancer control and quality of life following anatomical radical retropubic prostatectomy: results at 10 years. J Urol 152: 1831–1843
26. Zincke H, Oesterling JE, Blute ML, et al (1994) Long-term (15 years) results after radical prostatectomy for clinically localized (stage T2c lower) prostate cancer. J Urol 152: 1850–1859

8 Preoperative Staging

P. Hammerer, M. Graefen, A. Haese, J. Palisaar, J. Noldus,
S. Fernandez, H. Huland

8.1 Introduction

The detection of prostate carcinoma is currently based on three parameters: digital rectal examination (DRE), serum prostate-specific antigen (PSA), and transrectal ultrasound of the prostate (TRUS) (although TRUS is mainly used as a guide for biopsies) [26, 46]. Definitive treatment for localized prostate cancer is most effective when the cancer is organ-confined or specimen-confined at the time of treatment [57].

It has been shown that the use of PSA measurements and DRE findings leads to early detection and has increased the percentage of organ-confined disease [42]. But clinical T1- T2 prostate carcinomas are heterogeneous in respect to pathologic stage and outcome [20, 29]. In addition to DRE and PSA concentration, imaging procedures such as TRUS, computed tomography (CT), magnetic resonance imaging (MRI), positron emission tomography (PET), and radio isotope bone scan are used to stage prostate cancer.

An exact preoperative staging should identify patients who will be cured by radical prostatectomy or radiation therapy. The identification of an organ-confined disease will also help to select men who are candidates for a nerve-sparing procedure [29].

8.2 Nomograms

Nomograms, which predict pathologic stage and outcome probabilities for individual patients, can be very useful for counseling the individual patient and for making decisions for treatment. These nomograms may limit the necessity of using imaging procedures for staging purposes [32].

There are numerous pitfalls to nomogram development; chief among them is failure of validation. A nomogram may not predict well when applied to future patients if the predictor variables are not reproducible and available [55]. If the sample size used for nomogram development is small or contains short follow-ups, the estimates may not be accurate. In addition, the statistical model behind the nomogram may not be a proper fit. Validation is an essential step in the process of developing nomograms [25].

8.2.1 Prediction of Pathological Stage

In recent years several pretreatment nomograms have been developed that help in predicting when radical prostatectomy will fail [12, 45].

While these tools have reported reasonable predictive accuracy for their specific patient population, the only one published to date that has been validated on an external multi-institutional dataset is the Partin nomogram [46]. Its authors combined clinical stage, Gleason sum, and PSA to predict pathologic stage. In a multi-institutional update combining data from the Johns Hopkins Hospital, Baylor College of Medicine, and the University of Michigan School of Medicine the Partin nomogram was validated [46]. It allows prediction of organ-confined disease, capsular penetration, seminal vesicle involvement, and lymph node involvement. While useful for predicting pathologic stage, this nomogram does not indicate the probability of recurrence or need for further cancer treatment since organ confinement (or lack thereof) is not synonymous with surgical cure (or failure).

Most men with organ-confined disease will have improved disease-free survival compared to men with capsular penetration, though some patients with capsular penetration may be cured by radical prostatectomy. In addition, a preoperative identification of unilateral capsular penetration may allow a nerve-sparing approach on the contralateral side. This information is not given by the Partin nomogram.

The Hamburg classification and regression tree analysis (CART) based on the analysis of the prostate biopsy results and preoperative PSA has improved our preoperative staging and selection for patients who are candidates for a nerve-sparing-radical prostatectomy (NSRP) [20–22] (Fig. 8.1). Because the neurovascular bundle runs outside the prostate, a nerve-sparing procedure can be considered safe with respect to surgical margins in patients with organ-confined (pT2) tumors.

Hence, selection criteria that predict organ-confined growth of the cancer offer a useful tool for determining whether NSRP is indicated. The combination of Gleason score, clinical stage, and PSA concentration allows estimation of organ-confined prostate cancer as shown above [46]. However, many patients are left in an intermediate risk group, so little additional information can be expected from those characteristics for prediction of organ-confined disease. In addition, it would be most helpful to predict not only whether a tumor has penetrated the prostate capsule, but also if the penetration is unilateral or bilateral. A few studies have used the information from systematic biopsies to indicate a NSRP, but they did not use a multivariate approach and did not yield prospective evaluation of selection criteria [5].

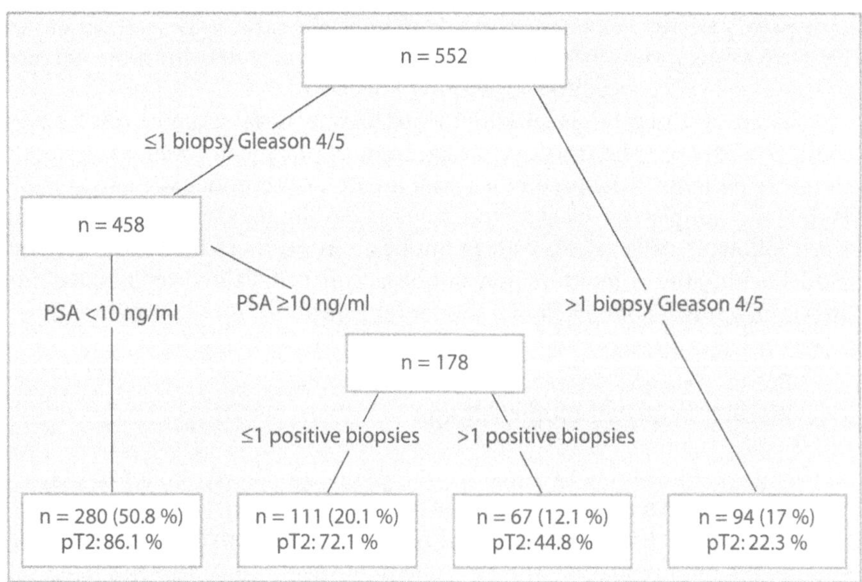

Fig. 8.1. Preoperative nomogram for predicting pathologic stage. *PSA*, prostate-specific antigen

In patients who met the criteria of high likelihood of organ-confined disease in the validation of our retrospective analysis, the likelihood increased from 86% (training data set) to 88.5% (validation data set). This increase was also apparent in the other risk groups. That reflects our experience of stage migration between 1992 and 2000. By using the tree-structured regression analysis for selecting patients for NSRP, we overestimate the likelihood of capsular penetration when it is applied to future patients in whom, in general, non-organ-confined cancer is less likely because of stage migration. We believe that this conservatism is acceptable; it will not affect the cure rate. Instead, it will lead to wide excision of nerves in some patients who have organ-confined disease.

In our analysis we deliberately resolved to use parameters that are not routinely obtained for the diagnosis of prostate cancer to make our discrimination rule applicable for a day-to-day use. We developed a discrimination rule that is reliable, valid, and impressive because of its simplicity. Combined with prospective validation, it was demonstrated that the method derived from these results can be applied to patients in the future. In our computerized patient database, the likelihood of organ-confined tumor is expressed for each lobe of the prostate as soon as preoperative data are obtained.

Using the results of systematic biopsies of the prostate and quantifying the total cancer and high-grade cancer found will add useful information to predictive tools for organ-confined disease.

We performed a semiquantitative analysis of cancer and high-grade cancer found in the biopsies by simply counting the cores positive for cancer, high-grade cancer, and predominantly high-grade cancer. These parameters were included in the regression-tree analysis and allow an estimation of the amount of those tumor entities in the prostate specimen. The fact that the Gleason grade was rejected by our multivariate analysis while the number of cores positive for cancer (of any grade) and the number of cores positive for high-grade cancer were accepted as independent predictors demonstrate their superiority for prediction of organ-confined disease.

Our results are similar to those of other recent studies that have reinvestigated the predictive power of tumor extent from needle biopsies. Sebo et al. demonstrated in a series of 207 patients that the percentage of cores positive for cancer in prostate needle biopsy specimens and surface area positive for cancer were the strongest predictors of pathologic stage and cancer volume on multivariate analysis [53]. Egawa et al. [14] reported that the number of cores with cancer is jointly predictive of extraprostatic extension in a model that incorporates PSA, clinical stage, and Gleason score.

Using the percentage of poorly differentiated cancer and serum PSA in a study of 190 patients, Goto et al. showed that the total core length of cancer in all needle biopsies was predictive of advanced stage disease on multivariate analysis [19].

In a series of 113 patients, Wills et al. identified high Gleason score and number of cancer positive cores as the two variables most predictive of pathologic stage [61].

In a recent editorial comment, Klein and Zippe [33] suggested that the number of cores that contain cancer should be incorporated into models that predict pathologic stage. They assumed that this might ultimately alter therapeutic approaches, making TRUS-guided biopsy not only essential for diagnosis, but also a standard clinical diagnostic tool necessary for planning therapy. In all the above-mentioned studies, it was demonstrated that quantification of the tumor found in the biopsy outperforms the traditionally used Gleason score in multivariate analysis. Although authors use different ways of quantifying tumor in the biopsy, combining methods of quantification can enhance the amount of information. In our univariate analysis, the number of positive biopsies was the most useful single parameter, with a positive predictive value (ppv) of 83% in 274 lobes and a negative predictive value of 55% followed by millimeters of cancer in the biopsy. As our multivariate analysis considered the number of cores positive for high-grade cancer as an independent factor, we believe that this semiquantitative assessment should be incorporated into discrimination rules. It might be even more accurate to measure the length of high-grade cancer, however, the above mentioned way of a semiquantitative assessment is more practical and can be easily performed by each pathologist. In addition, we could not enhance the predictive power of our multivariate analysis by measuring millimeters of cancerous tissue in the biopsies, and we suspect that measuring millimeters of high-grade cancer would lead to a corresponding result. The multivariate approach with the two most favorable risk groups achieved a ppv of 82%. The advantage of this approach is that more prostate lobes ($n = 391$) could be assigned to those favorable risk groups compared to the univariate approach ($n = 329$ prostate lobes if number of positive biopsies is considered).

Sebo et al. evaluated the percentage of prostate surface area and needle biopsy cores positive for cancer in addition to the Gleason score, but no quantification of high-grade cancer was added to their multivariate analysis. Further information about the tumor is lost if the Gleason score is used instead of the Gleason grade, as demonstrated by Chan et al. [6], who found significant prognostic differences in tumors between Gleason score 3+4 and 4+3. Egawa et al. used a quantification of the tumor by counting the number of cores positive for cancer. Again, no quantification of high-grade cancer was performed. We believe that the predictive power of discrimination rules can be improved by taking the amount of high-grade cancer into consideration.

8.2.2
Prediction of Lymph Node Status

A semiquantitative assessment of high-grade cancer in the preoperative biopsies enhances the predictive power of algorithms with respect to lymph-node status and outcome after radical retropubic prostatectomy (Fig. 8.2). In our

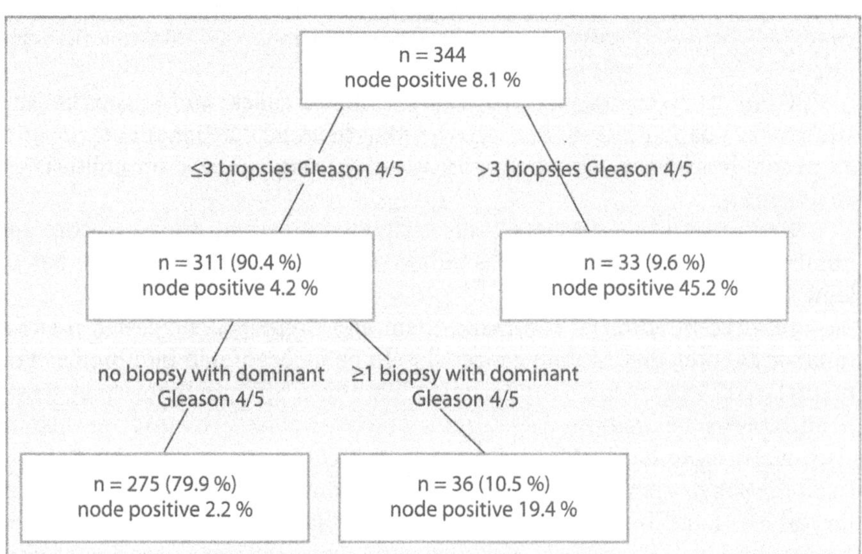

Fig. 8.2. Preoperative nomogram for predicting lymph node status

patients, we demonstrated in a multivariate analysis incorporating eight preoperative tumor characteristics that the amount of high-grade cancer in preoperative biopsies had the greatest influence on the likelihood of lymph-node metastasis and early PSA relapse [10, 20]. The importance of high-grade cancer for prognosis of prostate cancer was demonstrated by Stamey et al. [57]. The quantitative assessment of high-grade cancer in prostate biopsies we have presented offers a practicable way of transforming this information into preoperative diagnostic tools.

As promising markers emerge that might enhance the predictive accuracy of preoperative findings related to the likelihood of organ-confined tumor growth, they must be considered in a multivariate fashion with a quantified result of systematic biopsy. To our knowledge, no molecular or angiogenetic marker so far has been shown to be superior to quantified analysis of histologic findings of biopsy specimens.

8.2.3 Prediction of Outcome

The data from the Hamburg prostate cancer registry were also used to validate the Baylor nomogram which predicts disease progression, the information of most concern to the patient [21, 22]. This nomogram considers pretreatment serum PSA, clinical stage, and Gleason grade of the biopsy as predictor variables [31] (Fig. 8.3). Disease progression was categorized as biochemical, clinical, administration of adjuvant therapy, or death from prostate cancer.

Preop. Nomogram for PSA progression

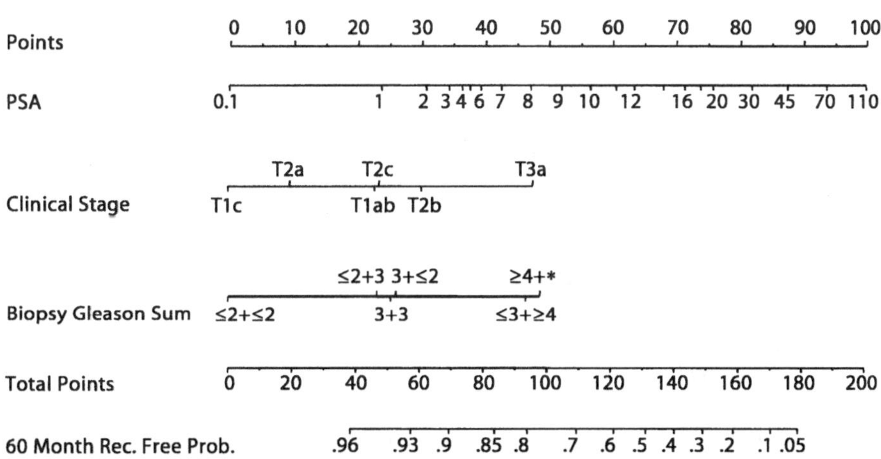

Instructions for Physician: Locate the patient's PSA on the **PSA** axis. Draw a line straight upwards to the **Points** axis to determine how many points towards recurrence the patient receives for his PSA. Repeat this process for the **Clinical Stage** and **Biopsy Gleason Sum** axes, each time drawing straight upward to the **Points** axis. Sum the points achieved for each predictor and locate this sum on the **Total Points** axis. Draw a line straight down to find the patient's probability of remaining recurrence free for 60 months assuming he does not die of another cause first.

Note: This nomogram is not applicable to a man who is not otherwise a candidate for radical prostatectomy. You can use this only on a man who has already selected radical prostatectomy as treatment for his prostate cancer.

Instruction to Patient: "Mr. X, if we had 100 men exactly like you, we would expect between <predicted percentage from nomogram – 10%> and <predicted percentage + 10%> to remain free of their disease at 5 years following radical prostatectomy, and recurrence after 5 years is very rare."

Scott Department of Urology

Fig. 8.3. Preoperative nomogram based on 983 patients treated at The Methodist Hospital, Houston, TX, for predicting prostate-specific antigen (*PSA*) recurrence after radical prostatectomy

We have obtained data from seven other treatment centers that feature a variety of surgeons, pathologists, and PSA assays (Departments of Urology and Biostatistics, Memorial Sloan-Kettering Cancer Center, University of Southern California, Los Angeles: Cleveland Clinic, Cleveland, Ohio; Garvan Institute of Medical Research, Sydney, Australia; Louisiana State University Medical Center, Shreveport, Louisiana; University of California at Los Angeles; and Erasmus University Rotterdam, Netherlands). We compared the nomogram's predictions with actual patient follow-up.

This was the first time that a nomogram using preoperative data to predict treatment failure after radical prostatectomy was validated on a multi-institutional dataset. The comparison of the predicted outcome and the actual incidence of recurrence for the prediction quadrants appeared to confirm the 10% margin of error. The general applicability of the Baylor nomogram was thus demonstrated.

The Baylor nomogram appears to be accurate when applied at treatment centers with similar patient selection and management strategies. It may be the most accurate tool currently available for preoperative prediction of disease recurrence following radical prostatectomy for clinically localized prostate cancer.

The area under the curve (AUC) for the multi-institutional dataset in the validation was 0.757 and varied among centers from 0.669 to 0827. It must be emphasized that differences in the AUC's merely reflect differences in the ability of the nomogram to predict outcome in a given group of patients and not an actual difference in patient outcome.

These results have important implications for the practicing urologist who needs a prediction of surgical efficacy for the individual patient. It appears that the use of the Baylor nomogram is an accurate tool for the prediction of recurrence. It is an accurate tool based on readily available parameters that are accepted as predictive tumor characteristics in the urologic community. Of course better nomograms may be developed as new predictor variables are found.

It allows accurate prediction of 5-year freedom from recurrence after radical prostatectomy even when minor variations of the input variables or differences in the patient selection are accepted.

8.3 Imaging Procedures

8.3.1 Transrectal Ultrasound

Since its introduction in 1968 [57] TRUS has developed significantly, and its application in evaluation of the prostate has been well established. The use of TRUS, however, for early detection and staging of prostate carcinoma is still controversial due to the non-uniform ultrasound appearance of malignancy.

8.3.1.2 Sonographic Appearance of Prostate Cancer

Clinically significant prostate cancer in the peripheral zone is hypoechoic on TRUS 60%–80% of cases. However, hypoechogenicity has a low specificity and, in addition, the extent of the hypoechoic lesion does not correspond to the total cancer volume [24, 36]. Some benign lesions such as laterally located venous structures, atrophic areas, muscular tissue, and granulomatous prostatitis are also hypoechoic on TRUS.

Fifteen to forty percent of peripheral zone prostate cancers are isoechoic or equally echogenic as compared to the remainder of the peripheral zone. These might be small cancers or large cancers with infiltration of the whole peripheral zone. Capsular bulging or asymmetry can identify these cancers.

Approximately 20% of all prostate cancers arise in the transition zone (TZ). No specific ultrasound appearance can be seen in these cancers. In TZ cancers asymmetry of the prostate or irregular boundaries to the bladder neck are noted in 10%–15%.

Criteria for capsular infiltration are irregular boundaries, bulging of the capsule, or hypoechoic lesions infiltrating the lateral aspects of the levator muscle. Seminal vesicle infiltration is assumed with asymmetric seminal vesicles, or, for example, with hypoechoic lesions at the base of the prostate with widening of angle between the seminal vesicle and the prostate.

While the sensitivity for detection of capsular infiltration or seminal vesicle infiltration is relatively low, TRUS detection of these features has a high specificity. In our Hamburg series we found specificities of 92% and 84% for capsular or seminal vesicle infiltration, and corresponding sensitivities of 42% and 54%, respectively. A ppv of 63% was reported by Presti et al. in 1996 [47].

Recent developments in computer technology have resulted in more powerful ultrasound machines with new technological modalities such as color Doppler, power Doppler, and 3D imaging [1, 54]. The promising improvements of Doppler ultrasound imaging by adding ultrasound contrast agents are being investigated as well.

8.3.2 Computer-Assisted Ultrasound Imaging of the Prostate

Computer-assisted TRUS of the prostate has been investigated as an objective tool to assess the gray scale ultrasound images, overcome the interobserver variability, and improve the low predictive value of TRUS [18, 39]. Computer interpretation can improve the reproducibility of gray scale and may reveal information not perceptible by the human eye.

In the patients analyzed, a sensitivity of 75% and a specificity of 78% was obtained with the use of the automated cancer detection. The diagnostic accuracy achieved was 75% [18].

Artificial neural networks (ANN) are being developed to improve the diagnosis of prostate cancer with the use of ultrasound. Recent studies proclaim high sensitivity and specificity. The ANN described by Ronco et al. using 14 ultrasound variables achieved a ppv of 82% and a negative predictive value of 97% [39, 49]; and they reported a 79% correctly classified pathologic stage.

One problem with neural networks is the reproducibility of the results. Each ultrasound scanner has its own specific set-up for the different gray scales and the frequencies used, and of course the personal preference for settings of the physician working with the system must be taken into account, all of which limit the value of the neural network for prostate cancer staging. For routine use in staging prostate cancer these methods may be of limited help.

8.3.3 Three-Dimensional Ultrasound of the Prostate

The development of three-dimensional (3D) scanners enables storage of whole volumes of gray scale ultrasounds of the prostate, allowing the physician to assess the whole prostate even when the patient has left the office.

3D ultrasonography of the prostate seems to be of additional value for staging of prostate cancer [11, 17, 54]. 3D ultrasound could also be of value in enhanced ultrasound like Doppler and contrast enhanced ultrasound. With the use of the 3D mode, the architecture of the blood vessels can be reconstructed and can be visualized in every plane desired. This could provide an extra imaging possibility to assess the vascularity of the prostate. The 3D technique will add additional information when evaluating the cranial aspects of the prostate as well as seminal vesicle and/or vas deferens infiltration. It will not provide greater sensitivity, however, for identification of capsular infiltration.

8.3.4 Doppler Ultrasound

It is known that vascularization in prostate cancer alters during the development of the tumor [4].

It is reported that power Doppler ultrasonography (PDU) has several advantages over color Doppler ultrasound (CDU) [35, 51]. PDU is essentially angle independent, it should increase the usable dynamic range of the Doppler imager, and in contrast to CDU it gives information on direction or velocity. With all these advantages PDU is more sensitive than CDU in detecting slow and/or low flow.

Lavoipierre et al. indicated that CDU complements gray scale imaging and should become a routine part of TRUS imaging of the prostate for improved detection and staging [35].

However, some authors compared gray scale ultrasound, color Doppler, and power Doppler in the detection and staging of prostate cancer, and found no additional value of power over color Doppler [16]. The ultrasound evaluation of blood flow offers additional information, but it remains controversial whether this information can be translated into improvement in staging.

8.3.5 Contrast-Enhanced Imaging

With the introduction of an ultrasound contrast agent, it has become possible to enhance the acoustic properties of the blood and thus improve the detection of blood flow. This works even in organs with mostly small blood vessels such as the prostate.

The use of ultrasound contrast in combination with CDU or PDU can provide important additional information for visualizing changes in blood flow.

Ragde et al. [48] concluded that contrast-enhanced ultrasound promises to be a useful technique for better imaging of prostatic blood flow and might allow for more accurate staging.

Contrast ultrasound seems to be an ideal imaging tool. New contrast agents also appear capable of improving the duration of contrast enhancement in the small blood vessels of the prostate. Up to now only a small series on prostate cancer staging was reported with controversial results [13, 15].

8.3.6 Positron Emission Tomography

The value of 18-fluoro-2-deoxyglucose (FDG) PET studies for staging of patients with organ-confined prostate cancer is limited because of excretion of the isotope into the urine, thus masking possible lower urinary tract lesions.

Liu et al. [38] evaluated PET using hydration, furosemide, and bladder emptying for more rapid evacuation of the nonspecific isotope in the urine on 24 patients diagnosed with clinically organ-confined prostate cancer. FDG PET scans were performed 1 h after injection of 15 mCi of FDG. Patients were scanned from the base of the skull through the inguinal region (including the pelvis). Additional signal attenuation-corrected images of the inguinal region were acquired 30 min after intravenous injection of 40 mg of furosemide. They found FDG PET studies negative in 23 of the 24 organ-confined prostate cancers and the study was only faintly positive in one tumor (4.0% sensitivity); they therefore concluded that FDG PET is not a useful test in the evaluation of clinically organ-confined prostate cancer.

8.3.7 MRI for Local Staging

MRI allows imaging of the zonal anatomy of the prostate and evaluation of malignant lesions of the prostate. Prostatic MRI should be performed no earlier than 2 weeks after prostatic biopsy, as hemorrhage decreases the accuracy of staging [60].

Prostatic MRI is performed using coils which can transmit radiofrequencies and receive MR signals; these coils improve the spatial resolution. Three types of coils can be used for prostatic MRI [62]. Initially a body coil was used, which is integrated in most MRI scanners. More recently surface coils have been used; these are placed on the patient over the anatomical region of interest [3, 28].

In prostatic MRI the pelvic phased-array coil (PPA) and the endorectal (ER) coil are used. The PPA coil is positioned above and below the patient's pelvis,whereas the ER coil is inserted into the rectum.

Prostate cancer usually shows a low-signal-intensity lesion in a bright peripheral zone on the T2-weighted image. By using the T1-weighted images, hemorrhage can be differentiated by its hyperintense appearance from cancer [52].

Criteria for extracapsular extension (ECE) of prostatic cancer are asymmetry of the neurovascular bundle, obliteration of the rectoprostatic angle, and tumor bulging with an accuracy of 58%–90%, a specificity of 70%–90%, and a sensitivity of 15%–68%. These large ranges can be attributed to differences in imaging protocols, inexperience of interpretation, in patient selection, and in criteria for diagnosis of ECE [16]. Prostatic MRI is not able to detect microscopic ECE [7, 44].

The detection of seminal vesicle invasion (SVI) is generally good using the ER coil, with accuracies of 81%–96% [50].

May et al. [40] published their results on 54 patients with biopsy-confirmed prostate cancer who underwent endorectal MRI (eMRI) before radical retropubic prostatectomy. The images were prospectively interpreted by two radiologists with special expertise in this field. Evaluated in each patient were ECE and SVI, and the results were correlated with the histopathological findings after radical prostatectomy. They reported an overall accuracy of eMRI in defining local tumor stage of 93% by radiologist A and 56% by radiologist B. The authors found that eMRI tended to over-stage prostate cancer and concluded that treatment decisions should not be based on eMRI findings alone.

Sonnad et al. [56] analysed 27 studies for the effect of high magnetic field strength, the ER coil, fast spin-echo (SE) imaging, and study size on staging accuracy, comaparing MRI to a pathologic standard in patients with clinically limited prostate cancer. A characteristic receiver-operating curve for all studies had a maximum joint sensitivity and specificity of 74%. At a specificity of 80% on this curve, sensitivity was 69%. Subgroup analyses showed that fast SE imaging was with statistical significance more accurate than conventional SE techniques ($P<.001$). Unexpectedly, studies employing a high magnetic field strength or an ER coil were less accurate. They concluded that small technologic advances may influence test accuracy. Early and small studies, however, may overstate accuracy because of publication bias, bias in small samples, or because early studies tend to be performed by those who developed the technology, and are thus more proficient than latecomers in using it.

8.4 Staging for Metastatic Disease

If metastatic lymph nodes or hematogenous metastases are present, local treatment will not be curative.

Albertsen et al. [2] analyzed the freqency of usage and positive yield of imaging studies in men with newly diagnosed prostate cancer. In 1995 a bone scan was ordered for approximately 2/3 of patients with newly diagnosed prostate cancer and CT for 1/3. They reported a very low rate of positive findings on CT and bone scan in men with low risk and concluded that these imaging studies should be performed only in men at risk for advanced disease.

8.4.1 CT and MRI

CT and MRI are noninvasive methods of detecting pelvic lymph node involvement. An important limitation of CT and MRI in the evaluation of nodal metastasis is that both methods depend on the enlargement of lymph nodes as the criterion for metastasis. The problem is that metastases may also be present in normal-sized nodes.

CT can identify enlarged lymph nodes with any node >1 cm being considered abnormal [44]. The sensitivity of diagnosing lymph node metastasis based on this threshold is only 25%–78%, while specificity is in the range of 90%.

MRI can also identify enlarged lymph nodes. Sensitivities and specificities vary from 20% to 100%; they differ depending on the selection of the threshold [30, 62].

MRI with a 3D technique can produce an accuracy up to 90% in highly selected cases in detecting nodal metastasis from prostate cancer [30]. Because of their high cost, CT and MRI should only be used to detect nodal metastases in a selected group of patients at high risk, as predicted by DRE, PSA, and biopsy Gleason score [45].

Lymph node-specific MR contrast agents with ultrasmall superparamagnetic iron oxide particles may improve accuracy in detecting metastases in normal-sized nodes [59].

8.4.2 Bone Scan

Although radionuclide bone scan (BS) is frequently recommended as part of the staging evaluation for newly diagnosed prostate cancer, most scans are negative for metastases. Before PSA testing, use of BS imaging was certainly reasonable, even in the asymptomatic patient. However, several clinical studies have shown that a radionuclide BS should not be obtained in staging the asymptomatic, newly diagnosed prostate cancer patient with a serum PSA level less than or equal to 10 ng/ml.

In a retrospective review of 521 patients with newly diagnosed, untreated prostate cancer the ability of PSA to predict BS findings was analyzed [9]. The median serum PSA concentration in patients with a positive BS was 158.0 ng/ml, whereas men with a negative BS had a median serum PSA level of 11.3 ng/ml. In 306 men with a serum PSA level of 20 ng/ml or less only one (PSA 18.2 ng/ml) had a positive BS (negative predictive value 99.7%). This suggests that a staging BS in a previously untreated prostate cancer patient with a low serum PSA is not necessary.

In a recent study by Lee et al. univariate and multivariate analyses were performed to assess their ability to predict a positive BS. Of the 631 consecutive patients, 88 (14%) had positive BS. Multivariate analysis showed Gleason score, PSA, and clinical stage to be significant independent predictors for positive radionucleotide BS in newly diagnosed prostate cancer patients. The odds ratios were 5.25 for PSA >50 vs. 0–15 and 2.25 for Gleason of 8–10 vs. 2–6. Only three of 308 (1%) had a positive BS in patients with Gleason 2–7, PSA of 50 or less, and clinical stage of T2b or less. In patients with PSA greater than 50, 49/99 (49.5%) had positive BS, thus disclosing PSA as the major predictor for positive BS. About one-half of the patients analyzed were in the low-risk group (Gleason 2–7, PSA ≤50, clinical stage ≤T2b); elimination of BS in these patients will result in considerable cost savings.

8.4.3 Radio-immunoscintigraphy

Radiolabeled antibodies directed against prostate antigens are being developed to detect metastatic disease in lymph nodes, viscera, and bone. The monoclonal antibodies against prostate-specific membrane antigen (PSMA) are highly restricted to normal, benign growth, and malignant epithelium of the prostate, with over-expression in both primary and metastatic prostatic carcinomas [27].

Both ^{111}In and ^{99m}Tc have been used to label the anti-PSMA antibody – termed CYT-356 when labeled with ^{111}In, and CYT 351 when labeled with ^{99m}Tc.

Having received Federal Drug Administration approval in 1998, 111 In-capromab pendetide (Prostascint 1) is now commercially available [35].

Obvious enlargement with focal uptake in an obturator node definitely indicates involvement. Several studies demonstrated a sensitivity of 60% and a specificitiy of 70% for detecting positive lymph nodes [35]. However, the probability of having positive nodes in theses studies ranged from 40% to 60%, which is much higher than the incidence in men with newly diagnosed prostate cancer. The value of Prostascint for detecting extraprostatic disease is still controversial, and most of the published data do not support its use in routine clinical managment.

8.5 Conclusion

Preoperative parameters can stratify patients according to risk groups for extraprostatic tumor extension or metastasis. The most important information is still based on the analysis of systematic biopsies in combination with PSA and clinical stage. Validated nomograms will help to optimize the use of the currently available imaging modalities. The new developments in ultrasound technology and MRI technology are expected to improve the identification of tumor localization and extension in the prostate.

References

1. Aarnink RG, Beerlage HP, De La Rosette JJ, Debruyne FM, Wijkstra H (1998) Transrectal ultrasound of the prostate: innovations and future applications. J Urol 159:15668–1579
2. Albertsen PC, Hanley JA, Harlan LC, Gilliland FD, Hamilton A, Liff JA, Stanford JL, Stephenson RA (2000) The positive yield of imaging studies in the evaluation of men with newly diagnosed prosatate cancer: a population based analysis. J Urol 163:1138–1143
3. Bartolozzi C, Menchi I, Lencioni R, et al (1996) Local staging of prostate carcinoma with endorectal coil MRI. Correlation with whole mount radical prostatectomy specimens. Eur Radiol 6:339–345
4. Bostwick DG, Iczkowiski KA (1998) Microvessel density in prostate cancer: prognostic and therapeutic utility. Semin Urol Oncol 16:118–123
5. Catalona WJ, Basler JW (1993) Return of erections and urinary continence following nerve sparing radical prostatectomy. J Urol 150:905
6. Chan TY, Partin AW, Walsh PC, Epstein JI (2000) Prognostic significance of Gleason score 3+4 versus Gleason score 4+3 tumor at radical prostatctomy [abstract]. J Urol 163 [Suppl 4]:1422
7. Chelsky MJ, Schnall MD, Seidmon EJ, Pollack HM (1993) Use of endorectal surface coil magnetic resonance imaging for local staging of prostate cancer. J Urol 150:391–395
8. Cho JY, Kim SH, Lee SE (2000) Peripheral hypoechoic lesions of the prostate: evaluation with color and power doppler ultrasound. Eur Urol 37:443–448
9. Chybowski FM, Keller JJ, Bergstralh EJ, Oesterling JE (1991) Predicting radionuclide bone scan findings in patients with newly diagnosed, untreated prostate cancer: prostate specific antigen is superior to all other clinical parameters. J Urol 145:313–318
10. Conrad S, Graefen M, Pichlmeier U, Hammerer P, Huland H (1998) Systematic sextant biopsies enhance the accuracy of predicting pelvic lymph node metatstasis in prostatic cancer. J Urol 159:2023
11. Cornud F, Hamida K, Flam T, Helenon O, Chretien Y, Thiounn N, Correas JM, Casanova JM, Moreau JF (2000) Endorectal color doppler sonography and endorectal MR imaging features of nonpalpable prostate cancer: correlation with radical prostatectomy findings. AJR Am J Roentgenol 175:1161–1168
12. D'Amico AV, Whittington R, Malkowicz SB, et al (1999) Pretreatment nomogram for prostate-specific antigen recurrence after radical prostatectomy or external beam radiation therapy for clinically localized prostate cancer. J Clin Oncol 17:168–172
13. de la Rosette JJ, Aarnink RG (2001) New developments in ultrasonography for the detection of prostate cancer. J Endourol 15:93–104
14. Egawa S, Suyama K, Matsumoto K, Satoh T, Ucida T, Kuwao S, Koshiba K (1998) Improved predictibility of extracapsular extension and seminal vesical involvment based on clinical and biopsy findings in prostate cancer in Japanese men. Urology 52:433
15. El-Gabry EA, Halpern EJ, Strup SE, Gomella LG (2001) Imaging prostat cancer: current and future applications. Oncology 15: 325–336
16. Engelbrecht MR, Barentsz JO, Jager GJ, van der Graaf M, Heerschap A, Sedelaar JP, Aarnink RG, de la Rosette JJ (2000) Prostate cancer staging using imaging. BJU Int 86 [Suppl 1]:123–134
17. Garg S, Fortling B, Chadwick D, Robinson MC, Hamdy FC (1999) Staging of prostate cancer using 3-dimensional transrectal ultrasound images:a pilot study. J Urol 162:1318–1321
18. Giesen RJ, Huynen AL, Aarnink RG, de la Rosette JJ, v d Kaa C, Oosterhof GO, Debruyne FM, Wijkstra H (1995) Computer analysis of transrectal ultrasound images of the prostate for the detection of carcinoma: a prospective study in radical prostatectomy specimens. J Urol 154: 1397–1400
19. Goto Y, Ohori M, Scardino PT (1998) Use of systematic biopsy results to predict pathologic stage in patients with clinically localized prostate cancer: a preliminary report. Int J Urol 5:337
20. Graefen M, Noldus J, Pichlmeier U, Haese A, Hammerer P, Fernandez S, Conrad S, Henke R-P, Huland E, Huland H (1999) Early PSA relapse after radical retropubic prostatectomy: prediction on the basis of preoperative and postoperative tumor characteristics. Eur Urol 36:21
21. Graefen M, Haese A, Pichlmeier U, Hammerer PG, Noldus J, Butz K, Erbersdobler A, Henke RP, Michl U, Fernandez S, Huland H (2001) A validated strategy for side specific prediction of organ confined prostate cancer: a tool to select for nerve sparing radical prostatectomy. J Urol 165:857–863
22. Graefen M, Karakiewicz PI, Cagiannos I, Klein E, Kupelian PA, Quinn DI, Henshall SM, Grygiel JJ, Sutherland RL, Stricker PD, de Kernion J, Cangiano T, Schroder FH, Wildhagen MF, Scardino PT, Kattan MW (2002) Validation study of the accuracy of a postoperative nomogram for recurrence after radical prostatectomy for localized prostate cancer. J Clin Oncol 20(4): 951–956
23. Hammerer P, Huland H, Sparenberg A (1992) Digital rectal examination, imaging, and random biopsies in identifying lymph-node-negative prostatic carcinoma. Eur Urol 22:281–286
24. Hammerer P, Huland H (1994) Systematic sextant biopsies in 651 patients referred for prostate evaluation. J Urol 151:99–102
25. Harrell FE, Califf RM (1982) Evaluating the yield of medical tests. JAMA 247:2543–2546

26. Hodge KK, McNeal JE, Terris MK, Stamey TA (1989) Random-systematic versus directed ultrasound guided transrectal core biopsies of the prostate. J Urol 142:71–74
27. Horoszewicz JS, Kawinski E, Murphy GP (1987) Monoclonal antibodies to a new antigenic marker in epithelial prostatic cells and serum of prostatic cancer patients. Anticancer Res 7: 927–935
28. Hricak H, White S, Vigneron DB, et al (1994) Carcinoma of the prostate gland: MR imaging with pelvic phased-array coils versus integrated endorectal-pelvic phased-array coils. Radiology 193:703–709
29. Huland H, Hübner D, Henke R-P (1994) Systematic biopsies and digital rectal examination to identify the nerve-sparing side for radical prostatectomy without risk of positive margin in patients with clinical stage T2, N0 prostatic carcinoma. Urology 44:211
30. Jager GJ, Barentsz JO, Oosterhof G, Witjes JA, Ruijs SHJ (1997) Pelvic adenopathy in prostatic and urinary bladder carcinoma: MR imaging with a three-dimensional T1-weighted magnetization-prepared rapid gradient-echo sequence. AJR Am J Roentgenol 167:1503–1507
31. Kattan MW, Stapleton AMF, Wheeler TM, Scardino PT (1997) Evaluation of a nomogram for predicting pathological stage of men with clinically localized prostate cancer. Cancer 79: 528–537
32. Kattan MW, Eastham JA, Stapleton AMF, Wheeler TM, Scardino PT (1998) A preoperative nomogram for disease recurrence following radical prostatectomy for prostate cancer. J Natl Cancer Inst 90:766–771
33. Klein EA, Zippe CD (2000) Transrectal ultrasound guided prostate biopsy – defining a new standard [editorial]. J Urol 163:179
34. Lange PH (2001) PROSTASCINT scan for staging prostate cancer. Urology 57:402–406
35. Lavoipierre AM, Snow RM, Frydenberg M, Gunter D, Reisner G, Royce PL, Lavoipierre GJ (1998) Prostatic cancer: role of color Doppler imaging in transrectal sonography. AJR Am J Roentgenol 171:205–210
36. Lee F, Torp-Pedersen ST, Siders DB, Littrup PJ, McLeary RD (1989) Transrectal ultrasound in the diagnosis and staging of prostatic carcinoma. Radiology 170:609–615
37. Lee N, Fawaaz R, Olsson CA, Benson MC, Petrylak DP, Schiff PB, Bagiella E, Singh A, Ennis RD (2000) Which patients with newly diagnosed prostate cancer need a radionuclide bone scan? An analysis based on 631 patients. Int J Radiat Oncol Biol Phys 48:1443–1446
38. Liu IJ, Zafar MB, Lai Y, Segall GM, Terris MK (2001) Fluorodeoxyglucose positron emission tomography studies in diagnosis and staging of clinically organ-confined prostate cancer. Urology 57:108–111
39. Loch T, Leuschner I, Genberg C, Weichert-Jacobsen K, Kuppers F, Yfantis E, Evans M, Tsarev V, Stöckle M (1999) Artificial neural network analysis (ANNA) of prostatic transrectal ultrasound. Prostate 39:198–204
40. May F, Treumann T, Dettmar P, Hartung R, Breul J (2001) Limited value of endorectal magnetic resonance imaging and transrectal ultrasonography in the staging of clinically localized prostate cancer. BJU Int 87:66–69
41. Montie JE, Wei JT (2000) Artificial neural networks for prostate carcinoma risk assessment: an overview. Cancer 88:2655–2660
42. Noldus J, Graefen M, Hammerer P, Henke R-P, Huland H (1998) Entwicklung der Tumorselektion anhand des pathologischen Stadiums beim klinisch lokalisierten Prostatakarzinom. Urologe A 37:195
43. Outwater E, Petersen RO, Siegelman ES, Gomella LG, Chernesky CE, Mitchell DG (1994) Prostate carcinoma: assessment of diagnostic criteria for capsular penetration on endorectal coil MR images. Radiology 193:333–339
44. Oyen RH, Van Poppel HP, Ameye FE, Van de Voorde WA, Baert AL, Baert LV (1994) Lymph node staging of localized prostatic carcinoma with CT and CT-guided fine-needle aspiration biopsy: prospective study of 285 patients. Radiology 190:315–322
45. Partin AW, Yoo J, Ballentine Carter JY, et al (1993) The use of prostate specific antigen, clinical stage and Gleason score to predict pathological stage in men with localized prostatecancer. J Urol 150:110–115
46. Partin AW, Kattan MW, Subong EN, et al (1997) Combination of prostate specific antigen, clinical stage, and Gleason score to predict pathological stage of localized prostate cancer. A multi-institutional update. JAMA 277:1445
47. Presti JC Jr, Hricak H, Narayan PA, Shinohara K, White S, Carroll PR (1996) Local staging of prostatic carcinoma: comparison of transrectal sonography and endorectl MR imaging. AJR Am J Roentgenol 166:103–108
48. Ragde H, Kenny GM, Murphy GP, Landin K (1997) Transrectale ultrasound microbubble contrast angiography of the prostate. Prostate 32:279–283
49. Ronco AL, Fernandez R (1999) Improving ultrasonographic diagnosis of prostate cancer with neural networks. Ultrasound Med Biol 25:729–733
50. Rùrvik J, Halvorsen OJ, Albrektsen G, Ersland L, Daehlin L, Haukaas S (1999) MRI with an endorectal coil for staging of clinically localised prostate cancer prior to radical prostatectomy. Eur Radiol 9:29–34
51. Sakarya ME, Arslan H, Unal O, Atilla MK, Aydin S (1998) The role of power Doppler ultrasonography in the diagnosis of prostate cancer: a preliminary study. Br J Urol 82:386–388

52. Schiebler ML, Schnall MD, Pollack HM, et al (1993) Current role of MR imaging in the staging of adenocarcinoma of the prostate. Radiology 189:339–352
53. Sebo TJ, Bock BJ, Cheville JC, Lohse C, Wollan P, Zincke H (2000) The precent of cores positive for cancer in prostate needle biopsy specimens is strongly predictive of tumor stage and volume at radical prostatectomy. J Urol 163:174
54. Sedelaar JPM, Aarnink RG, van Leenders GJLH, Beerlage HP, Debruyne FMJ, Wijkstra H, de la Rosette JJMCH (2000) The application of three-dimensional contrast-enhanced ultrasound to measure volume of affected tissue after HIFU treatment for localized prostate cancer. Eur Urol 37:559–568
55. Snow PB, Smith DS, Catalona WJ (1994) Artificial neural networks in the diagnosis and prognosis of prostate cancer: a pilot study. J Urol 1525:1923–1926
56. Sonnad SS, Langlotz CP, Schwartz JS (2001) Accuracy of MR imaging for staging prostate cancer: a meta-analysis to examine the effect of technologic change. Acad Radiol 8:149–157
57. Stamey TA, McNeal JE, Yemoto CM, Sigal BM, Johnstone IM (1999) Biological determinants of cancer progression in men with prostate cancer. JAMA 15:1395
58. Watanabe H, Igari D, Tanahasi Y, Harada K, Saito M (1974) Development and application of new equipment for transrectal ultrasonography. J Clin Ultrasound 2:91–98
59. Weissleder R, Elizondo G, Wittenberg J, Lee AS, Josephson L, Brady TJ (1990) Ultrasmall superparamagnetic iron oxide: an intravenous contrast agent for assessing lymphnodes with MR imaging. Radiology 175:494–498
60. White S, Hricak H, Forstner R, et al (1995) Prostate cancer: effect of postbiopsy hemorrhage on interpretation of MR images. Radiology 195:385–390
61. Wills ML, Sauvageot J, Partin AW, Gurganus R, Epstein JI (1998) Ability of sextant biopsies to predict radical prostatectomy stage. Urology 51:759
62. Yu KK, Hricak H, Alagappan R, Chernoff DM, Bacchetti P, Zaloudek CJ (1997) Detection of extracapsular extension of prostate carcinoma with endorectal and phased-array coil MR imaging: multivariate feature analysis. Radiology 202:697–702

9 Preoperative Staging of Prostate Cancer: The Role of Molecular Markers

J.W. Moul, A.S. Merseburger

9.1 Introduction

With the advent of prostate-specific antigen (PSA) screening programs and increased public awareness of the disease, the incidence of prostate cancer (PC) has dramatically increased over the past decade. It has now leveled off at approximately 180,000 cases per year [53]. An equally significant stage migration toward earlier stages has also occurred, allowing radical prostatectomy to take on a more prominent role [53, 69]. Despite this stage migration toward clinically organ-confined disease, a significant portion (40%–60%) of patients are found to have extracapsular disease after radical prostatectomy. Furthermore, approximately 40% have been found to recur within 10 years if no postoperative adjuvant therapy is used [21, 60, 63]. Ideally, tests would be available to clinicians for selecting men for surgery whose disease is definitely confined to the organ and thus have a high probability of cure with prostatectomy. From the above statistics it is obvious we do not yet have an ideal method of selection. Conversely, perhaps our goal of selecting candidates for radical prostatectomy is not to eliminate those with moderate or high risk of not being cured by surgery alone. Candidates may also be selected who may be expected to benefit from radical prostatectomy plus adjuvant therapies.

In 2002, urologic surgeons have a variety of tools to help them select candidates for surgery or surgery plus adjuvant therapy. These, including age, overall health, and co-morbidities, will not be discussed further here. All urologists use the PSA value, the biopsy tumor grade, and the digital rectal examination (DRE) on which to base the clinical stage from which surgical candidates are selected. The goal of this chapter is to review the contemporary value of molecular markers as a preoperative staging tool in the evaluation of radical prostatectomy candidates. We will discuss the emerging concept of molecular marker tests on prostate biopsy material or other body samples, such as blood, bone marrow, or semen, as an aid in the better assessment of micrometastases or risk of recurrence.

The opinions and assertions contained herein are the private views of the authors and are not to be construed as reflecting the views of the U.S. Army, U.S. Navy, the Department of Defense, or the U.S. Government.

Judd W. Moul is supported by a grant from the Center for Prostate Disease Research, a program of the Henry M. Jackson Foundation for the Advancement of Military Medicine (Rockville, MD), funded by the U.S. Army Medical Research and Material Command.

9.2 Molecular Markers: Reverse Transcriptase Polymerase Chain Reaction

The reverse transcriptase polymerase chain reaction (RT-PCR) assay in clinical oncology was first reported in 1988 when it was used to detect the *bcr/abl* messenger RNA (mRNA) sequence present in chronic myelogenous leukemia cells [35]. The RT-PCR assay has since been employed in the identification of tumor cell-specific unique mRNA sequences in the blood, bone marrow, or other tissue sites that yield information about disease activity. For prostate cancer (PC), detection of PSA-expressing cells by the RT-PCR method was first conceived in 1992 and reported in samples from patients with metastatic PC in 1992 [52]. In 1994, Katz et al. were the first to report a large series of RT-PCR assays of PSA-expressing cells in the peripheral blood of patients undergoing radical prostatectomy (RP), and these authors coined the term "molecular staging" [32, 33]. Twenty-six percent of their patients with clinically localized disease had positive PSA expression by RT-PCR assay, and positivity correlated with pathologic extraprostatic disease. Although later studies by this group continued to show that a positive RT-PCR reaction for PSA expression correlated with extraprostatic disease and recurrence [34, 55], other investigators have been unable to confirm the clinical value of RT-PCR in the molecular staging of patients with PC using RT-PCR assays for the detection of either PSA or prostate-specific membrane antigen (PSMA) [17, 22, 24, 25, 27, 29, 43, 49, 61, 67, 72].

Mejean et al. recently found that circulating prostate-derived cells detected by RT-PCR assay in patients with prostate adenocarcinoma are an independent risk factor for tumor recurrence [48]. Their results demonstrate that a highly controlled, carefully performed RT-PCR procedure may represent a noninvasive way of predicting the clinical course and stage of prostate cancer. The group assessed four different methods for isolating nucleated cells from peripheral blood, concluding that the density gradient separation method is the most efficient.

Our group subjected preoperative peripheral blood to RT-PCR assay for PSA-expressing cells in 85 radical prostatectomy patients. We found no correlation to pathological stage or early recurrence [22].

In contrast to the detection of PSA- or PSMA-expressing cells in blood, only a limited number of studies have evaluated PSA-expressing cells in bone marrow of patients undergoing radical prostatectomy [22, 49, 76, 77]. Wood et al. first reported that 29 of 55 prostate cancer patients (53%) had PSA-expressing cells in bone marrow before treatment, including 43% before radical prostatectomy [77]. In their initial report, 20% of organ-confined cases (pT2) were RT-PCR positive compared to 15 of 23 (65%) with extraprostatic extension (pT3 or greater) [77]. In a follow-up study Wood and Banerjee reported on 86 patients and showed an RT-PCR positive rate of 29% versus 62% comparing organ-confined to extraprostatic disease [76]. Furthermore, at a mean follow-up period of 15.4 months only two of 47 patients (4%) with a negative bone marrow RT-PCR had recurrence compared to 10 of 39 (26%) with recurrence when the bone marrow RT-PCR was positive (log rank, $p = 0.004$) [76]. However, in multivariate analysis, including pretreatment PSA level, bone marrow RT-PCR was not an independent predictor of recurrence. Melchior et al. also studied bone marrow RT-PCR (and peripheral blood RT-PCR) in 71 radical prostatectomy patients, 14 advanced disease patients, and 30 control subjects [49]. Bone marrow RT-PCR PSA was positive in 56% of organ confined, 73% extraprostatic extension, and 86% advanced disease cases. Furthermore, a subset of 24 cases had preoperative and postoperative bone marrow samples taken, and those which remained positive after surgery had a higher rate of extracapsular disease, although no definite association with recurrence could be ascribed due to short follow-up. Finally, Melchior et al. examined unilateral versus bilateral bone marrow aspiration and found that bilateral aspiration increased RT-PCR positivity from 57% to 74% in a group of 71 patients with clinically localized disease and 14 patients with advanced-stage carcinoma of the prostate before radical prostatectomy [49].

Our group has studied preoperative anterior unilateral iliac crest bone marrow aspirates for RT-PCR of PSA-expressing cells in 116 radical prostatectomy patients [23]. We found no correlation to pathologic stage, but the 2-year disease-free survival rate was 96.9% in RT-PCR negative patients versus 77.5%

in RT-PCR positive patients ($P = 0.054$). The RT-PCR test of the bone marrow in this study was an independent predictor of recurrence in multivariable analysis of PSA, Gleason grade, and pathologic stage.

Several studies have described the immunocytochemical detection of disseminated bone marrow cells for localized prostate cancer. Immunohistochemistry (IHC) has been used to evaluate the frequency of occult carcinoma cells in bone marrow. Neither the preoperative number of cells nor IHC positivity showed a statistically significant correlation with early relapses [37, 41]. Since the β subunit of human chorionic gonadotropin (β-hCG) has been detected in prostate cancer by immunologic and RT-PCR techniques, Daja et al. studied beta-hCG protein messenger RNA expression by RT-PCR in both prostate cancer cell lines and human ejaculate. The authors hoped that this could provide a noninvasive procedure for prostate cancer detection since prostate cells have been detected in human ejaculate. However, the low percentage of detection in ejaculate suggested that β-hCG in semen does not provide a useful marker for discovery of early prostate cancer [16].

At the present time, RT-PCR assays of the blood, bone marrow and semen are strictly research tools [80]. Before this test is used in routine clinical practice, it must be shown to be reproducible and must be made cost-effective. Furthermore, unless RT-PCR of the bone marrow becomes a strong predictor in longer-term follow-up, there will be no practical reason to subject patients to bone marrow aspiration. The future holds great promise for RT-PCR technology. Specifically, RT-PCR assessment of a panel of prostate cancer-specific genes may improve the prospects for "molecular staging" in surgical patients.

9.3 Molecular Markers: Tumor Tissue Markers

At the present time, there are no tumor tissue molecular biomarkers that are widely accepted for prostate cancer. Using molecular markers to select men for radical prostatectomy alone or to prompt neoadjuvant therapy requires prostate biopsy material. Three current dilemmas in prostate cancer are the heterogeneity of the neoplasm, the multifocality of the neoplasm, and the uncertainty that the needle biopsy sample available for study is reflective of the biology of the disease [68].

According to a literature review (February 2001), the following molecular markers have been studied in prostate needle biopsies: p53 and p27 tumor suppressor gene proteins, bcl-1 oncogene protein, Ki-67 proliferation index using MIB-1 antibody, microvessel density assessment, and E-cadherin, each determined by IHC analysis. (Various other proteins have been tested in early pilot investigations but are not discussed since they are many steps away from seeing clinical use.) The bottom line is that none of these biomarkers have shown consistent clinical utility for staging or prognosis prior to radical prostatectomy. However, there are a number of studies that are promising and point to the need for larger, multicenter biopsy biomarker investigations. We will briefly review these biomarkers individually.

The significance of p53 mutation in prostate cancer remains controversial. P53 protein is the product of expression of the p53 tumor suppresser gene [1]. It is involved in cell cycle regulation [31] and the apoptosis pathway [42, 44]. Mutation of the p53 gene can be a transforming event and is the most frequently reported mutation in human cancer [42]. Mutation in the p53 gene can also lead to an increase in the protein's normally short half-life, allowing detection by IHC techniques. Studies using different analytical tools besides IHC are single strand conformation polymorphism (SSCP) and DNA sequencing. All have yielded widely varying rates of p53 mutation in human prostate cancer specimens. Voeller et al. showed positive staining in only 4% of untreated cancers [75], while Van Veldhuizen et al. found positive immunostaining in 79% of untreated prostate cancers [74]. Mirchandani et al. showed through careful analysis that within radical prostatectomy specimens there was widespread heterogeneity of p53 mutations from tumor to tumor and within single tumors [50]. They proposed that this may be responsible, at least in part, for the wide variations reported in mutation rates.

Over the last 2 years, a number of important studies have shed more light on p53 as a prognostic marker in prostate cancer. Quinn et al. have reported the largest study to date with 263 radical prostatectomy patients followed for a mean of 55 months [56]. Two strong independent predictors of recurrence after surgery were determined to be focal staining status and P53 nuclear accumulation as revealed by IHC analysis of radical prostatectomy specimens, as measured by the percentage of malignant cells that were either stained or clustered. In patients who received neoadjuvant hormonal therapy, p53 cluster positivity carried a 90% risk of relapse within 36 months. All six patients who died of prostate cancer during the follow-up interval had p53 positivity in their radical specimen. This work confirms the study of Bauer et al. of 175 radical prostatectomy cases, where p53 in the removed specimen was also an independent predictor of recurrence [3]. Similarly, Theodorescu et al. studied 71 radical prostatectomy patients followed for 15 years, finding p53 status in the specimen to be a strong independent predictor of disease-specific survival [71]. Leibovich et al. also studied 72 locally advanced cases and found p53 IHC analysis of the radical specimen to provide independent prognostic information [40]. Borre et al. recently found that p53 nuclear protein accumulation was an independent adverse prognostic factor in patients with prostate cancer undergoing watchful waiting after retrospective evaluation of material obtained at transurethral resection of the prostate (TURP) [8].

Despite a growing consensus that p53 IHC assessment in radical prostatectomy specimens is clinically useful, studies of p53 assessment in prostate needle biopsy have been conflicting. The BIOMED-II Marker for Prostate Cancer Study Group based in Nijmegen, Netherlands, systematically studied 47 prostatectomy specimens and their corresponding needle biopsies for p53 and E-cadherin IHC expression [59]. Finding poor correlation due to prostate tumor heterogeneity and multifocality, this group questioned the utility of these biomarkers in needle biopsies. Similarly, Stackhouse et al. studied radical prostatectomy and corresponding needle biopsies for p53 and bcl-2 IHC in 129 patients [68]. Biopsy expression of these biomarkers did not correlate with prostatectomy expression or recurrence. On the other hand, a number of recent studies have suggested that p53 is an important biomarker in biopsy material. Brewster et al. studied 76 patients for p53, bcl-2, CD44, and E-cadherin expression by IHC in pretreatment prostate needle biopsies [10]. Multivariate analysis revealed that only Gleason score and biopsy p53 were independent predictors of relapse after radical prostatectomy. In the radical specimen, both p53 and bcl-2 IHC were predictors of relapse. Similarly, in separate studies of pretreatment needle biopsy of patients treated by external beam radiotherapy, four groups have shown that p53 IHC is an independent predictor of relapse [26, 28, 45, 64]. It is possible that these radiation patients, in general, had more extensive local disease and the needle biopsy was more reflective of the disease compared to surgical patients, noted above, where disease was of smaller volume and the needle biopsy was not representative. A prospective, multicenter study is needed to confirm the value of p53 assessment in needle biopsy prior to radical prostatectomy. Until this is performed, p53 assessment in needle biopsy must be considered investigational.

The proto-oncogene bcl-2 encodes a protein product which functions to inhibit apoptosis [65]. Transforming mutation leads to overexpression, which has been implicated in tumorigenesis [2]. Bcl-2 has been less thoroughly studied in prostate cancer than p53. Prior studies have suggested that it is often undetectable in most hormone-dependent prostate cancers, but elevated levels are seen in hormone-independent tumors [15, 47]. Overexpression by IHC is seen in a lower percentage of primary prostate tumors than p53 expression. Bauer et al. show a positive correlation between bcl-2 expression in the radical prostatectomy specimen and biochemical (PSA) recurrence [3]. Similarly, Keshgegian et al. studied 208 consecutive radical prostatectomy specimens, finding that bcl-2 and Ki-67 (MIB-1) by IHC were independent predictors of recurrence [36]. However, the value of bcl-2 even in radical specimens is controversial. Johnson et al. [30] found that bcl-2 expression was infrequent and not prognostic and Bylund et al. [13] actually found that bcl-2 overexpression was associated with a better outcome. In needle biopsy samples, Stackhouse et al. [68] and Brewster et al. [10] could not confirm clinical utility in predicting radical prostatectomy recurrence, but Scherr et al. [64], Huanq et al. [28], and Matsushima et al. [45] suggested that bcl-2 IHC had value in predicting failure after radiation. Borre et al. found that men with high p53 immunoreactivity and bcl-2 negative disease had a significantly better prognosis than men with bcl-2 positive disease [8]. As with p53, more study of bcl-2 in needle samples is needed.

While not truly a molecular genetic marker, Ki-67 expression, using the antibody MIB-1 which works in archival tissue, is being studied alone or in combination with p53, bcl-2, or other markers in radical prostatectomy and needle biopsy specimens [4, 5]. Bettencourt et al. studied radical prostatectomy specimens from 180 patients for MIB-1 staining to assess the Ki-67 proliferation index [5]. This biomarker was found to be an independent predictor of recurrence. Similarly, Bubendorf et al. studied needle biopsies from 111 consecutive patients who were followed for a mean of 5.0 years finding the Ki-67 proliferation index an independent predictor of tumor-specific survival [11]. Matsuura et al. suggest Ki-67 as a useful biomarker for predicting disease progression with patients after endocrine treatment. Ki-67 expression may be an efficient parameter for classifying patients with advanced prostate cancer into different prognostic groups [46]. Recently another group compared the expression of Ki-67 with normal tissue, high-grade prostatic intraepithelial neoplasia, and prostate carcinoma and showed an increase from benign to malignant tissue. These investigators further found no discernible difference in expression of Ki-67 between the radical prostatectomy specimens and biopsy samples [54]. Similarly, MIB-1 staining in biopsy material was an independent predictor of recurrence after radiation therapy in one study [62]. Dunsmuir et al. found that MIB-1, estrogen receptor, and cyclin D1 provide prognostic information but question their true clinical value since they are expressed mainly in the most advanced lesions. They therefore did not recommend any of these markers for use in routine histological preparations [19]. Proliferation index assessed by Ki-67 using the MIB-1 IHC stain deserves further study as a useful biomarker in needle biopsy prior to radical prostatectomy.

Also not a molecular genetic marker, microvessel density (MVD) assessment by vascular endothelial staining techniques has recently received attention as a biomarker in prostate cancer. For both radical prostatectomy and biopsy specimens the results are conflicting. Brawer et al. originally reported that MVD in radical specimens was a predictor of pathologic stage [9]. He also implied that MVD assessment in needle biopsy would be clinically useful [9].

Similarly, Rogatsch et al. studied 36 radical prostatectomy and corresponding needle biopsies for MVD, finding that the measurements correlated well between biopsy and prostatectomy and that it correlated with pathologic stage [57]. In four studies of MVD in radical specimens to predict recurrence, Silberman et al. [66] and Strohmeyer et al. [70] found independent correlation while Bettencourt et al. [6] and Rubin et al. [58] could not confirm independent prognostic value. Borre et al. [7] studied 221 patients on a watchful waiting protocol and found that MVD assessed by Factor VIII IHC in needle biopsy or TURP was a strong predictor of disease-specific survival. More study of MVD is clearly needed in needle biopsy prior to radical prostatectomy. In our opinion, it remains investigational.

The molecular marker p27 has recently been studied in radical prostatectomy specimens by a number of groups. The p27 gene is a member of the CIP/KIP family of cyclin-dependent kinases and encodes a protein that negatively regulates cell proliferation [39]. Studies in multiple tumors, including breast, colon, and prostate, have found that decreased p27 protein expression is associated with poor prognosis. Yang et al. [79] and Kuczyk et al. [39] found decreased p27 expression was an independent predictor of recurrence after radical prostatectomy when using the surgical specimen. Conversely, Erdamar et al. [20] did not find that p27 expression in radical specimens was associated with pathologic stage or recurrence. Recently, Thomas et al. [73] assessed p27 in prostate needle biopsies which correlated with subsequent radical prostatectomy p27, Gleason grade, and pathological stage and found that it may be a useful marker. These results suggest that p27 may help identify high-risk patients preoperatively. A prospective multicenter study of p27 is needed prior to clinical use.

Despite the fact that the molecular markers studied to date in prostate biopsy are not yet validated for clinical use, the potential of molecular risk assessment is great. As a principal example of the possibilities, Bauer et al. [4] combined p53 and bcl-2 expression along with traditional prognostic factors to develop a risk equation for recurrence. Although p53 and bcl-2 assessment was performed on the radical specimen, the concept of combining multiple biomarkers will be a key strategy in the future. The use of artificial neural networks, which are computer-based statistical models that can be used to imitate biologic neural processes, might help to recognize and model nonlinear relationships between the data [18]. It is envisioned that future prostate biopsy material will be assessed for multiple gene expression analysis. Gene chips already exist that can assess thousands of gene expression profiles using robotic and computerized data analysis software [12, 14, 78]. The group of Xu et al. identified human prostate cancer- and tissue-specific genes using complementary DNA (cDNA) library subtraction in conjunction with high throughput microarray screening [78]. In the future, commercial gene chips for prostate cancer will provide a molecular profile for individual patients and undoubtedly will rely on biopsy material to better assess the radical prostatectomy patient. The use of tissue arrays, where small tumor biopsies are retrieved from selected regions of archival tissue blocks and hundreds of such cylindrical samples are subsequently precisely arrayed in a new paraffin block, have already been established by Kononen et al. and are now in use [38, 51]. The combination of cDNA, tissue microarray technologies, and neural networks enables rapid identification of genes of prostate cancer and may facilitate analysis of the role of the encoded gene products in the pathogenesis of human prostate cancer.

9.4 Summary

For the typical newly-diagnosed prostate cancer patient in 2002 with clinically organ-confined disease, of moderate grade, and having a PSA of less than 10 ng/ml, the current role of molecular biomarkers is limited. RT-PCR testing of blood or bone marrow for prostate-specific or prostate-cancer-specific gene expression, or for "molecular staging" is a promising technique whose current use is still investigational. Much useful information may be gained by careful study of prostate needle biopsy material. However, aside from current Gleason grading and the number and/or percentage of cores involved with cancer, no molecular biomarker is approved for clinical use. P27, p53, bcl-2, Ki-67 (MIB-1), and assessment of neovascularity hold promise, but prospective multicenter studies are needed. In the long term, multiple-gene-expression profiling of biopsy material using gene chips may revolutionize the care of prostate cancer patients, including those who elect radical prostatectomy.

References

1. Baker SJ, Markowitz S, Fearon ER, Willson JK, Vogelstein, B (1990) Suppression of human colorectal carcinoma cell growth by wild-type p53. Science 249:912–915
2. Bakhshi A, et al (1985) Cloning the chromosomal breakpoint of t(14;18) human lymphomas: clustering around JH on chromosome 14 and near a transcriptional unit on 18. Cell 41:899–906
3. Bauer JJ, et al (1996) Elevated levels of apoptosis regulator proteins p53 and bcl-2 are independent prognostic biomarkers in surgically treated clinically localized prostate cancer. J Urol 156:1511–1516
4. Bauer JJ, et al (1997) Biostatistical modeling using traditional variables and genetic biomarkers for predicting the risk of prostate carcinoma recurrence after radical prostatectomy. Cancer 79:952–962
5. Bettencourt MC, et al (1996) Ki-67 expression is a prognostic marker of prostate cancer recurrence after radical prostatectomy [see comments]. J Urol 156:1064–1068
6. Bettencourt MC, Bauer JJ, Sesterhenn IA, Connelly RR, Moul JW (1998) CD34 immunohistochemical assessment of angiogenesis as a prognostic marker for prostate cancer recurrence after radical prostatectomy. J Urol 160:459–465
7. Borre M, Offersen BV, Nerstrom B, Overgaard J (1998) Microvessel density predicts survival in prostate cancer patients subjected to watchful waiting. Br J Cancer 78:940–944
8. Borre M, Stausbol-Gron B, Overgaard J (2000) p53 accumulation associated with bcl-2, the proliferation marker MIB-1 and survival in patients with prostate cancer subjected to watchful waiting. J Urol 164:716–721
9. Brawer MK, Deering RE, Brown M, Preston SD, Bigler SA (1994) Predictors of pathologic stage in prostatic carcinoma. The role of neovascularity. Cancer 73:678–687
10. Brewster SF, Oxley JD, Trivella M, Abbott CD, Gillatt DA (1999) Preoperative p53, bcl-2, CD44 and E-cadherin immunohistochemistry as predictors of biochemical relapse after radical prostatectomy. J Urol 161:1238–1243
11. Bubendorf L, et al (1998) Ki67 labeling index in core needle biopsies independently predicts tumor-specific survival in prostate cancer. Hum Pathol 29:949–954
12. Bubendorf L., et al (1999) Hormone therapy failure in human prostate cancer: analysis by complementary DNA and tissue microarrays. J Natl Cancer Inst 91:1758–1764
13. Bylund A, Stattin P, Widmark A, Bergh A (1998) Predictive value of bcl-2 immunoreactivity in prostate cancer patients treated with radiotherapy. Radiother Oncol 49:143–148
14. Carlisle AJ, et al (2000) Development of a prostate cDNA microarray and statistical gene expression analysis package. Mol Carcinog 28:12–22
15. Colombel M, et al. Detection of the apoptosis-suppressing oncoprotein bc1–2 in hormone-refractory human prostate cancers. Am J Pathol 143:390–400
16. Daja MM, et al (2000) Beta-human chorionic gonadotropin in semen: a marker for early detection of prostate cancer? Mol Urol 4:421–427
17. De Cremoux P, et al (1997) Value of the preoperative detection of prostate-specific-antigen-positive circulating cells by nested RT-PCR in patients submitted to radical prostatectomy. Eur Urol 32:69–74
18. Douglas TH, Moul JW (1998) Applications of neural networks in urologic oncology. Semin Urol Oncol 16:35–39

19. Dunsmuir WD, et al (2000) Molecular markers for predicting prostate cancer stage and survival. BJU Int 86:869–878
20. Erdamar S, et al (1999) Levels of expression of p27KIP1 protein in human prostate and prostate cancer: an immunohistochemical analysis. Mod Pathol 12:751–755
21. Ferguson JK, Oesterling JE (1994) Patient evaluation if prostate-specific antigen becomes elevated following radical prostatectomy or radiation therapy. Urol Clin North Am 21:677–685
22. Gao CL, et al (1999) Blinded evaluation of reverse transcriptase-polymerase chain reaction prostate-specific antigen peripheral blood assay for molecular staging of prostate cancer. Urology 53:714–721
23. Gao CL, et al (1999) Detection of circulating prostate specific antigen expressing prostatic cells in the bone marrow of radical prostatectomy patients by sensitive reverse transcriptase polymerase chain reaction. J Urol 161:1070–1076
24. Ghossein RA, et al (1995) Detection of circulating tumor cells in patients with localized and metastatic prostatic carcinoma: clinical implications. J Clin Oncol 13:1195–1200
25. Ghossein RA, et al (1997) Prognostic significance of detection of prostate-specific antigen transcripts in the peripheral blood of patients with metastatic androgen-independent prostatic carcinoma. Urology 50:100–105
26. Grignon DJ, et al (1997) p53 status and prognosis of locally advanced prostatic adenocarcinoma: a study based on RTOG 8610. J Natl Cancer Inst 89:158–165
27. Henke W, et al (1997) Increased analytical sensitivity of RT-PCR of PSA mRNA decreases diagnostic specificity of detection of prostatic cells in blood [see comments]. Int J Cancer 70:52–56
28. Huang A, et al (1998) p53 and bcl-2 immunohistochemical alterations in prostate cancer treated with radiation therapy. Urology 51:346–351
29. Ignatoff JM, Oefelein MG, Watkin W, Chmiel JS, Kaul KL (1997) Prostate specific antigen reverse transcriptase-polymerase chain reaction assay in preoperative staging of prostate cancer. J Urol 158:1870–1874
30. Johnson MI, et al (1998) Expression of Bcl-2, Bax, and p53 in high-grade prostatic intraepithelial neoplasia and localized prostate cancer: relationship with apoptosis and proliferation. Prostate 37:223–229
31. Kastan MB, Onyekwere O, Sidransky D, Vogelstein B, Craig RW (1991) Participation of p53 protein in the cellular response to DNA damage. Cancer Res 51:6304–6311
32. Katz AE, et al (1994) Molecular staging of prostate cancer with the use of an enhanced reverse transcriptase-PCR assay. Urology 43:765–775
33. Katz AE, et al (1995) Enhanced reverse transcriptase-polymerase chain reaction for prostate specific antigen as an indicator of true pathologic stage in patients with prostate cancer. Cancer 75:1642–1648
34. Katz AE, et al (1996) Molecular staging of genitourinary malignancies. Urology 47:948–958
35. Kawasaki ES, et al (1988) Diagnosis of chronic myeloid and acute lymphocytic leukemias by detection of leukemia-specific mRNA sequences amplified in vitro. Proc Natl Acad Sci USA 85:5698–5702
36. Keshgegian AA, Johnston E, Cnaan A (1998) Bcl-2 oncoprotein positivity and high MIB-1 (Ki-67) proliferative rate are independent predictive markers for recurrence in prostate carcinoma. Am J Clin Pathol 110:443–449
37. Kollermann J, Heseding B, Helpap B, Kollermann MW, Pantel K (1999) Comparative immunocytochemical assessment of isolated carcinoma cells in lymph nodes and bone marrow of patients with clinically localized prostate cancer. Int J Cancer 84:145–149
38. Kononen J, et al (1998) Tissue microarrays for high-throughput molecular profiling of tumor specimens [see comments]. Nat Med 4:844–847
39. Kuczyk M, et al (1999) Predictive value of decreased p27Kip1 protein expression for the recurrence-free and long-term survival of prostate cancer patients. Br J Cancer 81:1052–1058
40. Leibovich BC, Cheng L, Weaver AL, Myers RP, Bostwick DG (2000) Outcome prediction with p53 immunostaining after radical prostatectomy in patients with locally advanced prostate cancer. J Urol 163:1756–1760
41. Leissner SLIJ, Steinbach F, Brenner W, Bürger RA, Stöckle M (1995) Immunozytologische Färbung des Knochenmarks bei Patienten mit scheinbar organbegrenzten Tumoren: Nachweismöglichkeit einer beginnenden Tumordisseminierung? Akt Urol 26
42. Levine AJ, Momand J, Finlay CA (1991) The p53 tumour suppressor gene. Nature 351:453–456
43. Llanes L, et al (2000) Detecting circulating prostate cells in patients with clinically localized prostate cancer: clinical implications for molecular staging [in process citation]. BJU Int 86:1023–1027
44. Lowe SW, Schmitt EM, Smith SW, Osborne BA, Jacks T (1993) p53 is required for radiation-induced apoptosis in mouse thymocytes [see comments]. Nature 362:847–849
45. Matsushima H, et al (1997) Combined analysis with Bcl-2 and P53 immunostaining predicts poorer prognosis in prostatic carcinoma. J Urol 158:2278–2283
46. Matsuura H, Hayashi N, Kawamura J, Shiraishi T, Yatani R (2000) Prognostic significance of Ki-67 expression in advanced prostate cancers in relation to disease progression after androgen ablation. Eur Urol 37:212–217

47. McDonnell TJ, et al (1992) Expression of the protooncogene bcl-2 in the prostate and its association with emergence of androgen-independent prostate cancer. Cancer Res 52:6940–6944
48. Mejean A, et al (2000) Detection of circulating prostate derived cells in patients with prostate adenocarcinoma is an independent risk factor for tumor recurrence. J Urol 163:2022–2029
49. Melchior SW, et al (1997) Early tumor cell dissemination in patients with clinically localized carcinoma of the prostate. Clin Cancer Res 3:249–256
50. Mirchandani D, et al (1995) Heterogeneity in intratumor distribution of p53 mutations in human prostate cancer. Am J Pathol 147:92–101
51. Moch H, Kononen T, Kallioniemi OP, Sauter G (2001) Tissue microarrays: what will they bring to molecular and anatomic pathology? Adv Anat Pathol 8:14–20
52. Moreno JG, et al (1992) Detection of hematogenous micrometastasis in patients with prostate cancer. Cancer Res 52:6110–6112
53. Moul JW (1998) Treatment options for prostate cancer. I. Staged, grade, PSA, and changes in the 1990s. Am J Managed Care 4:1031–1036
54. Mucci NR, et al (2000) Expression of nuclear antigen Ki-67 in prostate cancer needle biopsy and radical prostatectomy specimens [in process citation]. J Natl Cancer Inst 92:1941–1942
55. Olsson CA, et al (1996) Preoperative reverse transcriptase polymerase chain reaction for prostate specific antigen predicts treatment failure following radical prostatectomy [see comments]. J Urol 155:1557–1562
56. Quinn DI, et al (2000) Prognostic significance of p53 nuclear accumulation in localized prostate cancer treated with radical prostatectomy. Cancer Res 60:1585–1594
57. Rogatsch H, Hittmair A, Reissigl A, Mikuz G, Feichtinger H (1997) Microvessel density in core biopsies of prostatic adenocarcinoma: a stage predictor? J Pathol 182:205–210
58. Rubin MA, et al (1999) Microvessel density in prostate cancer: lack of correlation with tumor grade, pathologic stage, and clinical outcome. Urology 53:542–547
59. Ruijter E, et al (1998) Heterogeneous expression of E-cadherin and p53 in prostate cancer: clinical implications. BIOMED-II Markers for Prostate Cancer Study Group. Mod Pathol 11:276–281
60. Russell K.J, et al (1991) Prostate specific antigen in the management of patients with localized adenocarcinoma of the prostate treated with primary radiation therapy. J Urol 146:1046–1052
61. Sardi I, et al (1997) The use of RT-"nested" PCR of prostate specific antigen to detect hematogenous neoplastic cells in patients with prostate adenocarcinoma. J Mol Med 75:751–757
62. Scalzo DA, et al (1998) Cell proliferation rate by MIB-1 immunohistochemistry predicts postradiation recurrence in prostatic adenocarcinomas. Am J Clin Pathol 109:163–168
63. Schellhammer PF, el Mahdi AM, Wright GL Jr, Kolm P, Ragle R (1993) Prostate-specific antigen to determine progression-free survival after radiation therapy for localized carcinoma of prostate. Urology 42:13–20
64. Scherr DS, et al (1999) BCL-2 and p53 expression in clinically localized prostate cancer predicts response to external beam radiotherapy [published erratum appears in J Urol 162:503]. J Urol 162:12–16
65. Sentman CL, Shutter JR, Hockenbery D, Kanagawa O, Korsmeyer SJ (1991) bcl-2 inhibits multiple forms of apoptosis but not negative selection in thymocytes. Cell 67:879–888
66. Silberman MA, Partin AW, Veltri RW, Epstein JI (1997) Tumor angiogenesis correlates with progression after radical prostatectomy but not with pathologic stage in Gleason sum 5 to 7 adenocarcinoma of the prostate. Cancer 79:772–779
67. Sokoloff MH, et al (1996) Quantitative polymerase chain reaction does not improve preoperative prostate cancer staging: a clinicopathological molecular analysis of 121 patients [see comments]. J Urol 156:1560–1566
68. Stackhouse GB, et al (1999) p53 and bcl-2 immunohistochemistry in pretreatment prostate needle biopsies to predict recurrence of prostate cancer after radical prostatectomy [see comments]. J Urol 162:2040–2045
69. Stephenson RA, Stanford JL (1997) Population-based prostate cancer trends in the United States: patterns of change in the era of prostate-specific antigen. World J Urol 15:331–335
70. Strohmeyer D, et al (2000) Tumor angiogenesis is associated with progression after radical prostatectomy in pT2/pT3 prostate cancer. Prostate 42:26–33
71. Theodorescu D, Broder SR, Boyd JC, Mills SE, Frierson HF Jr (1997) p53, bcl-2 and retinoblastoma proteins as long-term prognostic markers in localized carcinoma of the prostate. J Urol 158:131–137
72. Thiounn N, et al (1997) Positive prostate-specific antigen circulating cells detected by reverse transcriptase-polymerase chain reaction does not imply the presence of prostatic micrometastases. Urology 50:245–250
73. Thomas GV, et al (2000) Preoperative prostate needle biopsy p27 correlates with subsequent radical prostatectomy p27, gleason grade and pathological stage [in process citation]. J Urol 164:1987–1991
74. Van Veldhuizen PJ, Sadasivan R, Garcia F, Austenfeld MS, Stephens RL (1993) Mutant p53 expression in prostate carcinoma. Prostate 22:23–30
75. Voeller HJ, Sugars LY, Pretlow T, Gelmann EP (1994) p53 oncogene mutations in human prostate cancer specimens. J Urol 151:492–495

76. Wood DP Jr, Banerjee M (1997) Presence of circulating prostate cells in the bone marrow of patients undergoing radical prostatectomy is predictive of disease-free survival. J Clin Oncol 15:3451–3457
77. Wood DP Jr, Banks ER, Humphreys S, McRoberts JW, Rangnekar VM (1994) Identification of bone marrow micrometastases in patients with prostate cancer. Cancer 74:2533–2540
78. Xu J, et al (2000) Identification of differentially expressed genes in human prostate cancer using subtraction and microarray. Cancer Res 60:1677–1682
79. Yang RM, et al (1998) Low p27 expression predicts poor disease-free survival in patients with prostate cancer. J Urol 159:941–945
80. Zippelius A, et al (1997) Limitations of reverse-transcriptase polymerase chain reaction analyses for detection of micrometastatic epithelial cancer cells in bone marrow [see comments]. J Clin Oncol 15:2701–2708

10 Preoperative Imaging Techniques in Prostate Cancer

R. Hofmann, A. Heidenreich, S. Wille, Z. Varga, R. v. Knobloch

10.1 Introduction

Prostate cancer now outnumbers lung cancer as the most common cancer in American men. Nearly 200,000 new cases are seen yearly, and prostate cancer is the cause of 31,000 deaths each year. A significant migration to prostate-confined disease has taken place in recent years, but 40%–60% of those with this cancer are still found to have extracapsular disease after radical prostatectomy [74]. Although the intent and hope of such surgery has been cure, overall survival of roughly half of them may be limited. Prostate cancer can vary widely in its aggressiveness. Some men die of prostate cancer, but most still die with rather than of their cancer.

Autopsy studies have disclosed that 42% of men over 50 years of age who died of other causes harbored prostate cancer. The lifetime risk of being diagnosed with prostate cancer is around 11%–13%; the risk of dying from it is "only" 3.6%. These figures reflect the varying biological behavior of the disease and to some extent the impact of curative therapies such as radical prostatectomy for localized disease [51, 86].

Stage-appropriate management, and especially management of each individual's cancer, requires risk definition. Information is required: will this cancer progress locally or systemically?; what side effects might therapy impose and what will be the risk-to-benefit picture?; and what improvements in localized or advanced disease can be expected during this patient's lifetime?[17].

Usually patients are referred for imaging and biopsy because of elevated serum PSA levels and/or an abnormal digital rectal examination (DRE). Besides imaging and staging of the tumor, can aggressiveness of the cancer be evaluated by preoperative imaging or molecular techniques?

Staging is currently being done by DRE, serum PSA, and imaging techniques such as transrectal ultrasound (TRUS) and bone scan. Decision analysis models and neural networks may help in assessing a patient's individual risk of progression and dying from the disease. Still, data from these models and matrices allow only calculation of a "statistical and average"; the figures reflect the prognosis for a pool of a large number of patients [47, 48, 76].

Findings by DRE can be correlated to prostate size and pathologic stage, but only relatively weakly to prognosis. Serum PSA seems to be the most accurate parameter for predicting outcome [11, 66, 77].

Although the production of PSA is not specific for cancer, the serum concentration correlates with the likelihood of a cancer in the prostate gland and its volume and stage. Serum PSA can diagnose tumors in general about 5 years before the natural history of their growth allows them to be palpable as a nodule [27, 39]. Serum PSA concentrations correlate significantly with pathologic stage and the probability of negative margins at surgery. Roughly 75% of men with PSA <4 ng/ml have organ-confined disease [67]. In an individual patient, on the other hand, PSA does not predict the presence of extracapsular disease, seminal vesicle infiltration, or lymph node involvement [71, 87]. PSA production varies due to grade and volume of the disease and the site of origin of the tumor (transitional zone tumor versus peripheral zone tumor). Regarding the latter, transitional cell cancers tend to grow larger and be diagnosed with higher PSA levels than peripheral zone tumors [3, 19, 85]. Despite its correlation with tumor volume, PSA correction for prostate gland volume (PSA density) does not improve prediction of pathologic stage. Other factors for PSA elevation are leakage of PSA into the serum by inflammation or by iatrogenic causes such as DRE and cystoscopy. These causes make PSA testing problematic in itself [13, 59]. Percent free PSA adds to the predictive ability of pathologic staging in intermediate PSA levels of 4–10 ng/ml [65, 84].

Clinical prognostic factors for cure and long-term cancer control are clinical stage, grade of the tumor, and PSA level before treatment [8, 23, 90].

Imaging studies for prostate cancer can be divided into three categories:

1. *Imaging* is mainly based on *anatomic alterations* of the tissue and macroscopic changes in organ structure; these can be displayed by various techniques [TRUS, computed tomography (CT) scan, magnetic resonance imagine (MRI), etc.].
2. *Functional imaging* is a refinement of anatomic imaging and adds information about lesions with regard to tissue properties such as membrane density and tumor blood flow (color Doppler TRUS, elastography, etc.).
3. Diagnosis may be dramatically improved if and when *molecular imaging* in vivo becomes a reality. This technique holds promise of quantifying tissue specificity and assessing tumor aggressiveness. Adding tissue markers such as p-53, bcl-2 to histologic probes or evaluating genetic markers would seem to be likely bases for molecular imaging.

Current imaging techniques and further prospectives in imaging of localized prostate cancer are reviewed.

10.2 Ultrasound

Eighty percent of prostate cancers originate in the peripheral zone. This area can be evaluated accurately by TRUS. This technique is not a primary means of diagnosing prostate cancer, however; in those men suspected of having cancer due to elevated PSA and/or positive DRE, TRUS may help clarify the diagnosis.

Lesions suspect for prostate cancer on the ultrasound image may be hypoechoic, mixed echogenic, or isoechoic [15, 52, 82].

Most common is the hypoechoic lesion, which is close to the capsule. These lesions can also be delineated because they are adjacent to the more echogenic areas outside the prostate (fat, muscle). Usually in elderly men, in whom prostate cancer is more common, the enlargement of benign prostatic hyperplasia (BPH) is also prevalent. BPH tissue displaces the peripheral zone outward and compresses the outer gland; and the enlarged inner gland usually is less echogenic than the compressed outer gland. . If one finds no difference in echogenicity between the outer and the inner gland of a prostate containing BPH, suspicion should be entertained that a tumor exists in the outer part of the gland. Hypoechoic areas can also be demonstrated near the ejaculatory ducts due to smooth muscle tissue here, making diagnosis of these especially aggressive hypoechoic tumors in this area difficult by TRUS (Figs. 10.1, 10.2) [14, 62].

Apical tumors can be difficult to distinguish on the axial sonogram. Longitudinal views help identify changes in apical echogenicity.

10.1
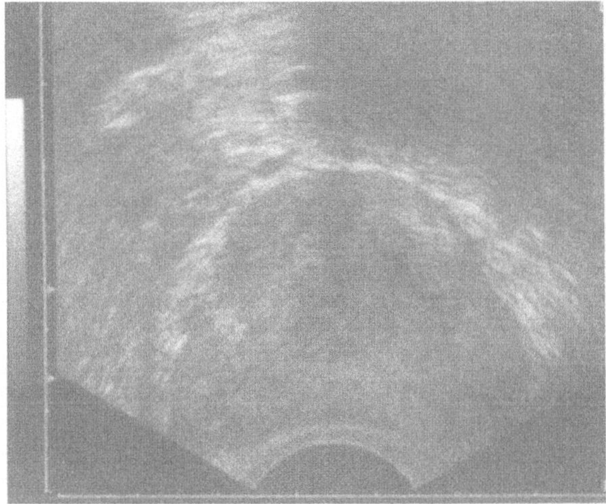

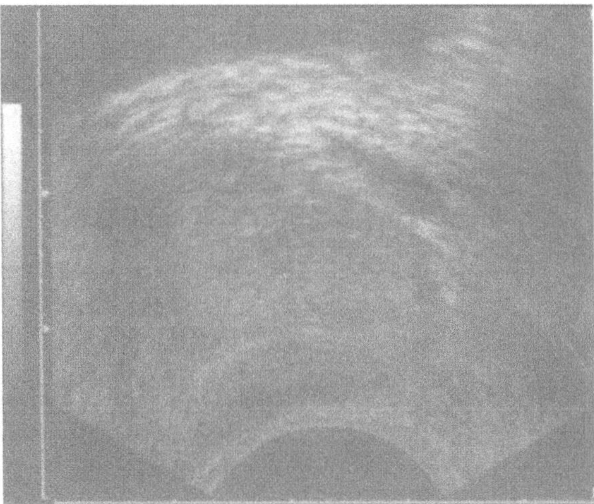
10.2

10.3
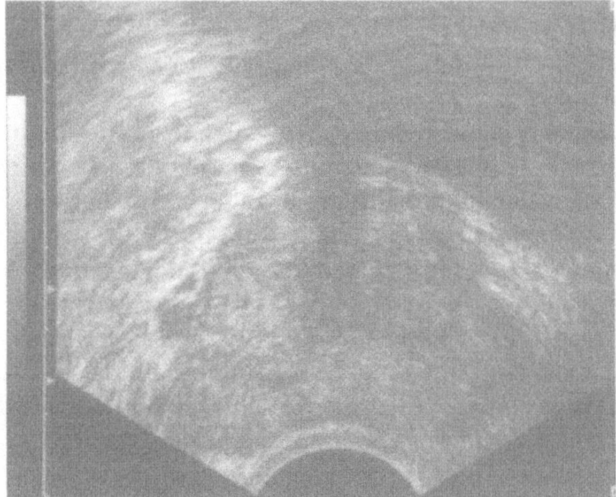

Fig. 10.1. Prostate with hypoechoic area close to the capsule in the right lobe. Histologically T2a, Gleason 3+4 cancer

Fig. 10.2. Prostate cancer with larger hypoechoic lesion close to the capsule. Histologically pT2b, Gleason 3+3 tumor

Fig. 10.3. Mixed hypoechoic and hyperechoic reflexes on the right side. Hypoechoic areas close to the capsule. Histologically pT3a Gleason 4+3 tumor

Mixed echogenic lesions can also harbor prostate tumors, with areas of hypoechognicity seen to be surrounded by hyperechoic tissue (Fig. 10.3).

Most difficult to distinguish is the isoechoic lesion, where only changes in the anatomy may hint at prostatic cancer. Some authors report that up to 50% of cancers cannot be visualized by gray scale ultrasound. Asymmetry of the gland, periprostatic fat infiltration, or a distinct bulge of the capsule can indicate prostate cancer.

In conclusion, hypoechoic lesions close to the capsule, asymmetry of the gland, capsular penetration of hypoechoic lesions, asymmetry of echo patterns and, more difficult to recognize, the lack of difference between the inner and the outer gland are signs of prostate cancer.

TRUS, however, lacks the sensitivity and specificity needed for early detection of cancer. Tumors detected by ultrasound can certainly be classified as at least T2 or T3 cancers. TRUS thus cannot replace biopsy as an accurate tool in the diagnosis of prostate cancer, but it can be useful in staging a known cancer and in determining the volume of the prostate gland.

TRUS images are used mostly as an aid in obtaining accurate biopsies. With TRUS, random biopsies are usually taken from both lateral lobes and the median lobe. The optimal sites for biopsies can be defined by TRUS – areas, including lateral ones, of ultrasonographic abnormality [2, 21, 89]. Besides making use of TRUS, diagnostic yield can be increased by increasing the number of biopsies. Ten biopsies obviously have the potential of discovering more cancer than the traditional six. Increasing the number of biopsies, however, reduces patients' tolerance of the procedure. Periprostatic local anaesthesia makes biopsy almost completely pain free, thus allowing an increased number of biopsies [83].

Improvements in TRUS for enhanced images of prostate cancer include:

1. Computer-assisted ultrasound imaging
2. Artificial neural networks (ANN) with TRUS parameters included
3. Color Doppler ultrasound
4. Power Doppler ultrasound
5. Contrast-enhanced Doppler ultrasound
6. Microbubble ultrasound
7. Ultrasound elastography

Computer-assisted ultrasound images analyze the gray scale ultrasound images and have been found to reduce interobserver variability and the low predictive value of gray scale TRUS. Despite an increased diagnostic accuracy with these systems, the diagnostic yield has not improved enough to allow their routine use as a primary tool in diagnosis.

Artificial neural networks are capable of improving diagnosis and staging of prostate cancer. They increase both specificity and sensitivity in predicting the presence of cancer, but reproducibility in different centers remains a problem. The ultrasound scanning device has to be adapted and the software of the artificial network improved by adding more information into the system so as to achieve optimal, standardized results.

Color Doppler ultrasound depicts blood flow within the prostate. Tumor vascularity is correlated to tumor aggressiveness, and it would be ideal if hypervascular areas in the prostate could be identified and biopsied under TRUS control. Color Doppler signal alone, however, does not add more specificity to the diagnosis [29].

Power Doppler ultrasound relies on evaluation of the integrated Doppler power spectrum. Power Doppler may have more sensitivity in low blood flow areas of prostate cancer thus being more informative than Color Doppler alone.

Contrast-enhanced Doppler ultrasound studies may help delineate tumors [1]. The agents used for these remain strictly in the vascular system and can better depict a tumor's vascularity. This technique does not provide more information on tissue specificity or echogenicity, but it may helpdiscover increased angiogenesis and hence increased aggressiveness of a tumor [25, 31].

Microbubble ultrasound contrast media may improve tumor-specific diagnosis. Harmonic and second harmonic images rely on the nonlinear backscatter signals of the contrast bubbles. *Intermittent imaging* used in conjunction with this technique can also detect a difference in tissue behavior. With ultrasound pulses, the microbubbles are destroyed in their flow through the vascularized area. However, when a second pulse comes a few seconds after the first, new bubbles arrive at the tissue to be studied, and thus microcirculation can be evaluated as it is seen with and without bubbles intermittently.

Ultrasonic elastography produces images based on the elastic properties of tissue. This new technique may better distinguish between tumor and benign tissue and even discriminate among different levels of tumor aggressiveness [63].

The value of TRUS in detecting local recurrence after radical prostatectomy is limited. Only tumor recurrences larger than 1 cm in the anastomotic area can be detected for biopsy.

Table 10.1. False-negative results of bone scans with different cut off values of prostate-specific antigen (PSA) [60]

PSA (ng/ml)	False-negative results (%)	95% confidence interval (%)
<4.0	0.0	0–1.9
<8.0	0.0	0–0.8
<10.0	0.5	0.1–1.6
<15.0	0.5	0.1–1.4
<20.0	0.8	0.3–1.7

10.3 Radionuclide Bone Scan

It is considered that nuclear medicine deals more with function than with anatomy. Bone scans, for example, provide poor spatial resolution, but are very sensitive to metabolic activity [46]. Currently less than 5% of all patients with prostate cancer have distant metastases at the time of diagnosis, which is a reduction from 30% 15 years ago. The era of bone scintigraphy started out in 1963 with the use of strontium-85, a highly energetic γ emitter with a long half-life. With a half life time of 6 h, Technetium-99m bound to polyphosphate has the advantage of rapid binding to bone structures. At the moment Technetium-99m diphosphonate is used predominantly; it has a rapid clearance from the serum and extracellular fluid, thus making for a high bone-to-soft tissue ratio. Patients with localized prostate cancer have little likelihood of bone metastases unless the PSA is higher than 20 ng/ml. Patients with a PSA of less than 10 ng/ml have no metastases, and patients with less than 20 ng/ml have them only 0.8% of the time [12, 60, 91] (Table 10.1). Thus, only patients with aggressive tumors, having a PSA of >20 ng/ml, Gleason sum >7 or an advanced local tumor stage (T3,T4), or patients with bone pain should undergo bone scintigraphy. Suspicous areas, which cannot be attributed directly to bone metastases or trauma, should be examined by routine skeletal radiographs or MRI.

At the moment about $50 million is spent for unnecessary bone scans each year. Adding to the cost of health care, bone scans also take at least 3 h to perform [61]. Thus, the American Urological Association states in its guidelines that bone scans are not indicated when PSA is less than 20 ng/ml in the absence of bone pain. Only 0.8% of all metastases of prostate cancer to bone would be missed by this recommendation. In radical prostatectomy patients with undectable or early rising PSA the value of bone scans is also very limited [10, 42, 45, 72].

10.4 Positron Emission Tomography

Fluorine-18-fluorodeoxyglucose positron emission tomography (FDG-PET) detects cancer within a tumor mass by assessing its metabolism. Uptake into most tumorous tissue is relatively specific in predicting the presence of cancer. However, uptake is very low in prostate cancer because glucose utilization of the malignancy is very similar to that of the benign prostatic tissue. It would seem that prostate cancer cells do not rely on glucose metabolism as much as do other cancer cells. Overlap of bladder activity due to renal clearance of FDG also makes it difficult to detect local recurrence.

The sensitivity of this technology in detection of bony metastases is low, only around 20% of such metastases taking up FDG. It can thus be seen that FDG-PET has not fulfilled its promises, especially for distant spread,since so many false-positive and, worse, false-negative results are encountered [81]. New positron-emitting pharmaceuticals such as choline or citrate/choline combinations may show promise, however, of use in conjunction with assessment of tumor vascularity for evaluation of tumor aggressiveness [32, 81].

10.5 Indium-11 Capromab Pendetide Antibody

Indium-11 capromab pendetide antibody (Prosta Scint, Cytogen Corp. Princeton, NJ) can be used for evaluation of soft tissue and bone metastases. A prostate-specific membrane antigen (PSMA)-antibody is radiolabeled and injected intravenously. Planar and cross sectional single photon emission computed tomography (SPECT) is performed. Repeat studies are done 72–120 h after injection until clearance from the vascular bed and intestines is complete [4].

Focal inflammatory lesions, nonspecific localization in the gastrointestinal tract, and high interobserver variability make the test of doubtful value. However, Prosta Scint seems to be useful in patients with untreated prostate cancer with high suspicion of distant metastases – PSA >20 ng/ml, Gleason >7 and stage T3 with a negative bone scan [43, 44]. In a study of 152 patients in this patient group, 64 had pelvic lymph node metastases. Forty scans were evaluated as positive and 38 patients had pathologically confirmed lymph node metastases (95%). The sensitivity realized here of 63% was superior to that of CT scan (4%) or MRI (15%). When considered together with PSA and Gleason score, Prostata Scint had a greater than 90% negative predictive value in patients with PSA<40 ng/ml and gleason score <7. For patients with PSA>40 ng/ml and a Gleason score >7, the positive predictive value was higher than 80% [54].

Thus, Prostascint may have its role only in newly diagnosed prostate cancers with a high risk profile.

10.6 Computed Tomography

Computed tomography (CT) scan cannot detect cancer in the prostate itself; differences between cancerous and benign tissue cannot be discriminated by this method. Sensitivity and specificity for local staging of the tumor is therefore very low – as low as 55%–75% and specificity 60%–73%, respectively, for extracapsular disease evaluation. Seminal vesicle involvement can only be detected in 19%–36% [36, 88].

CT scan is mostly used for staging of the lymph node status, though it can detect only lymph nodes larger than 1 cm at best [37, 53, 69]. Lymph nodes with micrometastases or even those grossly infiltrated by tumor but not enlarged thus cannot be detected by CT scan. False-positive results occur when lymph nodes are enlarged by inflammation, such as after prostate biopsy or hip replacement.

Lymph node metastases are very rare in newly diagnosed prostate cancer patients. In a screened population of 459 men in The Netherlands, positive nodes were found in only 1.7%. [73]. For a patient with a PSA <20 ng/ml, the likelihood of a positive lymph node is less than 1%. Only in patients at high risk for positive nodes or patients with an unfavorable histology (such as small cell or anaplastic prostate cancer) is CT scan of value in ruling out gross lymph node involvement. Micrometastases are not detectable by CT scan, and in the light of about 20% false-negative results of frozen sections and a favorable prognosis in patients with micrometastases undergoing radical prostatectomy, CT scan is unnecessary [24].

CT scan is likewise of little value in detecting local recurrences after radical prostatectomy [49].

10.7 Magnetic Resonance Imaging

MRI is not considered to be a primary screening tool for prostate cancer. The gland cannot be visualized very well by MRI or internal tissue differences graduated. On T1-weighted images, the prostate, seminal vesicle, and the periprostatic venous plexus appear homogeneous, while the surrounding soft tissue (fat) has a high signal. T2-weighted images, however, allow a limited evaluation of the internal structures of the prostate and the prostatic capsule [5, 6]. The peripheral zone shows a high contrast intensity compared to the central and transitional zones. Prostate cancer usually is demonstrated by higher signal intensity in the peripheral zone [55, 64, 41].

A primary goal in dealing with prostate cancer is to detect extracapsular spread. However, the same diagnostic dilemma posed by CT scan is again encountered with MRI: the 5% or so of nodes that are positive are usually not enlarged or otherwise different from normal nodes, and thus escape detection. Moreover, with microscopic disease in the lymph nodes, the patient usually undergoes prostatectomy anyhow as most urologists do not want to deny the patient a potentially curable resection [26, 56]. Thus MRI examinations preoperatively usually do not change operative regimens unless they find grossly enlarged nodes that are histologically proven positive (after laparascopic nodectomy or fine needle biopsy).

New lymphographic contrast media may help in better imaging of pelvic nodes [7871]. Meanwhile, MRI should only be used in men with a high probability of extracapsular disease, based on Gleason score, PSA, and high T-stage. Another indication for MRI is a history of abdomino-perineal rectum amputation where the prostate is inaccessible to the palpating finger and TRUS.

10.8 Endorectal Coil MRI

High resolution of the prostate can be obtained by endorectal coil MRI. In comparison with external MRI, endorectal surface coils show a decreased sensitivity and an increased signal-to-noise ratio, so that a high sensitivity (80%–90%) for the detection of extracapsular disease – e.g. seminal vesicle infiltration – can be expected. Fast spin echo pulses and multicoil array techniques improve image quality [79, 80].

A limitation of the endorectal MRI seems to be that the resolution cannot be brought to less than about a 3-mm discrimination. Capsular irregularities and minor infiltration of the tumor into the seminal vesicles are not distinguishable [9, 38, 70]. D'Amico studied 235 patients preoperatively with transrectal MRI coils and found this imaging technique to be an independent prognosticator for seminal vesicle involvement ($p<0.0001$) and extracapsular penetration ($p = 0.0001$) [18]. Independent prognostic factors such as pretreatment

PSA, Gleason score, and number of positive biosies are available anyhow before radical prostatectomy [68].

It would be desirable to image T1c prostate cancer and distinguish it from stage T2. Endorectal MRI imaging provides a more comprehensive cross-sectional image than TRUS or CT scan [20, 58]. In a study of 124 patients before radical prostatectomy, MRI findings were compared to pathohistologic data. Capsular irregularities were seen in 3.2% and seminal vesicle involvement in 3.1%. Preoperative PSA values and endorectal MRI were both predictive for seminal vesicle infiltration ($p<0.05\%$), whereas the percentage of positive (multiple) biopsies was predictive for positive surgical margins and extracapsular extension ($p<0.005$) [57]. Thus endorectal MRI may not be very helpful in this subgroup of patients in augmenting the information already available before surgery.

10.9 Other Techniques

Electron paramagnetic resonance imaging relies on the emission of electrons instead of positrons, as with PET. The signal produced is of higher frequency and lower intensity than the positron signal. This feature could make it more advantageous than PET save for the necessity that the lesion be no more than 1–2 cm away from the receiver. Electrons cannot be recovered farther away. With an endorectal coil tissue hypoxia in the prostate could potentially be mapped with such an electron-emitting device [30, 75].

Dynamic contrast-enhanced MRI may have a place in the evaluation of microvessel density (tissue vascularity) and together with T2-weighted imaging, the state of oxygenation in the tumor tissue could be assessed [22, 40].

Nodal involvement can be detected by injecting small iron particles into the prostate and imaging with MR [33].

MRI has not yet entered the field of molecular imaging in prostate cancer. However, paramagnetic substances such as iron chelate or gadolinium bound to antibodies, receptors, or proteins (to be transferred intracellularly) could improve functional imaging. Cell-cycle-regulating proteins such as p-16 could be used for molecular imaging. P-53 and p-21, however, are not related to prognosis and thus are not suitable [7].

Positron spectra of the prostate could be used for imaging. Depletion of citrate relative to creatine and choline seems to be characteristic for cancer tissue [16]. Color encoded, these areas could demonstrate cancer tissues, as on a tumor map. A limitations of this technique could be poor spatial resolution, making judgment of capsular involvement or seminal vesicle infiltration difficult (both of these being strong prognosticators of metastatic disease) [34, 50].

10.10 Sentinel Lymph Node Scintigraphy

Standard lymphadenectomy is limited to obturator and external iliac lymph nodes. Internal iliac nodes are not routinely removed, and yet this area is the primary metastatic site [28, 92, 94]. Extended pelvic lymphadenectomy (including external iliac, internal iliac, common iliac, obturator, and presacral nodes) has been reported to demonstrate mostly internal iliac spread in 26% of patients despite negative obturator lymph nodes [35]. A high-risk group for atypical metastases was defined as patients with preoperative PSA >10 ng/ml, Gleason score >7, and stage >cT2a.

Lymph node staging can be perfomed by preoperative injection of Technetium-99m colloid into the prostate under TRUS guidance [93]. During surgery nodes are then scanned with a γ probe optimized for technetium. Our own results on histopathologic evaluation of nodes from an extended pelvic lymphadenectomy were compared to sentinel lymph node scintigraphy (SLNS). Gamma probe during operation revealed that 54/517 were sentinel lymph nodes, but only 11 of them (20.4%) revealed metastases. Nine patients who did not accumulate radioactivity had 12 additional metastases that were undetected by SLNS. Sensitivity and specificity of the γ probe procedure were 55% and 91.3%, respectively, whereas the positive and negative predictive values were 20.4% and 97.8%, respectively. Diagnostic accuracy of the extended pelvic lymph node disection was not increased by SLNS. Based on the high sensitivity and high negative predictive value, preoperative dynamic lymph node scintigraphy coupled with intraoperative SLNS could be useful in ruling out occult lymph node metastases in high-risk patients.

References

1. Aarnink RG, Beerlage HP, de la Rosette JJMCH, et al (1998) Transrectal ultrasound of the prostate: innovations and future applications. J Urol 159:1568–1579
2. Altman AL, Resnick MD (2001) Ultrasonographically guided biopsy of the prostate. J Ultrasound Med 20:159–167
3. American Urological Association (AUA) (2000) Prostate-specific antigen (PSA) best practice policy. Oncology (Huntingt) 14:267–286
4. Babaian RJ, Sayer J, Podoloff DA, et al (1994) Radioimmunoscintigraphy of pelvic lymph nodes with 111-indium-labeled monoclonal antibody CYT-356. J Urol 152:1952–1955
5. Bezzi M, Kressel HY, Allen KS, et al (1998) Prostatic carcinoma: staging with MR imaging at 1.5 T. Radiology 169:339–346
6. Biondetti PR, Lee JKT, Ling D, et al (1987) Clinical stage B prostate carcinoma: staging with MR imaging. Radiology 162:325–329
7. Bryant LH Jr, Brechbiel MW, Wu C, Bulte JW, Herynek V, Frank JA (1999) Synthesis and relaxometry of high-generation (G=5, 7, 9 and 10) PAMAM dendrimer-DOTA-gadolinium chelates. J Magn Reson Imaging 9:348–352
8. Catalona WJ (1995) Surgical management of prostate cancer. Cancer 75:1903–1906
9. Chelsky MJ, Schnall MD, Seidmon EJ, et al (1993) Use of endorectal surface coil magnetic resonance imaging for local staging of prostate cancer. J Urol 150:391–395
10. Cher ML, Bianco FJ, Lam JS, et al (1998) Limited role of radionucleotide bone scintigraphy in patients with prostate specific antigen elevations after radical prostatectomy. J Urol 160:1387–1391
11. Chodak GW, Keller P, Schoenberg HW (1989) Assessment of screening for prostate cancer using the digital rectal examination. J Urol 141:1136–1138
12. Chybowski FM, Keller JJ, Bergstrahl EJ, et al (1991) Predicting radionuclide bone scan findings in patients with newly diagnosed, untreated prostate cancer: prostate specific antigen is superior to all other clinical parameters. J Urol 145:313
13. Conrad S, Graefen M, Pichlmeier U, et al (1998) Systematic sextant biopsies improve preoperative prediction of pelvic lymph node metastases in patients with clinically localized prostatic carcinoma. J Urol 159:2023–2029
14. Cooner WH (1992) Rectal examination and ultrasonography in the diagnosis of prostate cancer. Prostate Suppl 4:3–10
15. Cooner WH, Mosley BR, Rutherford CL Jr, et al (1990) Prostate cancer detection in a clinical urological practice by ultrasonography, digital rectal examination and prostate specific antigen. J Urol 143:1146–1152
16. Costello LC, Franklin RB, Narayan P (1999) Citrate in the diagnosis of prostate cancer. Prostate 38:237–245
17. Crawford ED, Batuello JT, Snow P, et al (2000) The use of artificial intelligence technology to predict lymph node spread in men with clinically localized prostate carcinoma. Cancer 88: 2105–2109
18. D'Amico AV, Whittington R, Malkowicz SB, et al (1994) A multivariable analysis of clinical factors predicting for pathological features associated with local failure after radical prostatectomy for prostate cancer. Int J Radiat Oncol Biophys 30:293–302

19. D'Amico AV, Whittington R, Malkowicz SB, et al (1998) Biochemical outcome after radical prostatectomy, external beam radiation therapy of interstitial radiation therapy for clinically localized prostate cancer. JAMA 280:969–974
20. D'Amico AV, Schnall M, Whittington R, et al (1998) Endorectal coil magnetic resonance imaging identifies locally advanced prostate cancer in select patients with clinically localized disease. Urology 51:449–454
21. Djavan B, Waldert M, Zlotta A, Dobronski P, Seitz C, Remzi M, Borkowski A, Schulman C, Marberger M (2001) Safety and morbidity of first and repeat transrectal ultrasound guided prostate needle biopsies: results of a prospective European prostate cancer detection study. J Urol 166:856–860
22. Dresner MA, Rose GH, Rossmann PJ, et al (1998) Magnetic resonance elastography of the prostate [abstract]. Radiology 209:181
23. Eastham JA, Scardino PT (2000) Radical prostatectomy for clinical stage T1 and T2 prostate cancer. In: Vogelzang NJ, Scardino PT, Shipley WU, et al (eds) Comprehensive textbook of genitourinary oncology, 2nd ed. Lippincott Williams & Wilkins, Baltimore, pp 722–728
24. Flanigan RC, McKay TC, Olson M, et al (1996) Limited efficacy of preoperative computed tomography scanning for the evaluation of lymph node metastasis in patients before radical prostatectomy. Urology 48:428–432
25. Forsberg F, Merton DA, Liu JB, et al (1998) Clinical applications of ultrasound contrast agents. Ultrasonics 36:695–701
26. Frazier HA, Robertson JE, Paulson DF (1994) Does radical prostatectomy in the presence of positive pelvic lymph nodes enhance survival? World J Urol 12:308–312
27. Gann PH, Hennekens CH, Stampfer MJ (1995) A prospective evaluation of plasma prostate-specific antigen for detection of prostatic cancer. JAMA 273:289–294
28. Golimbu M, Morales P, Al-Askari S, et al (1979) Extended lymphadenectomy for prostatic cancer. J Urol 121:617–620 Another copyeditor has arranged the list alphabetically
29. Goto Y, Ohori M, Arakawa A, et al (1996) Distinguishing clinically important from unimportant prostate cancers before treatment: value of systematic biopsies. J Urol 156:1059–1063
30. Hahn P, Smith ICP, Leboldus L, et al (1997) The classification of benign and malignant human prostate tissue by multivariate analysis of H-I magnetic resonance spectra. Cancer Res 57: 3398–3401
31. Halpern DJ, Verkh I, Fosberg F, et al (2000) Initial experience with contrast enhanced sonography of the prostate. AJR Am J Roentgenol 174:1575–1580
32. Hara T, Kosaka N, Kishi H (1998) PET imaging of prostate cancer using carbon-11 choline. J Nucl Med 39:990–995
33. Harisinghani MG, Saini S, Weissleder R, et al (1999) MR lymphangiography using ultrasmall superparamagnetic iron oxide in patients with primary abdominal and pelvic malignancies: radiographic-pathologic correlation. AJR Am J Roentgenol 172:1347–1351
34. Hebden JC, Arridge SR, Delpy DT (1997) Optical imaging in medicine. I. Experimental techniques. Phys Med Biol 42:825–840
35. Hofmann R, Heidenreich A, Engelmann U (2000) Radical pelvic lymphadenectomy in clinically localized prostate cancer: high frequency of atypical metastases. J Urol 163:294
36. Hricak H, Doms GC, Jeffrey RB, et al (1987) Prostate carcinoma: staging by clinical assessment, CT, and MRI. Radiology 162:331–336
37. Huncharek M, Muscat J (1996) Serum prostate specific antigen as a predictor of staging abdominal/pelvic computed tomography in newly diagnosed prostate cancer. Abdom Imaging 21: 364–367
38. Husband JE, Padhani AR, MacVicar DA, et al (1998) Magnetic resonance imaging of prostate cancer: comparison of image quality using endorectal and pelvic phased array coils. Clin Radiol 53:673–681
39. Jacobsen SJ, Katusic SK, Bergstralh EJ, et al (1995) Incidence of prostate cancer diagnosis in the eras before and after serum prostate-specific antigen testing. JAMA 274:1445–1449
40. Jager GJ, Ruijter ETG, vander Kaa CA, et al (1997) Dynamic turboFLASH subtraction technique for contrast-enhanced MR imaging of the prostate: correlation with histopathologic results. Radiology 204:645–652
41. Jager GJ, Severns JL, Thornbury JR, et al (2000) Prostate cancer staging: should MR imaging be used? A decision analytic approach. Radiology 215:445–451
42. Johnstone PAS, Tarman G, Riffenburgh R, et al (1997) Yield of imaging and scintigraphy assessing bNED failure in prostate cancer patients. Urol Oncol 3:108–112
43. Kahn D, Williams RD, Manyak MJ, et al (1998) 111-Indium capromab pendetide in the evaluation of patients with residual or recurrent prostate cancer after radical prostatectomy. The ProstaScint Study Group. J Urol 159:2041; discussion 2046–2047
44. Kahn D, Williams RD, Haseman MK, et al (1998) Radioimmunoscintigraphy with In-111 labeled capromab pendetide predicts prostate cancer response to salvage radiotherapy after failed radical prostatectomy. J Clin Oncol 16:284–289
45. Kane DJ, Amling CL, Johnstone PAS, et al (1999) Limited value of bone scintigraphy and computed tomography in assessing biochemical failure after radical prostatectomy [abstract no. 667]. J Urol 161 [Suppl]:176

46. Kane RD, Paulson DF (1977) Radioisotope bone scanning characteristics of metastatic skeletal deposits of prostate adenocarcinoma. J Urol 117:618–621
47. Kattan MW, Cowen ME, Miles BJ (1997) A decision analysis for treatment of clinically localized prostate cancer. J Gen Intern Med 12:299–305
48. Kattan MW, Beck JR, Miles BJ (2000) Quantitative approaches to diagnostic testing and decision making in genitourinary oncology. In: Vogelzang NJ, Scardino PT, Shipley WU, et al (eds) Comprehensive textbook of genitourinary oncology, 2nd edn. Lippincott Williams & Wilkins, Philadelphia, pp 22–30
49. Kramer S, Gorich J, Gottfried HW, et al (1997) Sensitivity of computed tomography in detecting local recurrence of prostate carcinoma following radical prostatectomy. Br J Radiol 70: 995–999
50. Kuppusamy P, Chzan M, Vij K, et al (1994) Three-dimensional spectral spatial EPR imaging of free radicals in the heart: a technique for imaging tissue metabolims and oxygenation. Proc Natl Acad Sci USA 91:3388–3392
51. Landis SH, Murray T, Bolden S, et al (1999) Cancer statistics. Cancer J Clin 49:8–31
52. Lee F, Gray JM, McLeary RD, et al (1985) Transrectal ultrasound in the diagnosis of prostate cancer: location, echogenicity, histopathology and staging. Prostate 7:117–129
53. Lee N, Newhouse JH, Olsson CA, et al (1999) Which patients with newly diagnosed prostate cancer need a computed tomography scan of the abdomen and pelvis? An analysis based on 599 patients. Urology 54:490–494
54. Manyak MJ, Javitt MC (1998) The role of computerized tomography magnetic resonance imaging, bone scan and monoclonal antibody nuclear scan for prognosis prediction in prostate cancer. Semin Urol Oncol 16:145–152
55. May P, Truemann T, Dettmar P, et al (2001) Limited value of endorectal magnetic resonance imaging and transrectal ultrasonography in a staging of clinically localized prostatic cancer. BJU Int 1:66–69
56. Messing E, Manola J, Sarosdy M, et al (1999) Immediate hormonal therapy compared with observation after radical prostatectomy and pelvic lymphadenectomy in men with node positive prostate cancer. New Engl J Med 341:1781–1788
57. Moul JW, Kane J, Malkowicz S (2001) The role of imaging studies and molecular markers for selecting candidates for radical prostatectomy. Urol Clin North Am 28:459–472
58. Nakashima J, Imai Y, Tachibana M, et al (1997) Effects of endocrine therapy on the primary lesion in patients with prostate carcinoma as evaluated by endorectal magnetic resonance imaging. Cancer 80:237–241
59. Noldus J, Graefen M, Huland E, et al (1998) The value of the ratio of free-to-total prostate specific antigen for staging purposes in previously untreated prostate cancer. J Urol 159:2004–2007
60. Oesterling JE (1995) Using prostate specific antigen to eliminate unnecessary diagnostic tests: significant worldwide economic implications. Urology 46 [Suppl 3A]:26–33
61. Oesterling JE, Martin SK, Bergstrahl EJ, et al (1993) The use of prostate specific antigen in staging patients with newly diagnosed prostate cancer. JAMA 269:57–60
62. Ohori M, Egawa S, Shinohara K, et al (1994) Detection of microscopic extracapsular extension prior to radical prostatectomy for clinically localized prostate cancer. Br J Urol 74:72–79
63. Ophir J, Garni B, Kallel F, et al (2000) Elastography imaging. Ultrasound Med Biol 26 [Suppl]: 23-29
64. Padbani AR, Gapinski CJ, MacVicar DA, et al (2000) Dynamic contrast enhanced MRI of prostate cancer: correlation with morphology and tumour stage, histological grade and PSA. Clin Radiol 55:99–109
65. Pannek J, Subong EN, Jones KA, et al (1996) The role of free/total prostate-specific antigen ratio in the prediction of final pathologic stage for men with clinically localized prostate cancer. Urology 48:51–54
66. Partin AW, Kattan MW, Subong EN, et al (1997) Combination of prostate-specific antigen, clinical stage, and Gleason score to predict pathological stage of localized prostate cancer. A multi-institutional update [see comments] (published erratum appears in JAMA (1997) 278:118). JAMA 277:1445–1451
67. Partin AW, Yoo J, Carter HB, et al (1999) The use of prostate specific antigen, clinical stage and Gleason score to predict pathological stage in men with localized prostate cancer. J Urol 150: 110–114
68. Perotti M, Kaufman RP, Jennings TA, et al (1996) Endorectal coil magnetic resonance imaging in clinically localized prostate cancer: is it accurate? J Urol 156:106–109
69. Platt JF, Bree RI, Schwab RE (1987) accuracy of CT in the staging of carcinoma of the prostate. AJR Am J Roentgenol 149:315–318
70. Pollack HM, Banner MP (1994) Diagnostic uroradiology. In: Hanno PM, Wein AJ (eds) Clinical manual of urology, 2nd edn. McGraw Hill, New York, pp 89–136
71. Pound CR, Partin AW, Epstein JI, et al (1997) Prostate-specific antigen after anatomic retropubic prostatectomy. Patterns of recurrence and cancer control. Urol Clin North Am 24:395–406
72. Pound CR, Partin AW, Eisenberger MA, et al (1999) Natural history of progression after PSA elevation following radical prostatectomy. JAMA 281:1591–1597

73. Reitbergen JBW, Hoedemaeker RF, Boeken Kruger AE, et al (1999) The changing pattern of prostate cancer at the time of diagnosis: characteristics of screen detected prostate cancer in a population based screening study. J Urol 161:1192–1198
74. PT, Weaver R, Hudson MA (1992) Early detection of prostate cancer. Hum Pathol 23:211–222
75. Scheidler J, Hricak H, Vigneron DB, et al (1999) Prostate cancer: localization with three-dimensional proton MR spectroscopic imaging: clinicopathologic study. Radiology 213:473–480
76. Scher HI, Heller (2000) Clinical states in prostate cancer: toward a dynamic model of disease progression. Urology 55:323–327
77. Scher HI, Isaacs JT, Zelefsky MJ, et al (2000) Prostate cancer. In: Abeloff MD, Armitage JO, Lichter AS, et al (eds) Clinical oncology, 2nd edn. Churchill Livingstone, New York, pp 1823–1835
78. Schiebler ML, Schnall MD, Pollack HM, et al (1993) Current role of MR imaging in the staging of adenocarcinoma of the prostate. Radiology 189:339–352
79. Schnall MD, Imai Y, Tomaszewski JE, et al (1991) Prostate cancer: local staging with endorectal surface coil MR imaging. Radiology 178:797–802
80. Schnall MD, Connick T, Hayes CE, et al (1992) MR imaging of the pelvis with an endorectal-external multicoil array. J Magn Reson Imaging 2:229–232
81. Seltzer MA, Barbaric Z, Belldegrun A, et al (1999) Comparison of helical computed tomography, positron emission tomography and monoclonal antibody scans for evaluation of lymph node metastases in patients with prostate specific antigen relapse after treatment for localized prostate cancer. J Urol 162:1322–1328
82. Shinohara K, Wheeler TM, Scardino PT (1989) The appearance of prostate cancer on transrectal ultrasonography: correlation of imaging and pathological examinations. J Urol 142:76–82
83. Soloway MS, Obek C (2000) Periprostatic local anaesthetic before ultrasound guided prostatic biopsy. J Urol 163:172–173
84. Southwick PC, Catalona WJ, Partin AW, et al (1999) Prediction of post-radical prostatectomy pathological outcome for stage T1c prostate cancer with percent free prostate specific antigen: A prospective multicenter clinical trial. J Urol 162:1346–1351
85. Stamey TA, Yang N, Hay AR, et al (1987) Prostate-specific antigen as a serum marker for adenocarcinoma of the prostate. N Engl J Med 317:909–916
86. Stanford JL, Stephenson RA, Coyle LM, et al (1999) Prostate Cancer trends 1973–1995, NIH Pub. No. 99–4543 edn. SEER Program. National Cancer Institute, Bethesda
87. Svatec D, Thompson IM (1998) PSA screening – current controversy. Ann Oncol 9:1283–1288
88. Tarkan T, Turkeri L, Biren T, et al (1996) The effectiveness of imaging modalities in clinical staging of localized prostate carcinoma. Int Urol Nephrol 28:773–779
89. Terris MK, McNeal JE, Freiha PS, et al (1993) Efficacy of transrectal ultrasound-guided seminal vesicle biopsies in the detection of seminal vesicle invasion by prostate cancer. J Urol 149:1035–1039
90. Thompson IM, Middleton RG, Optenberg SA, et al (1999) Have complication rates decreased after treatment for localized prostate cancer? J Urol 162:107–112
91. Vijayakumar VVijayakumar S, Quadri SF, et al (1994) Can prostate-specific antigen levels predict bone scan evidence of metastases in newly diagnosed prostate cancer? Am J Clin Oncol 17:432–436
92. Walsh PC (1980) Radical prostatectomy for the treatment of localized prostate carcinoma. Urol Clin North Am 7:583–589
93. Wawroschek F, Vogt H, Weckermann D, Wagner T, Harzmann R (1999) The sentinel lymph node concept in prostate cancer – first results of gamma probe-guided sentinel lymph node identification. Eur Urol 36:595–600
94. Zincke H, Utz DC, Myers RP, et al (1982) Bilateral pelvic lymphadenectomy and radical retropubic prostatectomy for adenocarcinoma of the prostate with regional lymph node involvement. Urology 19:238–247

11 Extended Pelvic Lymphadenectomy in Clinically Localized Prostate Cancer: High Frequency of Lymph Node Metastases

A. Heidenreich, Z. Varga, R. v. Knobloch, D. Brandt, R. Hofmann

11.1 Introduction

Systemic dissection of all lymph nodes located in the draining region of the primary tumor-bearing organ is a concept adopted in surgery of most malignant tumors as it allows for a better staging as well as reduction of regional recurrence rates. In patients with clinically organ-confined prostate cancer (PCA), standard pelvic lymphadenectomy including the external iliac artery and the obturator fossa is currently being performed if the preoperative prostate-specific antigen (PSA) serum level exceeds 10 ng/ml, biopsy Gleason score is greater than 7, and clinical stage is ≥2a [1–5]. The incidence of lymph node metastases found by pelvic lymphadenectomy is around 10% either as part of a radical prostatectomy or as part of pretreatment staging preceeding perineal prostatectomy [1–5]. Besides diagnostic information, lymphadenectomy in pN1 disease might be associated with prolonged progression-free periods and survival rates, as demonstrated in recent retrospective studies [6–8].

However, considering anatomical and lymphographic studies, the adequate extent of lymphadenectomy, and thereby its prognostic value in prostate cancer, is still under debate [9]. The prostate lymphatics drain into the periprostatic subcapsular network from which three groups of ducts originate: the ascending duct from the cranial gland draining into the external iliac nodes, the lateral duct running to the hypogastric nodes, and the posterior duct draining from the caudal gland to the subaortic sacral nodes of the promontory. The levels of nodal drainage are segregated into the hypogastric (primary), obturator (secondary), external iliac (tertiary), and presacral (quarternary) lymphatics. Based on these anatomical and lymphographic studies, it becomes evident that standard pelvic lymphadenectomy will miss primary and quarternary lymphatics of the prostate, thereby reducing the opportunity for adequate regional staging. This hypothesis is further substantiated by systemic recurrence rates of 6%–16% in pT1/2 and pT3a PCA, respectively, suggesting the presence of occult lymph node disease at time of ascending retropubic prostatectomy (RRP) [10].

Based on the discrepancies between anatomical considerations and clinical practice, we analyzed the incidence of lymph node metastases in clinically localized PCA, performing an anatomically extended regional lymphadectomy in 103 consecutive patients as compared to standard pelvic lymphadenectomy in 100 consecutive patients. Furthermore, we evaluated the clinical utility of various prognostic models in predicting low risk groups for metastatic lymph node disease which have been developed on the basis of standard pelvic lymphadenectomy (pLA) [1–5]. Furthermore, the clinical utility of prostatic lymphoscintigraphy to identify sentinel lymph nodes was tested in a subset of patients. We describe the technique, results, and the clinical significance of extended pLA (epLA) in the management of clinically localized PCA.

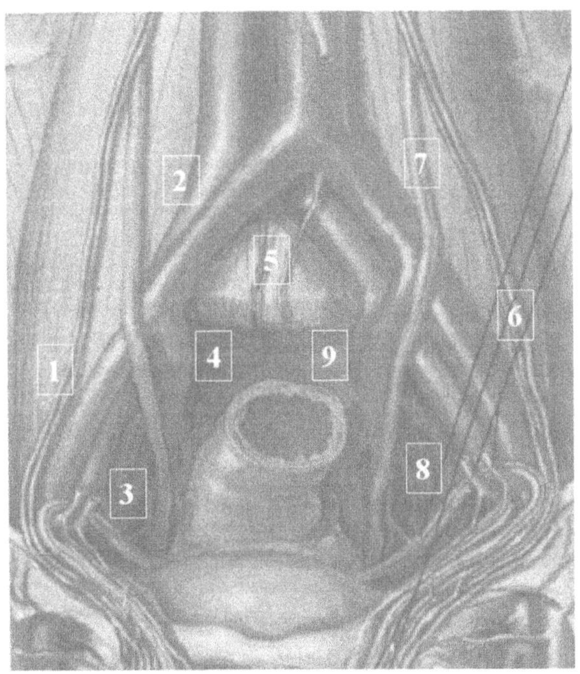

Fig. 11.1. Distribution and localization of the nine selective fields for extended pelvic lymphadenectomy, including external iliac nodes (*1*), common iliac nodes (*2*), obturator fossa nodes (*3*), and internal iliac nodes (*4*) on the right; presacral lymph nodes (*5*) and external iliac nodes (*6*), common iliac nodes (*7*), obturator fossa nodes (*8*) and internal iliac nodes (*9*) on the left

11.2 Patients and Methods

Between January 1999 and December 2000, 103 consecutive patients (group 1) with histologically proven, clinically localized PCA underwent RRP as described by Walsh [15] and epLA comprising nine distinct fields of dissection (Fig. 11.1).

The number of dissected lymph nodes, frequency of lymph node metastases, operating time, and associated complications were compared with a series of 100 consecutive patients undergoing RRP and standard pLA (group 2).

Furthermore, pathohistological and clinical parameters such as cT-stage (Whitmore-Jewett), preoperative PSA serum concentration (monoclonal assay, Tandem R, Hybritech), and preoperative biopsy Gleason sum were correlated with the presence and the number of positive lymph nodes in order to calculate groups at low versus high risk for the presence of occult lymph node disease at time of surgery.

Assessment of the clinical tumor stage was performed by digital rectal examination (DRE) and transrectal ultrasound (TRUS) using a 7.5-MHz scanner (Kretz GmbH, Gelsenkirchen, Germany). All patients with clinical stage 4 PCA were excluded from RRP and underwent radiation therapy or androgen deprivation. Preoperatively, patients underwent pelvic CT scans if serum PSA levels were higher than 40 ng/ml; all patients underwent bone scintigraphy if serum PSA levels exceeded 20 ng/ml.

11.2.1 Surgical Technique

EpLA was performed through an open extraperitoneal approach via a lower abdominal midline incision before RRP. The boundaries of the bilateral pelvic lymph node dissection were the aortic bifurcation cranially, the circumflex iliac vein and Cooper's ligament caudally, the external iliac vein laterally, and the ureter medially. Lymph nodes of each of the nine dissection fields were removed en bloc and subjected to histological examination. Frozen sections were only done when lymph nodes appeared grossly suspicious. If the cases dealt with pN1 disease, RRP was continued and patients received immediate adjuvant androgen deprivation therapy postoperatively, applying luteinizing hormone-releasing hormone (LHRH) analogues or performing subcapsular orchiectomy.

Standard pLA was performed through an open approach via a lower abdominal midline incision before RRP. Lymph nodes of the obturator fossa and the external iliac group were dissected en bloc and subjected to histological examination.

For histopathological analysis each of the lymph nodes was assessed for metastasis after hematoxylin and eosin (H&E) staining; immunohistochemical staining was performed only in case of negative H&E findings.

11.2.2 Risk Group Assessment and Statistical Analysis

To define a group of patients being at low risk for lymph node metastases of PCA, preoperative PSA values obtained at least 4 weeks after transrectal needle biopsy or transurethral resection of the prostate, histological grade according to the Gleason scoring system, and clinical tumor stage according to the Whithmore-Jewett classification were analyzed and correlated with the presence or absence of lymph node metastases. None of the patients received neoadjuvant hormonal therapy prior to the evaluation of serum PSA levels or prior to RRP.

Following the prospective documentation of clinical, surgical, and pathohistological data, the number of resected and metastatic lymph nodes was analyzed and correlated to various clinical and pathohistological factors. Statistical significance ($p<0.05$) was determined with the nonparametric analysis of variance according to Kruskal-Wallis.

Univariate and multivariate logistic regression models were used to predict the probability of positive pelvic lymph nodes as a function of patient age, prostate volume, PSA density, preoperative PSA, primary biopsy Gleason sum, and local clinical stage. For multivariate analysis all variables that were significant in univariate analysis ($p<0.05$) were considered. All models were fit using the LOGISTIC procedure of the SAS program.

Sensitivity and specificity were calculated with all theoretically possible cutoff scores as shown by a receiver operating characteristic analysis curve [12].

To verify our results, we compared the distribution of preoperative PSA levels and Gleason sum between those patients being classified as low risk for developing lymph node metastases who had lymph node metastases (false negatives) and those who did not (true negatives).

11.2.3 Technique of Lymphoscintigraphy

Dynamic lymphoscintigraphy was carried out preoperatively in 26 consecutive patients. On the day of surgery, a total volume of 2 ml Technetium-99m nanocolloid (Nancoll, Sorin Co., Italy) was applied by one or two injections into each lobe under transrectal sonographic guidance, making up a total activity of 100 MBq. At approximately 15 min and again at 2 h following injection, scintigraphies in the anteroposterior and dorsal projections were obtained with the prostate being covered during the procedure (Figs. 11.2, 11.3).

In all cases, epLA was performed as described using a γ-probe optimized for technetium as described by Wawroschek et al. [17] (C-trak; Car-Wise Medical Products, Morgan Hill, CA). The prostate was covered by a tungsten plate in order to block radiation derived from the prostate and interfering with the

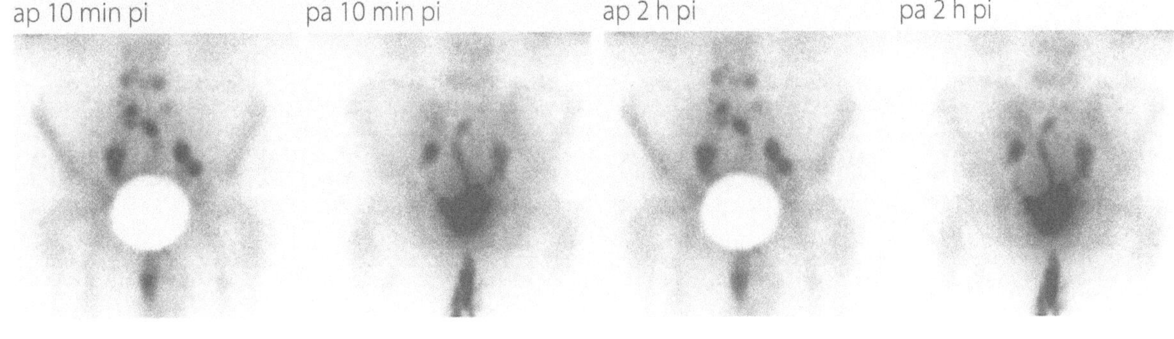

Fig. 11.2. Preoperative lymphoscintigraphy showing two radiating lymph nodes in the external iliac and the common iliac lymph node group; both lymph nodes were identified as harboring metastases from prostate cancer

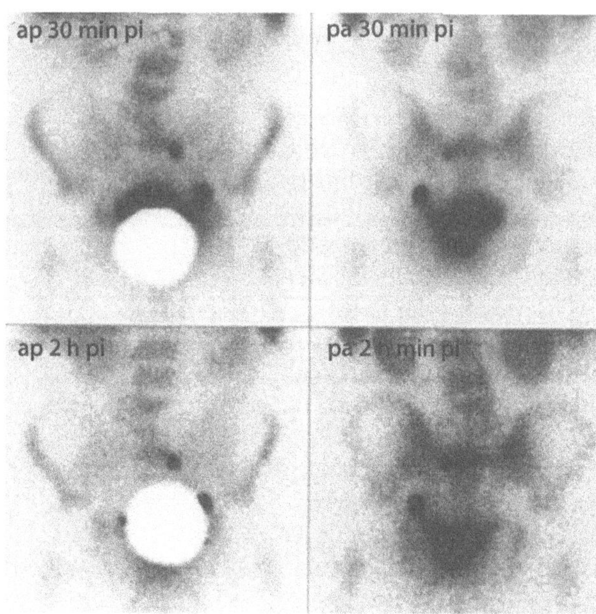

Fig. 11.3.
Preoperative lymphoscintigraphy 2 h post injectionem demonstrating multiple radiating lymph nodes in the external iliac, common iliac and internal iliac lymph nodes as well as in the presacral area. Histopathology revelaed lymph node metastases in the internal and common iliac region

accurate measurements of nodal activity. Using the γ-probe, those lymph nodes detected by preoperative lymphoscintigraphy or measurable radiation were identified and removed, followed by the dissection of the remaining lymphatic tissue of the designated dissection fields.

For histopathological analysis, each of the identified radiating lymph nodes was assessed for metastasis after H&E statining; immunohistochemical staining was performed only if H&E findings were negative.

11.3 Results

Mean age at time of RRP was 61.8 (51–71) years in group 1 and 63.5 (49–72) years in group 2 (n.s.). There was no significant difference in preoperative serum PSA concentrations, clinical stage, or preoperative biopsy Gleason score between group 1 and group 2 (Table 11.1). The mean follow-up of all patients was 10.5 (1–20) months.

The mean number of dissected lymph nodes was 28 (21–48) in group 1 and 11 (6–19) in group 2 ($p<0.01$). Operating time for RRP including epLA and pLA, respectively, was 179 (140–235) min and 125 (85–150) min, respectively ($p<0.03$).

The incidence of lymph node metastases was 26.2% (27/103) in group 1 and 12% in group 2 ($p<0.03$). In group 1, 15 patients (55.5%) demonstrated a single metastasis, nine patients (36%) exhibited two positive and one patient (4%) had three positive lymph nodes (Fig. 11.4); 42% of all lymph node metastases were located outside the regions of standard pelvic LA, which includes external iliac and obturator nodes only (Table 11.2, Fig. 11.3). The preoperative PSA range for these patients was 9.5–180 ng/ml, with a mean PSA of 59.9 ng/ml (Tables 11.1, 11.3). The range for Gleason sum was from 4 to 10, with a mean Gleason sum of 6.2 (Tables 11.1, 11.3). The clinical T stage was from cT1a to cT4a, with a mean cT-stage of 6.4 according to a developed scoring system (Table 11.1).

Table 11.1. Characteristics of patients undergoing extended pelvic lymphadenectomy (epLA) and standard pelvic lymphadenectomy (pLA)

	epLA	pLA
Number of patients	103	100
Mean age (years)	61.8 (51–71)	63.5 (49–72)
Preop. PSA (ng/ml)	15.9 (1.2–129)	14.9 (1.6–109)
Prostate weight	36.4 (22–195) g	32.5 (15–235)g
Dissected lymph nodes (*n*)	28 (21–42)	11 (6–19)
Surgical time (min)	179 (140–235)	125 (85–150)

PSA, prostate-specific antigen.

11.3.2 Intraoperative Complications

In two of 203 patients (0.9%) a rectal perforation occurred which was closed with a two-layer closing suture and by temporary colostomy being relocated 3 months later. Ureteric lesions, vessel injuries, or damage to the obturator nerve were observed in twocases (0.9%).

The mean intraoperative estimated blood loss was 650 (200–1950) ml in group 1 and 590 ml (150 – 2100) in group 2; in 85 patients (45.9%) the mean estimated blood loss was <500 ml (Table 11.3).

Postoperative complications developed in 9/103 patients (8.7%) of group 1 and in nine patients (9%) of group 2 (Table 11.3); in nine patients of each group a pelvic lymphocele was detected sonographically; percutaneous puncture and drainage was required in one patient in each group.

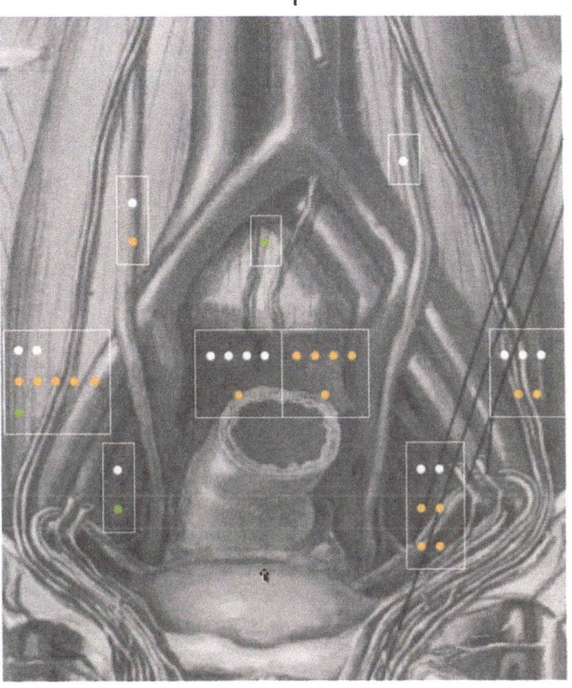

Fig. 11.4. Distribution and localization of lymph node metastases in patients with one positive (*white dot*), two positive (*orange dot*) and three positive (*green dot*) lymph nodes

11.3.3 Lymphoscintigraphy

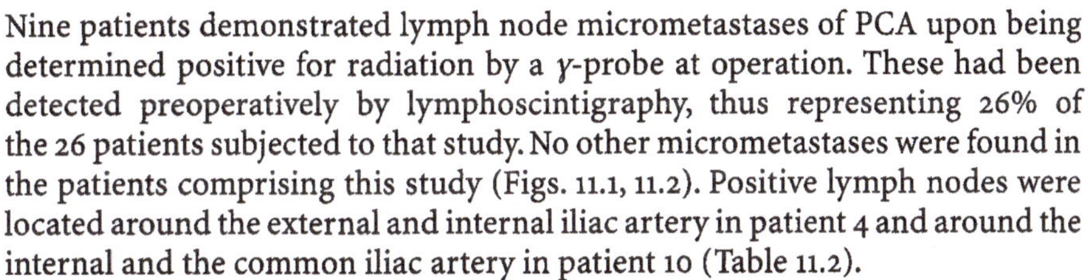

Nine patients demonstrated lymph node micrometastases of PCA upon being determined positive for radiation by a γ-probe at operation. These had been detected preoperatively by lymphoscintigraphy, thus representing 26% of the 26 patients subjected to that study. No other micrometastases were found in the patients comprising this study (Figs. 11.1, 11.2). Positive lymph nodes were located around the external and internal iliac artery in patient 4 and around the internal and the common iliac artery in patient 10 (Table 11.2).

In another patient, dynamic lymphoscintigraphy demonstrated multiple positive lymph nodes around the common and internal iliac artery preoperatively and confirmed at surgery by the use of the γ-probe. Pathohistology revealed multiple metastases from a non-Hodgkin's lymphoma in the radiating lymph nodes, all others being tumor free. Because of the unexpected histology, the patient was excluded from our study.

11.3.4 Risk Group Assessment

Based on the ROC analysis, PSA and Gleason cutoffs were defined as <10.6 ng/ml and ≤6, respectively, to define a low risk group for the development of lymph node metastases.

Of the 203 patients included in our study, 139 (68.5%) were classified as low risk for developing lymph node disease by using only PSA and Gleason sum. Of those patients in the low risk group, four patients had lymph node metastases giving a false-negative rate of 2.8%.

Adding the clinical stage score to the analysis did not improve the predictive value of our data.

Based on the preoperative serum PSA concentrations, Gleason sum, and clinical stage it was not possible to define a group of patients at high risk for the development of lymph node metastases (Fig. 11.5a–c). Over one fifth (22.1%) of the patients with PSA levels >10.5 ng/ml, 48.9% of the patients with Gleason sum of >6, and 66% of the patients with cT stage >cT2b demonstrated lymph node

Patient	PSA (ng/ml)	Gleason sum	pT stage	SM status	Fields with N+	Positive lymph nodes (n)
1	14.4	8	2b	Negative	1	1
2	11.0	8	3b	Negative	1,8	2
3	27.1	7	3b	Positive[a]	1, 3, 5	3
4	42.5	7	3c	Positive[a]	1, 9	3
5	16.1	5	3c	Negative	1, 6	2
6	41.0	6	3b	Negative	8	2
7	47.9	6	3b	Negative	3, 6	2
8	12.5	6	2c	Negative	8	1
9	9.5	5	2b	Negative	2	1
10	13.6	6	3b	Negative	2, 4	2
11	15.4	7	3c	Negative	8, 9	2
12	12.8	6	2b	Negative	6	1
13	18.7	7	3b	Negative	1, 9	2
14	18.3	7	3b	Negative	6	1
15	86.7	8	3a	Pos[b]	10[c]	1
16	15.1	8	3b	Negative	8, 9	2
17	14.5	6	3a	Negative	3	1
18	25.1	6	3b	Pos[a]	8, 9	2
19	18.0	9	3b	Pos[a]	4	1
20	40.0	7	3b	Negative	7	1
21	51.1	8	3b	Negative	4	1
22	17.5	7	3b	Negative	4	1
23	87.1	6	4	Negative	4	1
24	83.6	7	3b	Negative	1, 4	2
25	45.6	7	2b	Negative	1	1
26	27.6	7	3b	Negative	9	1

PSA, prostate-specific antigen; SM, surgical margins.
[a] Positive urethral margins.
[b] Positive vesicle margins.
[c] Atypical lymph node metastasis located at the dorsal venous plexus.

metastases. Sensitivity and specificity, however,were too low to adequately define prognostic parameters for positive lymph node involvement. Nevertheless, it may be worth noting that 26 of 27 patients (96.3%) with positive lymph nodes exhibited a preoperative PSA >10.5 ng/ml and biopsy Gleason sum ≥ 7.

11.3.5 Therapeutic Benefit of epLA

In order to analyze the potential therapeutic benefit of epLA combined with immediate androgen deprivation therapy in case of positive lymph node dis-

Table 11.3. Intra- and postoperative complications following extended pelvic lymphadenectomy (epLA) and pLA

	epLA	pLA
Number of patients	103	100
Blood loss, ml	650 (200–1950)	590 (150–2100)
Blood loss <500 ml	51 (53.7%)	48 (48%)
Rectal lesion	1 (1.1%)	1 (1%)
Ureteric lesion	1	0
Obturator lesion	1 (1.1%)	2 (2%)
Others	6 (7.1%)	6 (6%)
DVT	4 (4.2%)	6 (6%)
Pulmonary embolus	2 (2.1%)	2 (2%)
Pneumonia	2 (1.2%)	2 (2%)
Myocardial infarction	1 (0.6%)	2 (2%)
Lymphocele	9 (10.6%)	9 (9%)
Others	9 (10.6%)	6 (6%)

DVT, deep venous thrombosis.

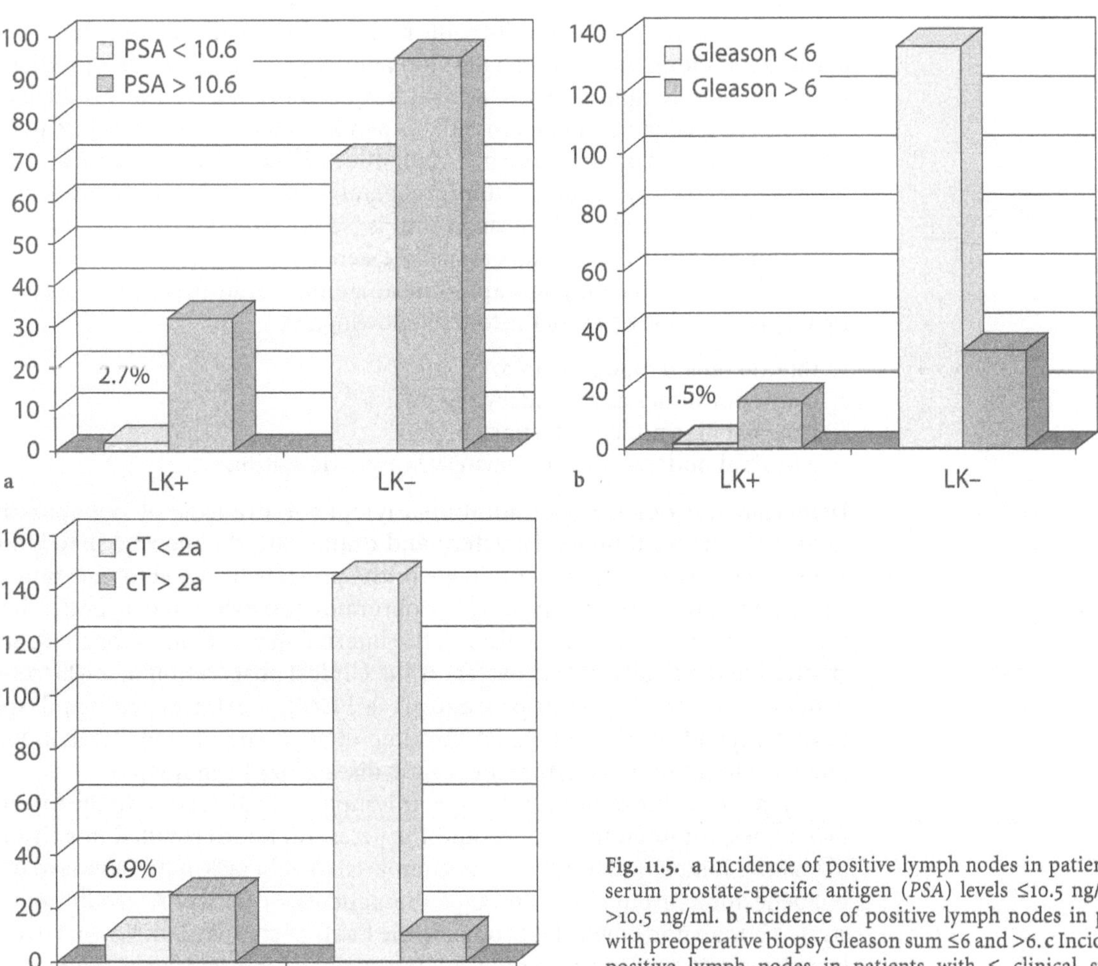

Fig. 11.5. **a** Incidence of positive lymph nodes in patients with serum prostate-specific antigen (*PSA*) levels ≤10.5 ng/ml and >10.5 ng/ml. **b** Incidence of positive lymph nodes in patients with preoperative biopsy Gleason sum ≤6 and >6. **c** Incidence of positive lymph nodes in patients with ≤ clinical stage 2a prostate cancer and >cT2a prostate cancer

ease, we retrospectively evaluated our data of 790 patients having undergone RRP since 1990. Eighty-four patients (10.6%) demonstrated lymph node metastases at time of RRP and underwent subcapsular orchiectomy (n=72) or medical castration (n=12). After a mean follow-up of 73.3 (2–130) months, 88% of the patients are still alive with 73.3% being without evidence of biochemical failure; the cancer-specific survival is 81%.

11.4 Discussion

The detection of micrometastases in PCA is of clinical importance since it has been demonstrated in earlier series that radical prostatectomy might result in prolonged survival for patients with less than three metastatic nodes [6, 7]. In addition, systematic dissection of all lymph nodes in the primary and secondary draining regions of PCA would be of clinical importance, for then a much better likelihood would be realized for detecting all metastatic lesions. With such enhanced knowledge a more informed consideration of adjuvant therapy is of course made possible. Messing et al. [8] and Zincke et al. [6] have demonstrated increased survival when immediate androgen deprivation follows RRP in patients with lymph node-positive disease as compared to patients who are treated when PSA progression occurs, or to patients without treatment.

In PCA, the clinical utility of regional lymphadenectomy has been debated for a long time, and the development of prognostic models predicting the absence of lymph node metastases has been pressed forward in order to find the criteria upon which omission of pelvic LA ican be based[1–5]. Current recommendations are to perform lymph node dissection of the obturator and external iliac artery regions if the preoperative serum PSA concentration is >10.5 ng/ml and the biopsy Gleason sum is >6 [5]. However, the primary lymphatic drainage of the prostate actually extends far beyond these regions. As revealed by prostatic lymphography and anatomical studies [9, 18], the prostate mainly drains along four paths to the following:

1. Internal iliac group as primary region
2. Obturator nodes as secondary region
3. External iliac nodes as tertiary region
4. Presacral nodes as the quarternary lymphatic station

DelRegato [13] describes an additional lymphatic drainage of the apex that follows the internal pudendal artery and drains into the internal iliac lymph nodes. The actual lymphatic drainage of the prostate brings into question the current practice of dissecting only the obturator and external iliac nodes, leaving the primary lymphatic station in the internal iliac region untouched. Substantiating the reality of this neglect is the clinical observation of a 6% to 16% systemic recurrence rate in pT2 and pT3a PCA [10, 11], respectively, despite negative lymph node findings at the time of RRP and standard pelvic lymphadenectomy, indicating that metastatic disease has been missed.

Extending the boundaries of pelvic lymph node dissection to the internal iliac nodes, common iliac nodes, and the presacral nodes resulted in a finding of positive lymph nodes in 25.3%, as compared to only 14% in the standard lymphadenectomy group. Two thirds of the patients in the epLA group demonstrated lymph node metastases outside the fields of standard pLA, which would have been left untreated if only the lesser dissection had been done. Based on the data of our series, epLA appears to be beneficial in patients with preoperative serum PSA concentrations >10.5 ng/ml, a Gleason sum >6, and a clinical stage >cT2a. In patients exhibiting a preoperative serum PSA level of <10.5 ng/ml, a Gleason sum <6, and a cT-stage <cT2, lymph node metastases are found in only 2.4% and epLA can be omitted.

The data of Frazier et al. [7] and Zincke et al. [6] indicate that, besides a mere diagnostic benefit, 21 of 24 (87.5%%) patients had two or fewer positive lymph nodes, resulting in a potential therapeutic benefit.

The concept of extended pelvic LA is not new and was described by a number of authors in the pre-PSA era. Golimbu et al. [18] demonstrated an 80% frequency of positive lymph nodes in 30 patients with more than 80% of the node-positive patients having metastatic nodes in the presacral region. Nicholson et al. [19] found 13% of 47 patients with clinically localized PCA to be lymph node positive with two thirds of the patients with positive nodes exhibiting metastases outside the fields of pLA. In another study of 93 consecutive patients with clinically localized PCA, Schubert et al. [20] performed an extended pelvic LA similar to our technique and removed a mean of 25 lymph nodes per patient. Thirty-eight percent of the patients had lymph node metastases with approximately 50% of the node-positive individuals exhibiting positive nodes outside the external iliac and obturator fossa fields. Similar observations were reported by Fujioka et al. [21], who found a 48% incidence of lymph node metastases in 31 patients, finding 100% of the node-positive patients with positive nodes in the internal iliac group, 67% with metastases in the external iliac group, and 47% with metastases in the common iliac group. The authors reported that they always included the internal iliac group when staging lymphadenectomy for PCA was performed These data are, however, vague in comparison with ours, since a high percentage of those patients of the pre-PSA era presented with locally advanced PCA.

Our results confirm the data of those studies from the pre-PSA era, and we now insist that the primary and secondary lymphatics of the prostate – that is, the internal iliac group, external iliac group, and the obturator fossa group – always be included for staging lymphadenectomy in order not to miss or leave lymph node metastases of PCA. Considering our data, it appears unnecessary to dissect the quarternary lymphatics also, since only three of 95 patients (3.1%) exhibited lymph node metastases in the presacral region and the common iliac group. Only one patient had a single metastasis in the external iliac group only (no other lymph node regions showing metastases); in all other patients lymphonodular disease was associated with metastases in the primary and secondary drainage stations. Therefore, the diagnostic benefit of lymphadenectomy including the presacral region would be only 1.2%. Our recommendations are in accordance with Brendler et al. [23], O'Donoghue et al. [24], and Zincke et al. [6] who demonstrated the identical diagnostic accuracy of a pelvic staging lymphadenectomy limited to the internal iliac and external iliac group and the obturator fossa as compared to an extended pelvic LA including the external group.

Arguments against performing routine epLA for staging purposes are decreasing incidence of lymph node metastasis in general, extensive operating time, more frequent complications, and financial considerations. The first argument can be dealt with by excluding patients at low risk for lymph node metastasis from staging LA based on clinical prognosticators to be discussed later. Operating roomtime was only 54 min longer in the RRP and epLA group than in the RRP and pLA group, and we consider this time not to be a significant extension of surgery.

Complications attributable to staging lymphadenectomy did not differ between the two groups, occurring in 9% of all patients; none of the complications were considered major, none prolonging the hospital stay more than 2 days. These data are in accordance with a recent study of Dillioglugil et al. [25] who demonstrated that approximately 7% of all complications developing after RRP are attributable solely to staging pelvic lymphadenectomy and mainly consist of symptomatic lymphocele, prolonged lymphatic drainage, and lower extremity edema. Thus, our personal experience and belief in the diagnostic benefit of the procedure leads us not to share in skepticism of epLA.

The incidence of lymph node metastases from PCA found by pLA is reported to be 10% or less; therefore, if that figure is to be taken as true, 90% of patients would undergo unnecessary pelvic lymphadenectomy and be exposed to potential morbidities associated with epLA. Prognosticators for identifying those patients with PCA who are at low risk for lymph node metastases by using clinical parameters that are currently obtained in the preoperative evaluation, such serum PSA levels, clinical stage, and Gleason sum, would be of tremendous clinical value. Partin et al. [3] developed nomograms for the prediction of lymph node involvement and found the risk to be less than 2% if the clinical stage was ≤cT2a, the preoperative PSA serum level was <10.1 ng/ml, and the Gleason sum was ≤6. Bishoff et al. [2] compared the preoperative parameters PSA, biopsy Gleason sum, and clinical stage to the risk of positive pelvic lymph nodes in 481 men with clinically localized PCA. Using logistic regression analysis, the authors demonstrated that up to 50% of the staging lymphadenectomies could have been omitted without any diagnostic disadvantage. Retrospective analysis of 1632 patients with localized PCA who underwent bilateral pLA identified the combination of preoperative PSA, biopsy Gleason sum, and clinical stage that would best estimate the probability of lymph node involvement. Using a cutoff point of less than 3% as an acceptable false-negative rate, Bluestein et al. [1] reported that 61% of patients with clinical stage cT1a to cT2b and 29% of the patients with cT1a to cT2c could have been spared pLA. Recently, Crawford et al. [5] employed artificial intelligence technology to predict lymph node spread in clinically localized PCA using a large data base of 4133 patients. Their decision-tree protocol derived cutoff values of ≤6 for biopsy Gleason sum, ≤10.6 ng/ml serum PSA level, and ≤cT2a clinical stage to identify the group of patients at low risk for lymph node metastases, with a false-negative rate <1%.

Since all prognostic models rely for their decision on results of standard pelvic lymphadenectomy, not including the primary lymphatic drainage of the prostate, the goal of our study was to assess the clinical utility of these models using pathohistological data of epLA. Even on the basis of our limited patient number, a low-risk group for positive lymph node disease could be defined with a false-negative rate of 2.7%, using preoperative serum PSA levels of less than 10.6 ng/ml, a biopsy Gleason sum of <6, and a clinical stage of ≤ cT 2a. However, it was not possible to define a high-risk group for lymph node involvement based on preoperative preclinical parameters: only 30 of 126 patients (23.8%) with preoperative serum PSA levels >10.6 ng/ml demonstrated lymph node metastases, 48.9% of the patients with a Gleason sum >6 were lymph node positive, and 66% of the patients with a clinical stage >cT2b had lymph node metastases. Although there was an increased risk for lymph node involvement, these clinical data were not able to provide criteria for identifying patients with positive lymph node disease.

Preoperative lymphoscintigraphy combined with intraoperative γ-probe evaluation of sentinel lymph nodes might be helpful in addition to the assessment of preoperative clinical parameters for detecting lymph node involvement. In eight patients studied by this method, lymphonodular micrometastases were accurately detected in all three patients who harbored metastases, and all five not exhibiting radioactive storage were lymph node negative. Based on our positive experience and the data recently reported by Wawroschek et al. [17], we have started a prospective evaluation of the clinical utility of lymphoscintigraphy in categorizing patients with clinically localized PCA at high or at low risk for lymph node metastases.

Besides being simply a diagnostic improvement, epLA might also have an impact on progression-free survival and survival rates in patients with N1 disease if immediate androgen blockade is performed. As demonstrated in our series, patients treated with immediate antiandrogen therapy following RRP have an excellent overall and cancer-specific survival rate of 88% and 81%, respectively, and a progression-free survival rate of 77% after a mean follow-up of more than 7 years. These data resemble the findings reported by Messing et al. [8], who report survival rates and progression-free rates of 84.2% and 77%, respectively, after immediate antiandrogen therapy in N1 disease as compared to 64.7% and 18%, respectively, in the observation group of their prospective randomized study.

In conclusion, extended pelvic staging lymphadenectomy in patients with clinically localized prostate cancer on the basis of anatomical lymphatic drainage detected lymph node metastases in 26.2% of the patients and resulted in a diagnostic benefit of 15% as compared to standard lymphadenectomy. When considered in conjunction with the therapeutic benefit of immediate adjuvant hormonal therapy, these data are of utmost clinical importance in avoiding systemic reccurrence in patients with pT2 PCA. Although our patients numbers were limited, a group of patients being at low risk for lymph involvement could be identified: preoperative serum PSA <10.6 ng/ml, a biopsy Gleason score ≤6, and clinical stage ≤2a were associated with an only 2% risk of lymph node metastasis. Staging pLA can be omitted in these patients, whereas all other patients should undergo epLA, to include lymph nodes of the external iliac group, the internal iliac group and the obturator fossa group; the routine dissection of the presacral nodes and the common-iliac nodes, however, can be eliminated.

References

1. Bluestein DL, Bostwick DG, Bergstrahl EJ, et al (1994) Eliminating the need for bilateral pelvic lymphadenectomy in select patients with prostate cancer. J Urol 151:1315–1320
2. Bishoff JT, Reyes A, Thompson IM, et al (1995) Pelvic lymphadenectomy can be omitted in selected patients with carcinoma of the prostate: development of a system of patient selection. Urology 45:270–275
3. Partin AW, Kattan MW, Subong ENP, Walsh PC, Wojno KJ, Oesterling JE, et al (1997) Combination of prostate-specific antigen, clinical stage, and Gleason score to predict pathologixcal stage of localized prostate cancer. A multiinstitutional update. JAMA 277:1445–1451
4. El-Galley RES, Keane TE, Petros JA, Sanders WH, Clarke HS, Cotsonis GA, Graham SD (1998) Evaluation of staging lympadenectomy in prostate cancer. Urology 52:663–667
5. Crawford ED, Batuello JT, Snow P, et al (2000) The use of artificial intelligence technology to predict lymph node spread in men with clinically localized prostate carcinoma. Cancer 88:2105–2109
6. Zincke H, Utz DC, Myers RP, et al (1982) Bilateral pelvic lymphadecectomy and radical retropubic prostatectomy for adenocarcinoma of the prostate with regional lymph node involvement. Urology 19:238–247
7. Frazier HA, Robertson JE, Paulson DF (1994) Does radical prostatectomy in the presence of positive pelvic lymph nodes enhance survival? World J Urol 12:308–312
8. Messing E, Manola J, Sarosdy M, et al (1999) Immediate hormonal therapy compared with observation after radical prostatectomy and pelvic lymphadenectomy in men with node-positive prostate cancer. N Engl J Med 341:1781–1788
9. Gil-Vernet JM (1996) Prostate cancer: anatomical and surgical considerations. Br J Urol 78:161–168
10. Raghavaiah NV, Jordan WP (1979) Prostatic lymphography. J Urol 121:178–181
11. Cerny JC, Farah R, Rian R, Weckstein ML (1975) An evaluation of lymphangiography in staging carcinoma of the prostate. J Urol 113:367–370

12. Amling CL, Blute ML, Bergstralh EJ, et al (2000) Long-term hazard of progression after radical prostatectomy for clinically localized prostate cancer: continued risk of biochemical failure after 5 years. J Urol 164:101–105
14. Metz CE (1978) Basic principles of ROC analysis. Semin Nucl Med 8:283
15. Walsh PC (1980) Radical prostatectomy for the treatment of localized prostate carcinoma. Urol Clin North Am 7:583–589
16. Hammerer P, Hübner D, Gonnermann D, Huland H (1995) Perioperative and postoperative complications in pelvic lymphadenectomy and radical prostatectomy in 320 consecutive patients. Urologe A 34:334–342
17. Wawroschek F, Vogt H, Weckermann D, Wagner T, Harzmann R (1999) The sentinel lymph node concept in prostate cancer – first results of gamma probe-guided sentinel lymph node identification. Eur Urol 36:595–600
18. Golimbu M, Morales P, Al-Askari S, et al (1979) Extended lymphadenectomy for prostatic cancer. J Urol 121:617–620
19. Nicholson TC, Richie JP (1977) Pelvic lymphadectomy for stage B1 adenocarcinoma of the prostate: justified or not? J Urol 117:199–201
20. Schubert J, Heidl G (1982) Lymphogenic metastases in prostatic cancer – operative and histopathologic investigations. Arch Geschwulstforsch 52:213–221
21. Fujioka T, Koike H, Aoki H, et al (1987) Significance of staging pelvic lymphadectomy for prostatic cancer. Urol Int 42:380–384
23. Brendler CB, Cleeve LK, Anderson EE, et al (1980) Staging pelvic lymphadenectomy for carcinoma of the prostate: risk versus benefit. J Urol 124:849–850
24. O'Donoghue EPN, Shridar P, Sherwood T, et al (1976) Lymphography and pelvic lymphadenectomy in carcinoma of the prostate. Br J Urol 48:689–696
25. Dillioglugli Ö, Leibman BD, Leibman NS, et al (1997) Risk factors for complications and morbidity after radical retropubic prostatectomy. J Urol 157:1760–17670

Operative Therapy of Clinically Localized Prostate Cancer

12 Anatomy: Surgical Aspects

R. Hofmann

12.1 Surgical aspects of non-nerve sparing ascending radical prostatectomy

The essential maneuvers in *ascending radical retropubic prostatectomy* will be

1. Opening the pelvic floor and separating the levator muscle
2. Controlling the dorsal vein complex (prostatic venous plexus)
3. Transecting the urethra
4. Separating the rectum along Denonvilliers' fascia
5. Isolating the seminal vesicles
6. Transecting the vasa deferentia
7. Switching to a descending mode by transecting the base of the bladder from the prostate, and
8. Dividing vascular pedicles to the prostate

The order of the steps can vary according to the size of the prostate, cancer location, and personal preference.

The retropubic space is exposed by removing fat. Care has to be taken not to injure periprostatic veins that lie within the thin sheet of fascia, which extends from the levator muscle fascia medially. Smaller veins are controlled by electrocautery, major bleeding by carefully placed stitches.

The endopelvic fascia or parietal pelvic fascia, which covers the levator muscle laterally is opened in the sulcus, or a few millimeters medial to the sulcus, thus dividing the pelvic floor from the visceral pelvic fascia that covers the medial and anterior surface of the prostate. The fusion of the two fasciae is thickened and called the tendinous arc of the pelvic fascia.

The levator muscle fibers are easily pushed away by a sponge stick dorsal to the prostate; however, these fibers can be adherent more cranial to the prostate. Wilson's muscle has to be gently mobilized and sometimes veins in this area have to be controlled by ligature or by electrocautery. Levator muscles fibers can also be strongly adherent at the apices of the prostate and have to be divided sharply.

Now the puboprostatic bands both laterally and cranially to the dorsal vein complex are exposed by a peanut dissector and incised close to the symphysis to avoid injury to the veins. Thus the prostate drops down from the symphysis, allowing the urethra to be exposed in a better manner later on.

The prostate is now still covered by its prostatic fascia, overlying the urethra, prostate, and neurovascular bundle. This fascia is also called lateral pelvic fascia or paraprostatic fascia.

Veins from the dorsum of the penis leave to the ventral aspect of the prostate forming a venous plexus on the prostate. Veins from this dorsal vein complex – also called Santorini plexus – drain into the internal iliac vein. Anterior to the striated sphincter a semicircular complex of veins surrounds the ventral rim of the prostate and the anterior urethra. Usually there are one or two major veins distributing blood into a varying arrangement of spreading veins on the anterior aspect of the prostate. A confluence of many veins results in a "lake of venous blood" close to the striated sphincter. Asymmetry of the veins is common. Most drain from on top of the prostate in a V-shaped manner laterally to either side of the prostate.

The venous complex can be subdivided by using a McDougal clamp; however, this maneuver can lead to severe bleeding if the venous lake is perforated. Preferably, the dorsal vein complex can be undermined by a curved needle and ligated. When cutting deeper to the urethra, the same needle can be used to suture the dorsal venous complex down to the striated sphincter. To avoid backbleeding from the cephalad portion, a medial stitch a few millimeters caudal to the bladder can be placed. Using a nerve sparing technique, either no stitch or oversewing the bleeders in a V-shaped manner avoids anterior displacement of the neurovascular bundles.

Dissection to the striated muscles of the urethra is now performed. Two pillars lateral to the urethra come into view. These fascial bands at the prostatic apex have to be separated sharply from the prostate to expose the urethral sphincter. Now a notch can be seen at the prostate where the apices protrude on both sides, while along the urethra the prostate retracts. At this stage of the operation a long urethral stump can be prepared by dissecting the urethra to the opening between the apices following dissection of both lateral fascial bands. Minimal venous plexus trauma and a long urethral stump are essential for maximum postoperative continence.

At the apex many forms and configurations are seen, but usually the prostate retracts at the entrance of the urethra into the prostate. However, the prostate usually forms a posterior notch, which can be entered and dissection carried out into the prostate.

First the urethra is divided half way, then anastomotic sutures are placed from inside out in the urethra and the striated sphincter. The sphincteric muscles can be avoided by suturing the urethra, avoiding the muscle, and then again suturing the oversewn dorsal vein complex. Three anastomotic sutures are placed at 12, 10, and 2 o'clock; then the catheter is mobilized out of the urethra and two more sutures are placed at 8 and 4 o'clock.

The verumontanum is transected at this stage. If a dorsal lip of the prostate protrudes, the "veru" sits at the edge of the cranial urethra in the prostate. With this anatomic configuration only a narrow margin exists for the maintenance of urethral continence.

The rectovesical fascia (Denonvilliers' fascia) is then separated straight down to the perirectal fat. Positive margins can result when Denonvilliers' fascia is separated too close to the prostate, thus cutting into the dorsal protruding notch of the prostate, which leaves a positive margin dorsal to the urethral stump.

Apical transection should not be done at the end of both apices, as urethral length is reduced compared to urethral-sparing preparation into the prostatic notch.

The prostatic apex can be held between the index and the middle finger of the left hand and pulled cranially. Thus the urethra is gently pulled out of the pelvic floor. This maneuver allows for a lengthening of the urethra prior to transection at the apex.

Ascending preparation of the prostate is performed by incising the soft perirectal fat at the dorsal aspect of the prostate. Laterally, fascial columns remain and can be generously undermined by a right angle clamp and clipped. Lateral to the seminal vesicles the prostatic pillars are clamped and ligated. The shining aspect of Denonvilliers' fascia is preserved and the rectum and perirectal fat are pushed down by a sponge stick. Opening of the rectovesical fascia a few millimeters below the bladder neck exposes the ductus deferens, which are separated and clipped. The tips of the seminal vesicles are exposed and clipped to control the small seminal vesicle arteries. In small prostates, sometimes the bladder neck can be exposed from the caudal aspect. The groove between the detrusor bladder muscles and the prostate can be exposed in a semicircular fashion.

Usually when done posteriorly this maneuver is too difficult to control due to prostate size and prerectal fat, so that in larger prostates separation of the bladder and prostate is more easily performed anteriorly.

Sphincteric loops of detrusor muscles can be preserved at the bladder neck by cutting close to the prostate. The first step is medial exposure of the fat and periprostatic venous plexus. Thereafter, muscle loops can be separated to preserve a narrow bladder neck. Muscle loops should only be preserved in small volume prostate cancers and in cancers not located cranially in order to avoid positive surgical margins at the bladder neck. However, soft perivesical fatty tissue and smooth muscle fibers can usually be distinguished from prostatic tissue by the surgeon. Preservation of the bladder neck has the advantage of allowing the possibility of fashioning a new and continent bladder neck. Early continence seems to be better in bladder neck sparing surgery, however definitive continence is not improved. Bladder neck preservation further avoids the production of tension on the anastomosis since no bladder tissue is lost.

Descending prostatectomy continues by median incision of the dorsal aspect of the bladder neck by cutting into smooth perivesical fat. Laterally, thicker prostatic bundles can be clipped or ligated. At the 10 and 2 o'clock positions venous backflow from the prostate is curtailed by ligation, and at 3 and 9 o'clock the superior prostatic artery is ligated.

Bladder neck sparing surgery has to be done with caution to avoid positive margins at the bladder neck. Only in small prostates -and in small tumors- it can be advised. Biopsies of the bladder neck help avoid positive margins. In larger prostates and larger tumors wide excision of the bladder neck and closure in a tennis racket fashion is preferable.

12.2 Neurovascular preservation

12.2.1 Neural innervation of the prostate

The prostate is innervated by sympathetic, parasympathetic, and somatic nerves. Sympathetic nerves arise from L1 and L2 and form the superior hypogastric plexus and the inferior pelvic plexus lateral to the bladder and prostate in the prerectal fat.

Parasympathetic innervation arises from S2–S4 forming the inferior pelvic plexus or inferior hypogastric plexus.

Thus the inferior hypogastric plexus – also called pelvic plexus – contains parasympathetic and sympathetic nerves and lies lateral and ventral to the rectum. The neurovascular bundle forms posterolaterally at the base of the prostate, where Denonvilliers' fascia and lateral pelvic fascia fuse. It proceeds along arteries and veins in the neurovascular bundle and ends as the cavernous nerve. The capsular arterial branches run posterolaterally and supply the prostate gland. During nerve sparing radical prostatectomy the endopelvic fascia (lateral pelvic fascia) has to be divided to allow lateral movement of the bundle. In perineal prostatectomy however, the plane of dissection is within the endopelvic fascia.

Autonomic innervation to the prostatic sphincters consists of sympathetic nerves from the superior hypogastric plexus located dorsal to the rectum, and from the pelvic plexus lateral to the rectum, prostate, bladder, and seminal vesicles. Somatic innervation is provided by the pelvic nerve, which also runs through the pelvic plexus, and, for the striated periurethral sphincter by branches of the pudendal nerve.

Urine is prevented from unintentionally escaping the bladder by fibers of the internal vesical sphincter at the bladder neck.

Somatic nerves also originate from S2-S4 and supply the external sphincters via the pudendal nerve.

Hypogastric and pelvic nerves form a plexus at the base of the prostate dorsal and lateral to the seminal vesicles. These then merge to become the cavernous nerves located at the dorso-lateral aspect of the prostate outside of Denonvilliers' fascia. These bundles hug at 5 and 7 o'clock on the outside of Denonvilliers' fascia and spread along from the base to the apex. At the apex the nerve bundle moves more cranially to the 3 and 9 o'clock positions and travels along the urethra laterally on both sides. Some fibers also spread more dorsally along the urethra and along the rectourethralis muscle.

12.2.2 Fascial layers

The prostatic venous plexus is embedded in the periprostatic fascia. The lateral aspect of the prostate is covered by a thin layer of fascia, separating it from the more lateral portion of fascia called endopelvic fascia (lateral pelvic fascia) which covers the pubococcygeus and internal obturator muscles.

The neurovascular bundle lies within the periprostatic fascia, enclosing the dorsal vein complex anteriorly, then proceeding laterally to the prostate and reaching Denonvilliers' fascia dorsally. The bundle is close to the prostate at the base (1–2 mm) and further away at the apex (2–3 mm). It can be separated from the prostate by entering the lateral periprostatic fascia and moving closer to the prostate gland.

Denonvilliers' fascia is composed of two layers. The anterior lamella covers the prostatic gland closely whereas the posterior lamella is the rectal fascia surrounding the anterior and lateral wall of the rectum. These two layers cannot always be separated when developing the prostate from the anterior surface of the rectum, so that both layers of Denonvilliers' fascia stay at the dorsal side of the prostate.

Laterally the prostate is covered by the prostatic sheath or by the lateral pelvic fascia. Dorsally the lateral pelvic fascia fuses with Denonvilliers' fascia and laterally with the endopelvic fascia covering the pelvic floor muscles. The periprostatic fascia also covers the neuromuscular bundle. Anteriorly and laterally this fascia fuses with the endopelvic fascia, also called lateral pelvic fascia.

12.2.3 Blood supply

The prostatovesical artery usually arises from the internal iliac artery; however, it also can branch off from the superior vesical artery or the internal pudendal artery. It runs on the surface of the levator muscle and divides to an inferior vesical and a prostatic artery. The prostatic artery itself is divided at the prostatic base into a bigger posterior lateral trunk that supplies most of the prostatic gland and a smaller anterior trunk for the anterior lateral part. The blood supply for the seminal vesicles arises from the superior vesical artery or in some cases from the inferior vesical artery. They send branches to the tip of the seminal vesicle and to the vasa deferentia.

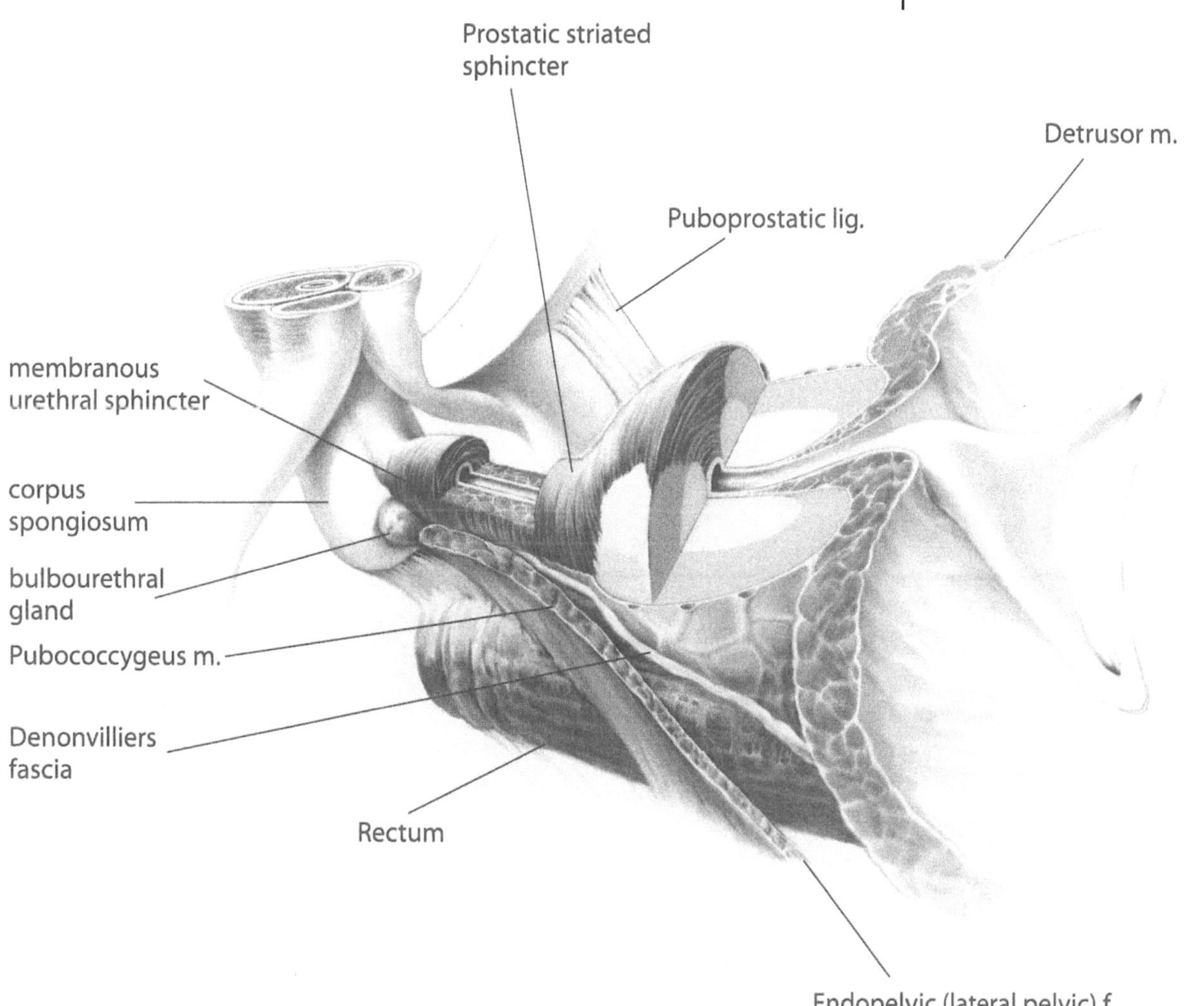

Structures related to the prostate

Laterally the prostate is covered by the prostatic sheath or lateral pelvic fascia. Dorsally it fuses with Denonvilliers fascia and laterally with the endopelvic fascia coverning the pelvic floor muscles. The periprostatic fascia also covers the neuromuscular bundle. Anteriorly and laterally it fuses with the endopelvic fascia, also called lateral pelvic fascia.

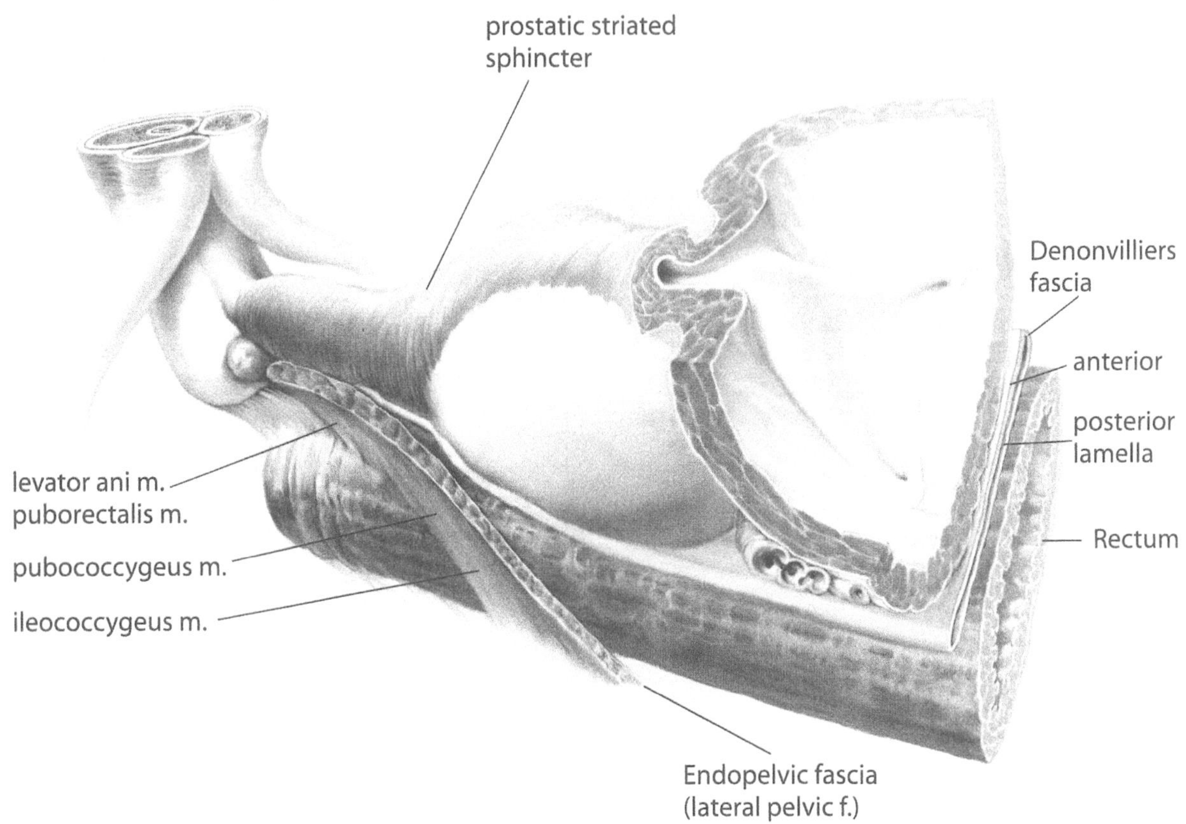

Configuration of Denonvilliers fascia

Denonvilliers fascia is composed of two layers. The anterior lamella covers the prostatic gland closely whereas the posterior lamella is the rectal fascia surrounding the anterior and lateral wall of the rectum. These two layers can not always be separated, when developing the prostate from the anterior surface of the rectum, so that both layers stay at the dorsal side of the prostate.

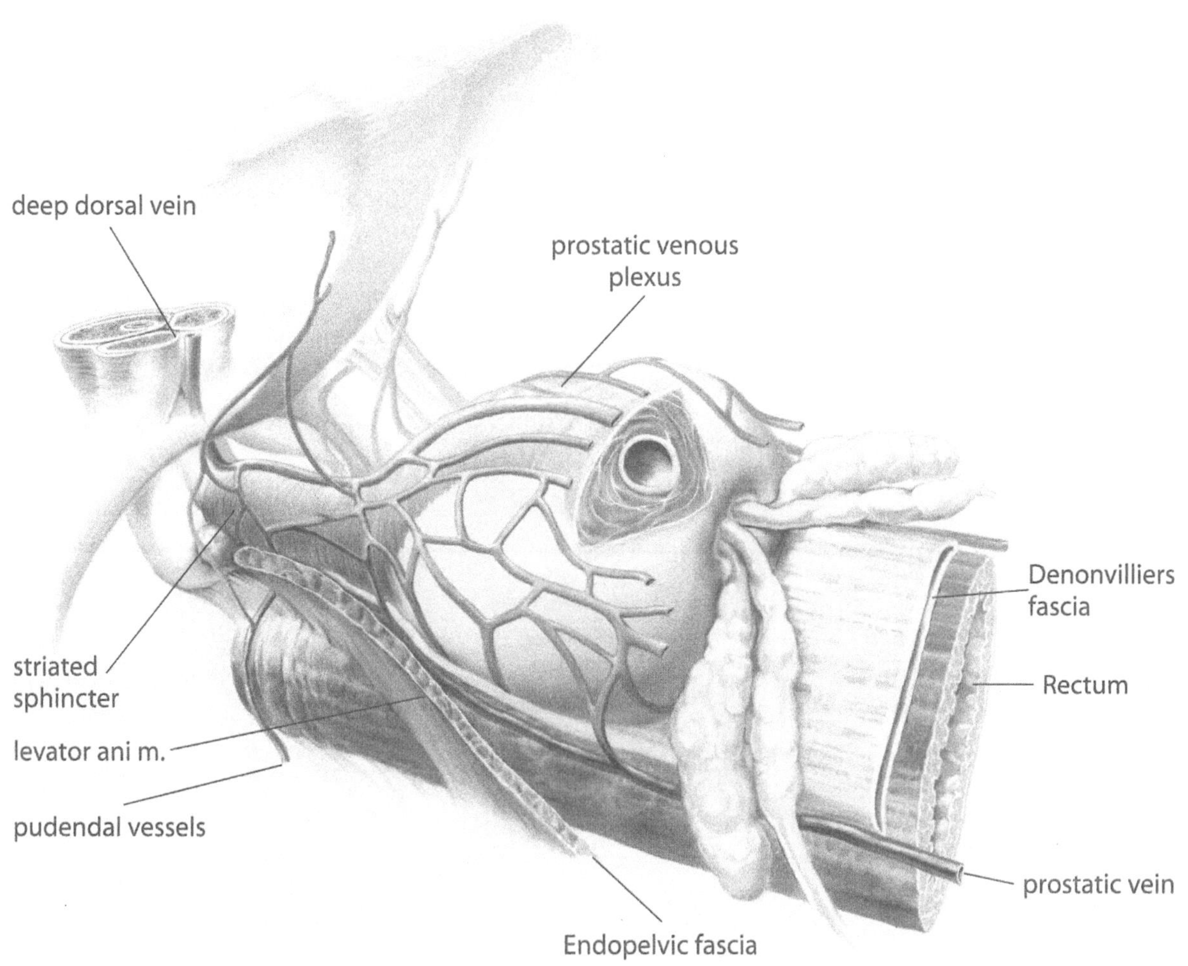

Venous drainage of the prostate

Veins from the dorsum of the penis leave to the ventral aspect of the prostate forming a venous plexus on the prostate. Veins from this dorsal vein complex – also called Santorini plexus – drain into the internal iliac vein. Anterior to the striated sphincter a semicircular complex of veins surrounds the ventral rim of the prostate and the anterior urethra.

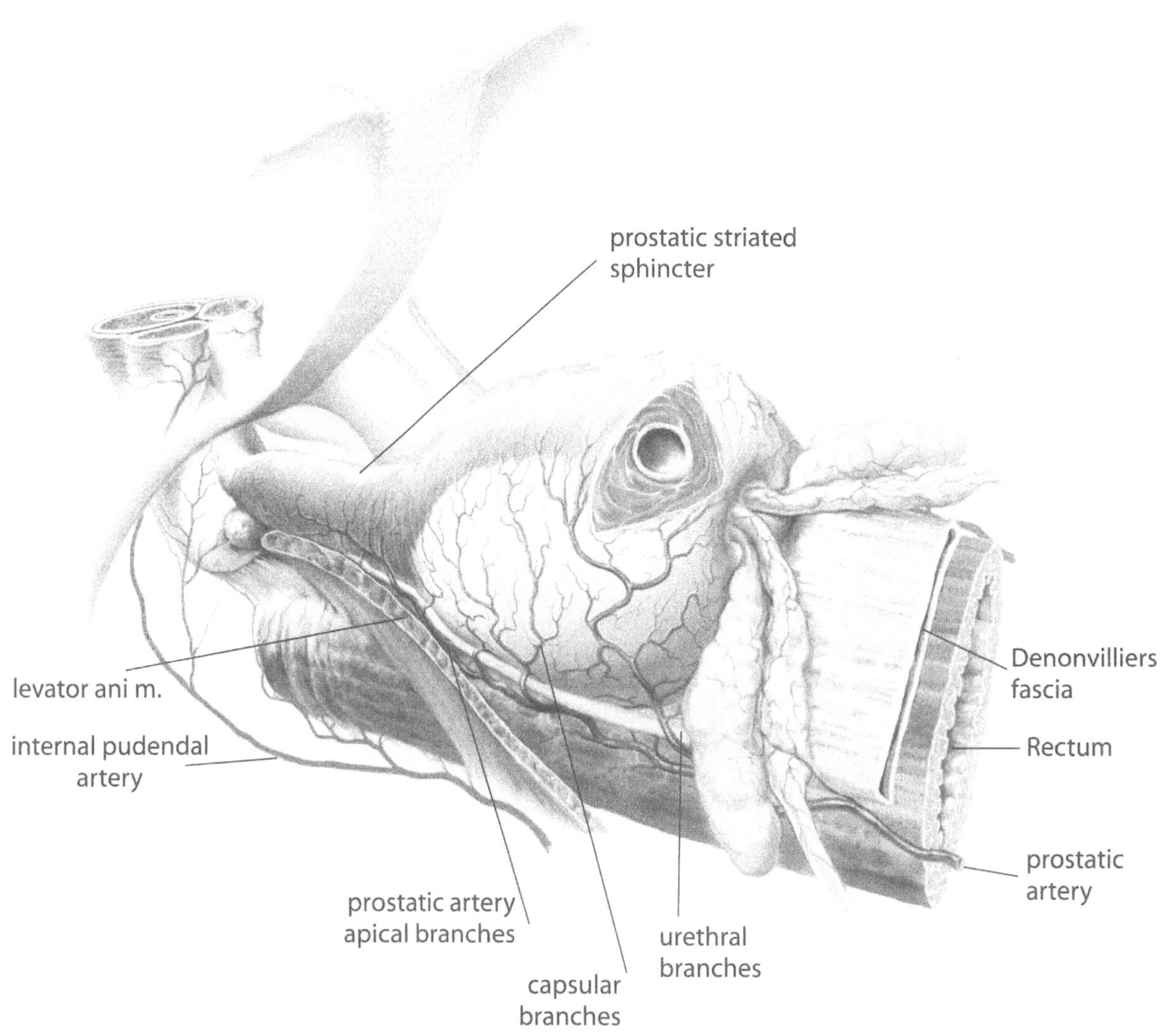

Arterial blood supply to the prostate

The prostatovescial artery usually arises from the internal iliac artery: however, it also can branch off from the superior vesical artery or the internal pudendal artery. It runs on the surface of the levator muscle and divides to an inferior vesical and a prostatic artery. The prostatic artery itself is divided at the prostatic base into a bigger posterior lateral trunk that supplies most of the prostatic gland and a smaller anterior trunk for the anterior lateral part. The blood supply for the seminal vesicles arises from the superior vesical artery or in some cases from the inferior vesical artery.

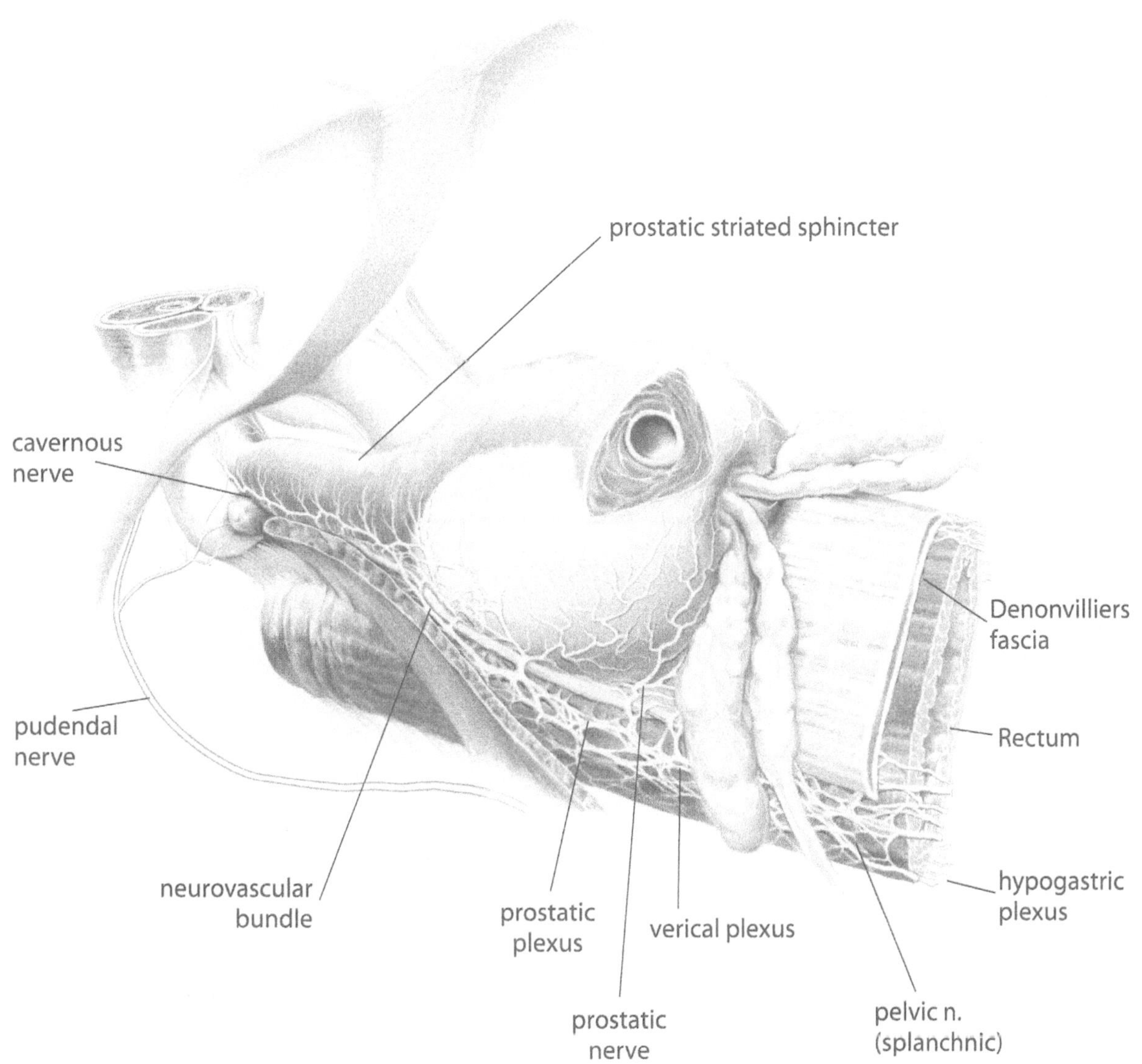

Innervation of the prostate

Autonomic innervation to the prostatic sphincters consists of sympathetic nerves from the superior hypogastric plexus located dorsal to the rectum, and from the pelvic plexus lateral to the rectum, prostate, bladder, and seminal vesicles. Somatic innervation is provided by the pelvic nerve, which also runs through the pelvic plexus, and, for the striated periurethral sphincter by branches of the pudendal nerve.

13 Extended Pelvic Lymphadenectomy

R. Hofmann

Standard lymphadenectomy is usually limited to obturator and external iliac lymph nodes. In a low risk group with PSA<10 ng/ml and a Gleason sum <7, a 2% risk of lymph node involvement is encountered and lymphadenectomy may be omitted before radical prostatectomy. However in patients with PSA >10 ng/ml, a biopsy Gleason sum >7 and a clinical stage greater than T2a, we found lymph node metastases in 26%. With extended pelvic lymphadenectomy, this resulted in a 15% diagnostic benefit over the standard lymphadenectomy approach. Lymphadenectomy including especially the internal iliac lymph nodes should be performed in a high risk patient group.

First the peritoneum is sharply dissected from the anterior abdominal wall, the ileopsoas region and the internal inguinal ring. The spermatic cord is freed. The fibrofatty tissue over the iliac artery is divided and the tissue between artery and vein resected. The lateral boundary of dissection is the iliac artery. The dissection is carried distally to reach the retrocrural lymph node of Cloquet near the inguinal canal. The circumflex iliac vein can be spared. Cranially the dissection is performed along the common iliac vessels to the bifurcation.

Dissection is carried along the bony surface of the pelvis and the levator fascia down to the obturator nerve. Care has to be taken to clip or ligate all afferent lymphatic vessels to prevent lymphocele formation.

Tissue is bluntly cleared dorsal to the iliac vein and along the obturator nerve to remove all obturator lymph nodes. Gentle lateral traction to the iliac vein with a peanut dissector or a vein retractor is performed. The obturator vessels may be either incorporated with the node package or left behind.

Fibrofatty tissue is resected from around the internal iliac artery and its branches to the pelvis.

Careful dissection, ligation or clipping of all afferent lymphatic channels and placement of a Redon drain left on suction for 24 h help to decrease the risk of prolonged lymphatic drainage.

Thus lymph nodes from the external iliac, common iliac, internal iliac and obturator region are obtained. With this technique a mean number of 30 lymph nodes are dissected with extended pelvic lymphadenectomy as compared to 11 nodes with standard lymphadenectomy.

The detection of micrometastases in a high risk group is of importance as a prolonged survival for patients with radical prostatectomy and less than three metastatic nodes has been found. Initiation of early adjuvant androgen deprivation in patients with minimal lymph node involvement may also result in a favourable prognosis. At the very least, patients with early antiandrogenic treatment have shown less morbidity than those being treated at the time of PSA progression or those without treatment.

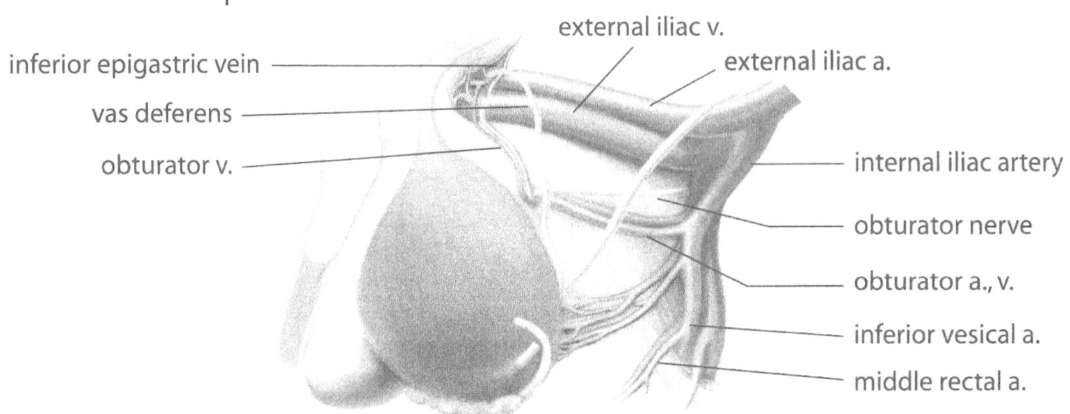

Anatomy of the lateral pelvic wall

Extended pelvic lymphadenectomy includes lymph nodes from the external iliac, common illiac, internal iliac and obturator region. Especially lymphadenectomy obtaining the internal iliac lymph nodes should be performed in a high risk patient group.

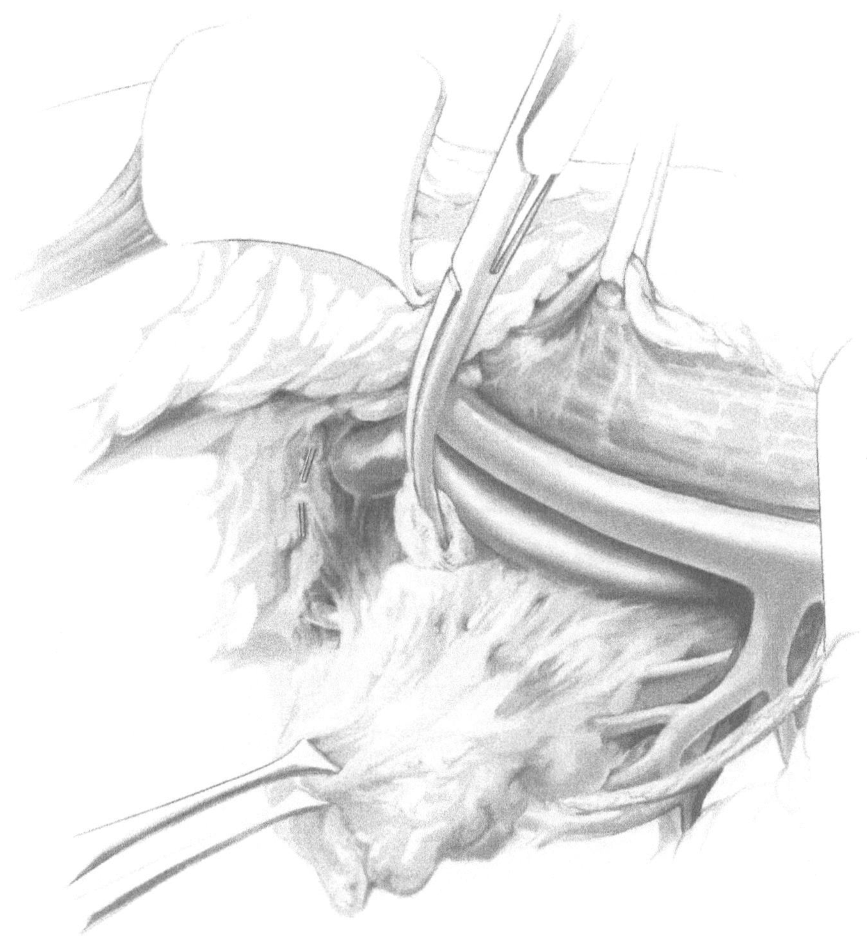

The fibrofatty tissue over the iliac artery is divided and the tissue between artery and vein resected. The lateral boundary of dissection is the iliac artery. The dissection is carried distally to reach the retrocrural lymph node of Cloquet near the inguinal canal. The circumflex iliac vein can be spared. Cranially the dissection is performed along the common iliac vessels to the bifurcation.

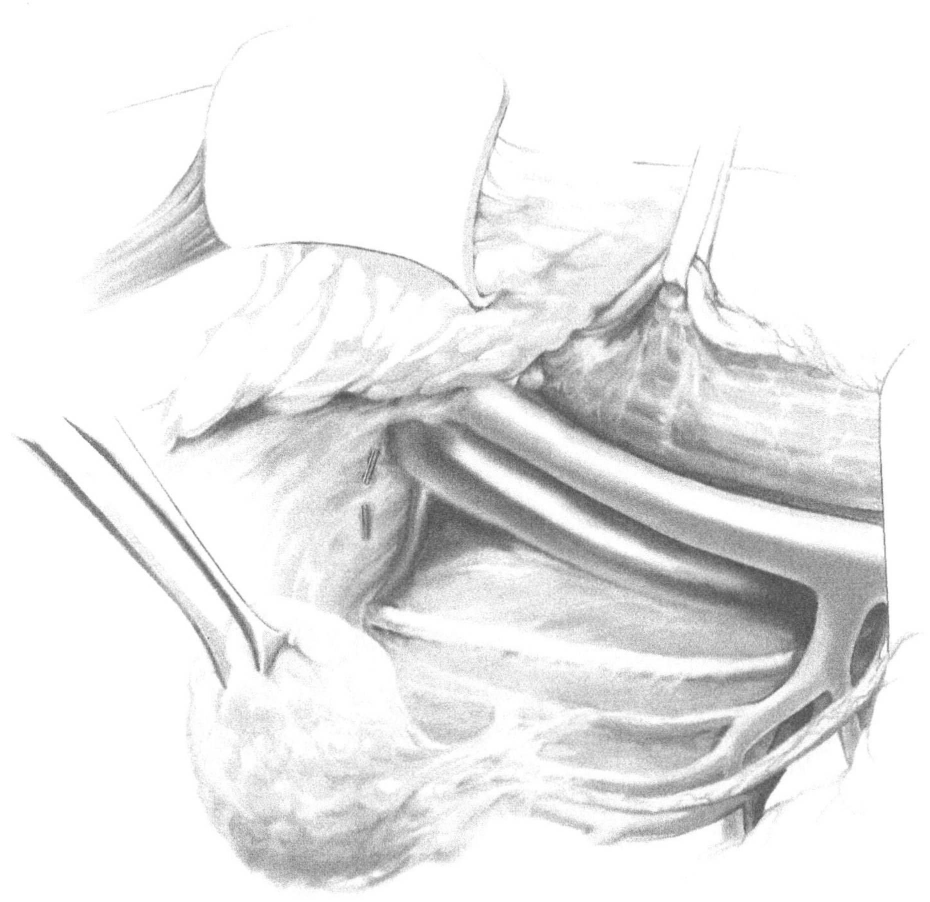

Tissue is bluntly cleared dorsal to the iliac vein and along the oburator nerve to remove all obturator lymph nodes. Gentle lateral traction to the iliac vein with a peanut dissector or a vein retractor is performed. The obturator vessels may be incorporated with the node package or may be left behind. Fibrofatty tissue is resected from around the internal iliac artery and its branches to the pelvis.

14 Radical Ascending Retropubic Prostatectomy

R. Hofmann

A suprapubic midline incision is made extending from the symphysis to the umbilicus. The rectus fascia is opened, the rectus abdominus muscles separated and the posterior transversalis fascia opened. The peritoneal sac is mobilized cranially beyond the external iliac vessels and a retractor placed underneath the peritoneum cranial to the iliac artery. Occasionally a cartilaginous protrusion from the symphysis is found, which can be easily shaved off by a scalpel. Fatty tissue on the pelvic fascia is removed gently, then the endopelvic fascia is opened. Cranial fibers of the levator muscle can be firmly attached to the prostatic capsule and are removed sharply, or bluntly with a swab. The puboprostatic ligaments should be exposed bluntly by teasing away fatty tissue and moving it sideways with a swab. Incision of the puboprostatic ligaments is done close to the symphysis to avoid the dorsal venous complex.

The superficial branch of the dorsal vein is not covered by the prostatic fascia, however the deep dorsal venous complex lies under the prostatic fascia.

A figure-of-eight suture is placed under the dorsal vein and its tributaries. The suture is tied and the needle left on the suture. The urethra is sharply prepared with scissors. Should there be more venous bleeding, the same suture can be used to suture the vein complex vertically down to the urethra.

Backbleeding is usually mild and can be controlled by a median suture about 0.5 cm cranial to the bladder neck, which also defines the site of bladder neck detachment from the prostate.

A gentle pull with two fingers at both prostatic apices cephalad brings the urethra out of the pelvic floor and exposes a 2–3 cm urethral length for separation from the apex.

The striated muscle is then sharply divided and the urethra exposed. With a peanut dissector, the urethra is freed from levator fibers laterally and the apex exposed.

The lateral pelvic fascia is opened a few millimeters cephalad to the apex on the lateral aspect of the prostate and extended down to the apex. Small vessels to the prostate are secured with miniclips and divided. Now the urethra is opened about 2–3 mm distal to the apex and the catheter exposed. From the inside out, 2-0 sutures are placed through the urethra, excluding the striated sphincter muscles but including the sutured dorsal vein complex and a few millimeters of the lateral pelvic fascia.

When dividing the urethra further, care should be taken not to cut into a protruding posterior apex, but to stay away and solely divide the striated sphincter by cutting straight down through Denonvilliers' fascia.

Apical dissection is made easier by pulling gently at the prostatic apices, hereby stretching the urethra out of the pelvic floor. Thus the prostatic notch can be seen and an additional length of the dorsal urethral stump saved.

The two-layered character of Denonvilliers' fascia being surgically insignificant, it can be divided. Both layers lie on the dorsal aspect of the prostate with a line of separation in the prerectal fat or immediately above the lamina propria of the rectum.

Upon dividing Denonvilliers' fascia, yellow fatty tissue is seen prerectally. Blunt movement with the finger cranially exposes the plane of dissection. Sometimes the prostate is firmly fixed to the rectum at this area making blunt dissection impossible. Scar tissue may have resulted from transrectal prostatic biopsies. At first, sharp dissection straight down through the rectourethralis muscle is done. If scar tissue is found, staying closer to the dorsal aspect of the prostate usually leads to softer prerectal tissue.

Lateral attachments of the prostate to Denonvilliers' fascia are separated by a right angle clamp and clipped.

For preparation of the seminal vesicles and the vasa deferentia, Denonvilliers' fascia has to be opened in the midline. The fascia should be mobilized as far cranially as possible and opened there.

The seminal vesicles are freed and the apex clipped for hemostasis at the seminal artery. The vasa deferentia are clipped and divided. Next the bladder neck is separated from the prostate, first by electrocautery then by scissors.

At the 3 and 9 o'clock positions arterial branches from the superior vesical artery are usually found and have to be ligated. The bladder is opened ventrally. Care has to be taken to avoid injury to the ureteral orifices. If a median lobe is found, the urothelium has to be incised around it, carefully sparing the trigone and ureteral crests. This can be made easier by lifting up the ventrally opened bladder with a lid hook.

Sharp division of the posterior bladder neck and straight-down careful exploration between the vasa deferentia and the dorsal bladder wall leads to the plane of dissection already opened from the caudal aspect. Usually the posterior lateral pedicle is still in place and can be separated with a right angle clamp. Ligation is advised.

The bladder neck is closed with interrupted 3–0 absorbable sutures. Then the bladder mucosa is everted and sutured outward with a running 4–0 polyglactin suture on both sides. The bladder neck should be narrowed to the width of the fifth finger for convenient passage of a 20-F catheter. Anastomotic sutures at the bladder neck are placed through the everted mucosa. During suturing, a forceps can be placed in the bladder to push the back wall and the trigone dorsally. After placing 5 and 7 o'clock sutures dorsally at the bladder neck, a 20-F catheter is positioned in the bladder, inflated with 15 ml and held between two fingers by the assistant. Further anastomotic sutures are placed.

Trendelenburg position is taken off and with gently pulling at the catheter, the anastomotic sutures can be tied without tension.

The bladder is filled with 100 cc of saline to be sure of a watertight anastomosis. Two suction drains are placed in the obturator fossa paravesically. The 10 F Redon drains remain on suction for one day; the drain removed at day three or four.

With larger prostates and those containing adenomatous hyperplasia, the apex lies higher and behind the anterior commissure, thus necessitating division of the urethra more cranially to avoid injuring the sphincter.

Saving the puboprostatic ligaments and securing the dorsal vein complex cranially to them is possible; however, one may then be left with less excessive surgical margins at the apex than is desirable.

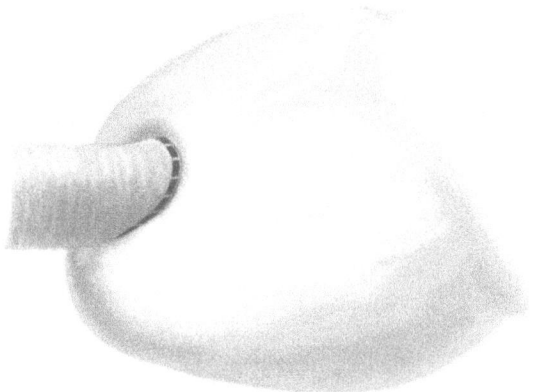

At the apex may forms and configuarations are seen, but usually the prostate retracts at the entrance of the urethra into the prostate. However, the prostate usually forms a posterior notch, which can be entered and transsection carried out into the prostate while separating the urethra from the prostate.

15 Radical Descending Retropubic Prostatectomy

R. Hofmann

Following exposure of the endopelvic fascia, one or more medial sutures are placed about 0.5 mm cephalad to the bladder neck in order to secure hemostasis. The vasa deferentia are exposed lateral to the bladder and divided. The bladder neck is opened at the sulcus between the bladder and the prostate. Palpation of the catheter balloon helps in identifying the area of dissection. By electrocautery, the detrusor fibers are separated from the prostate ventrally. Next, preparation is accomplished with scissors and the bladder opened sharply. With two pick-ups the bladder is held open and the ureteral orifices identified. The catheter is pulled out and divided. The dorsal aspect of the bladder neck is opened by scissors and divided straight down between vasa deferentia and bladder. The vasa deferentia are pulled through to the opening and lifted up to place tension on the seminal vesicles. Each seminal vesicle is mobilized close to its lateral aspect in a plane between the seminal vesicle and its overlying lateral fascia. If it is a nerve sparing procedure, the lateral neurovascular bundle and the lateral tissue containing the pelvic plexus is mobilized laterally. If the procedure is radical and not sparing of nerves, the lateral pedicles are undermined by a right angle clamp and ligated. Denonvilliers' fascia is opened in the midline and the dorsal aspect of the prostate is bluntly mobilized by finger dissection. By pulling the prostate up, prostate and prerectal fat can be separated by Satinsky scissors. The lateral pillars are clipped and divided.

The endopelvic fascia has to be opened and the prostate exposed laterally by gently separating the levator fibers away from the prostate with a peanut dissector. In a fashion similar to that of the ascending technique, the dorsal vein complex is controlled, the urethra divided, and anastomotic sutures placed. Pulling the catheter back into the urethra to help expose the lumen of the urethra can be useful, especially in placement of sutures at the 5 and 7 o'clock positions.

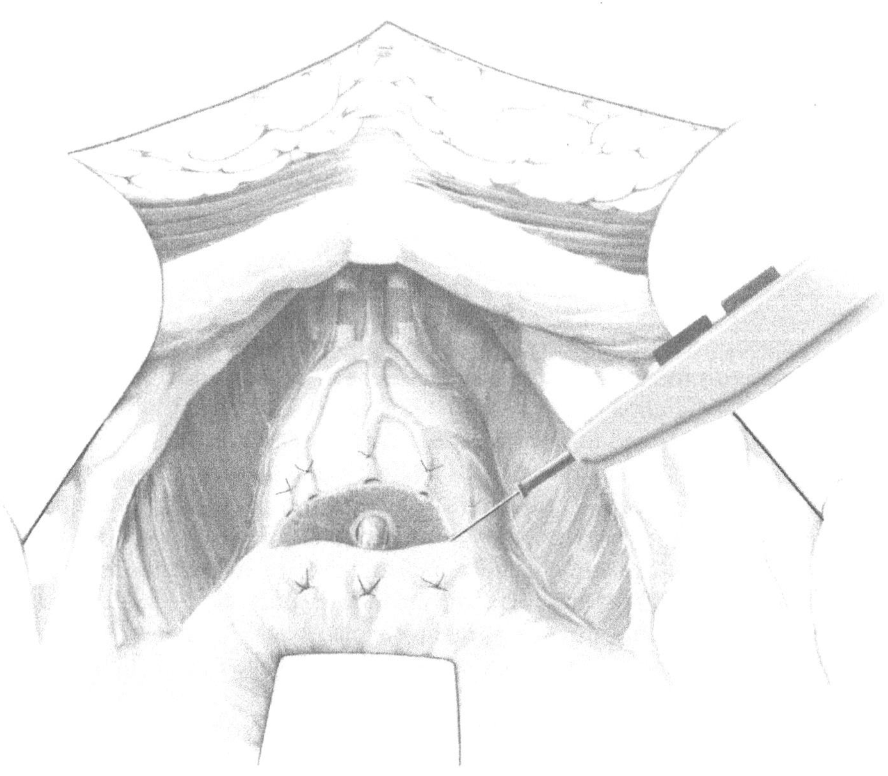

One or more medial sutures are placed about 0.5 mm cephalad to the bladder neck in order to secure hemostasis. The bladder neck is opened at the sulcus between the bladder and the prostate by electrocautery.

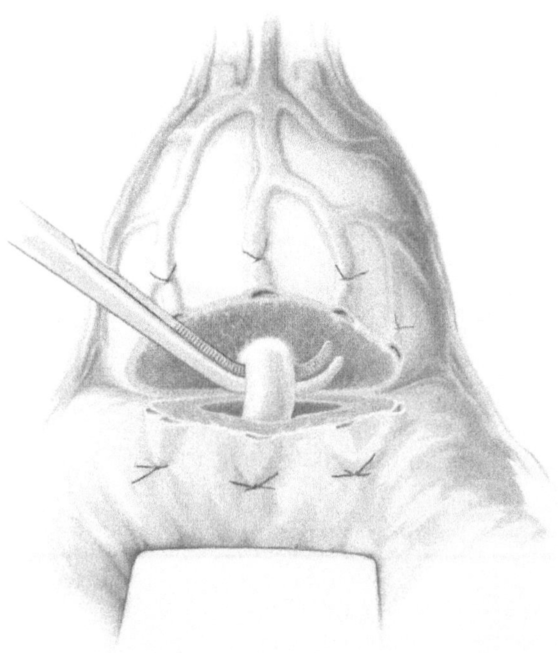

Further preparation is accomplished with scissors and the bladder opened sharply. The catheter is pulled out and divided.

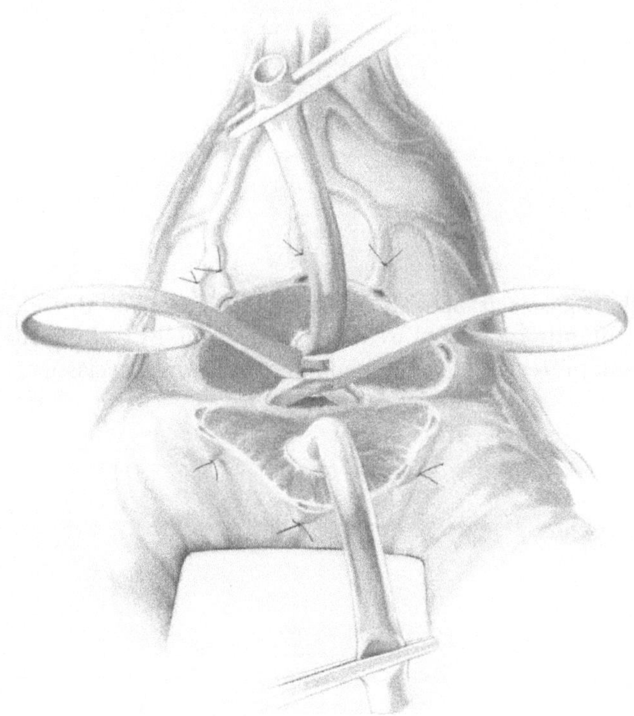

The dorsal aspect of the bladder neck is opened by scissors and divided straight down between vasa deferentia and bladder. The vasa deferentia are pulled through to the opening and lifted up to place tension on the seminal vesicles.

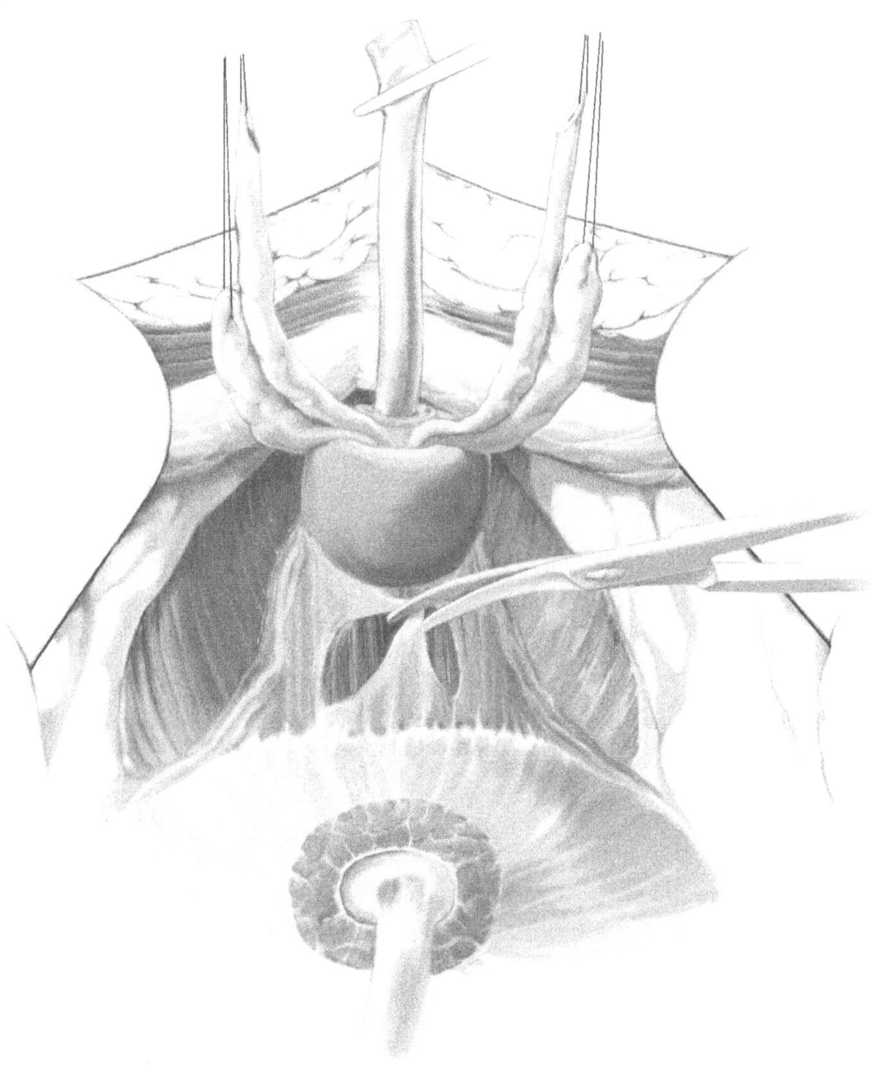

Denonvilliers fascia is opened in the midline and the dorsal aspect of the prostae is bluntly mobilized by finger dissection. By pulling the prostate up, prostate and prerectal fat can be separated by Satinsky scissors.

16 Radical Retropubic Nerve Sparing Prostatectomy

H. HULAND, R. HOFMANN

The neurovascular bundle contains nervi cavernosi, lymphatic vessels, arterial branches from prostatic arteries, nerve fibers from the pelvic plexus, and the deep dorsal penile vein. It is covered by a layer of the parietal plane of the pelvic fascia. The striated rhabdosphincter in the pelvic floor is innervated from branches from the pudendal nerve. This nerve runs underneath the levator muscle on the internal obturator muscle in a separate canal (Alcock's canal) and traverses the pelvic floor to reach the dorsal side of the penis.

During release of the dorsal vein complex it is not necessary to immediately oversew that structure. Control of bleeding can either be achieved by moderate direct stitching underneath the veins or by letting the divided veins bleed and simply compressing them with a sponge stick. After release of the urethra, the dorsal vein complex can be oversewn to provide stability for the sutures and control backbleeding. The wedge shaped proximal defect can either be left open or sutured in a V-shape. Prior medial stitches may lift up the lateral pelvic fascia covering the lateral aspect and the neurovascular bundle, leaving them prone to later injury. To avoid injury to the nerve bundle, the urethra and striated sphincter should be divided not too closely to the apex of the prostate, because in some patients the neurovascular bundle can be very close to the apex (whereas it runs parallel to the urethra a few millimeters further distally). There may be angulation of the neurovascular bundle medially at the apex of the prostate. For hemostasis, small hemoclips should be used or carefully placed sutures, whereas cautery may lead to nerve damage. The anastomotic sutures should be placed with care at the 4 to 6 and 6 to 8 o'clock positions. Sutures should not go too deep and care has to be taken to avoid the 5 and 7 o'clock positions. A right angle clamp is not used since its application may lead to inadvertent inclusion of the neurovascular bundle into the division of the posterior striated sphincter. For division of the dorsal venous complex it is best to directly place stitches underneath the venous complex and tie instead of undermining with a McDougal clamp.

Nerve sparing technique requires that the medial fascia lateral to the apices be opened and a plane dissected close to Denonvilliers' fascia. The bundles are moved away from the prostate and displaced laterally. Injury to the bundles occurs either by anastomotic sutures at the 5 and 7´o clock position being placed too deeply or by efforts to achieve hemostasis beneath the urethral stump. In nerve sparing procedures any hemostatic suturing below the urethra should be avoided.

In order to avoid injury to the prostatic plexus dissection proceeds along the prostate close to the seminal vesicles.

The fibers of the neurovascular bundle run cranially to Denonvilliers' fascia between the posterolateral surface of the prostate and the rectum. To mobilize the neurovascular bundle, which lies in the periprostatic fascia over the surface of the prostate, it is necessary to open the thin periprostatic fascia and expose the neurovascular bundle. This structure can be pushed downward after freeing and ligating small vessels originating from the bundle and leading upward to the prostate.

With a peanut dissector, the neurovascular bundle can be gently pushed downwards and laterally. Care has to be taken to stay close to the lateral aspect of the seminal vesicles and leave the DE fascia at the neurovascular bundle to avoid injuring the pelvic plexus.

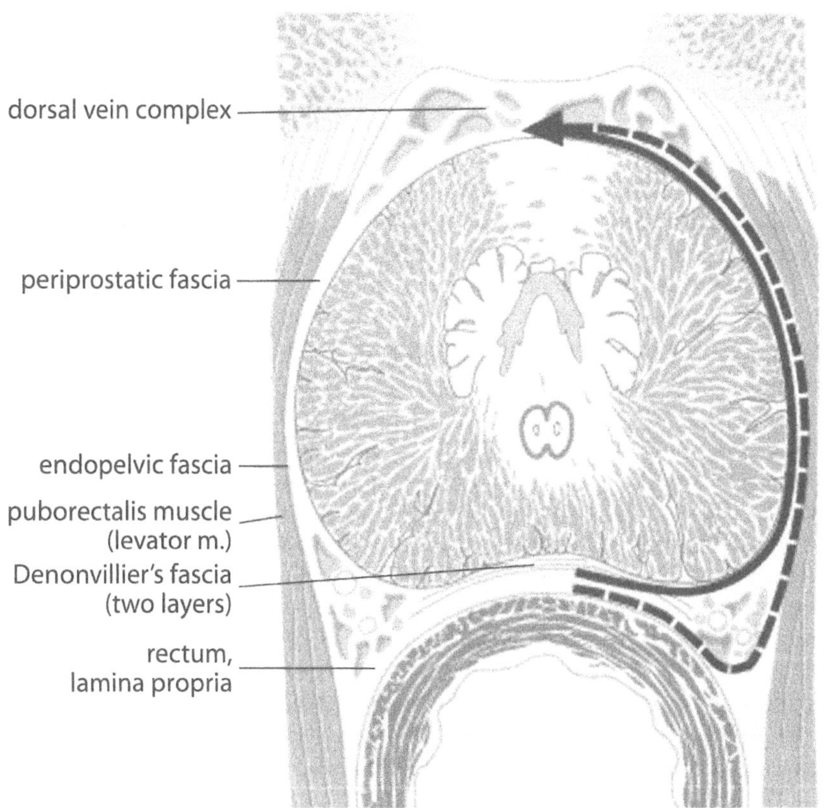

Axial section through mid prostate. Lines show dissection for retropubic nerve-sparing prostatectomy (——) and non-nerve-sparing radical prostatectomy (-----). The lateral leaf of the periprostatic fascia encases the neurovascular bundle. Anterior laterally it fuses with the endopelvic fascia.

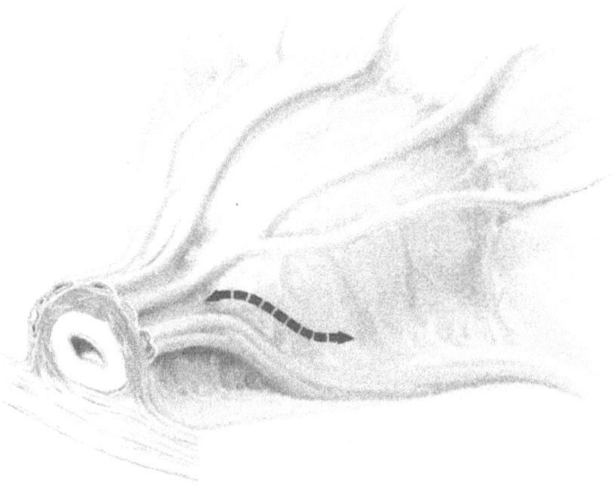

Location of the neurovascular bundle at the apex of the prostate. There may be angulation of the neurovascular bundle medially at the apex. The arrow indicates the plane of dissection.

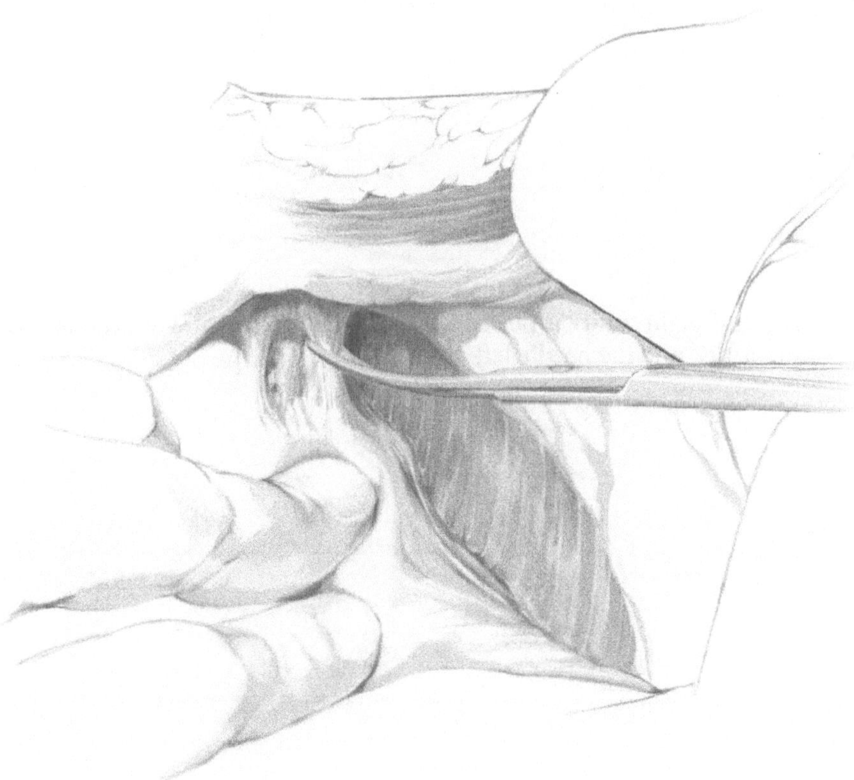

The puboprostatic ligaments should be exposed bluntly by teasing away fatty tissue with pick-ups. Incision is done close to the symphysis to avoid the dorsal vein complex.

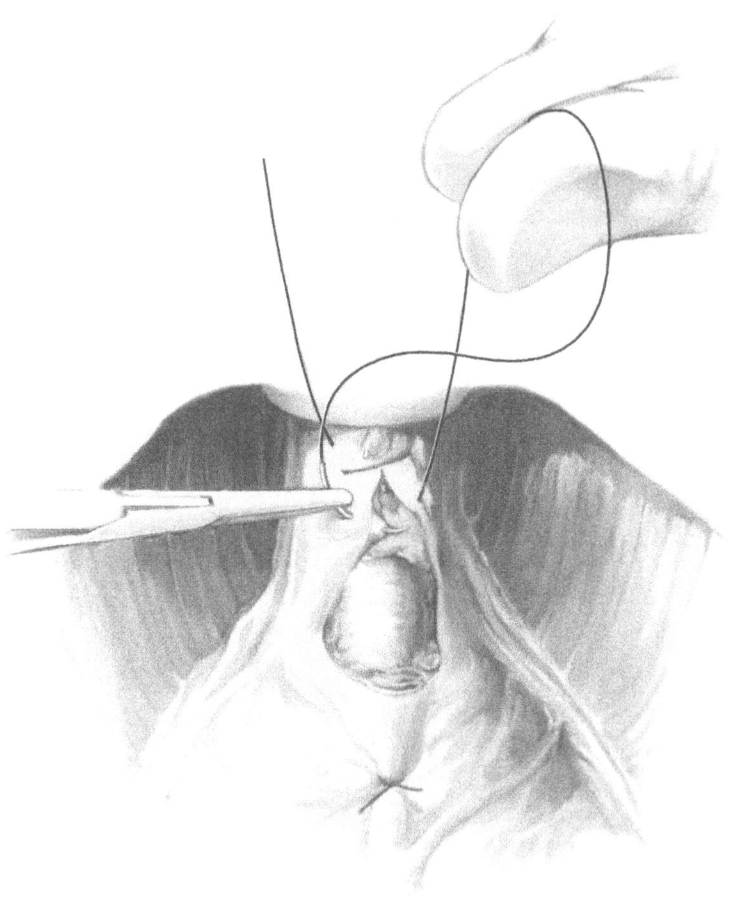

A figure-of-eight suture is placed under the dorsal vein and its tributaries. The suture is tied and the needle left on the suture.

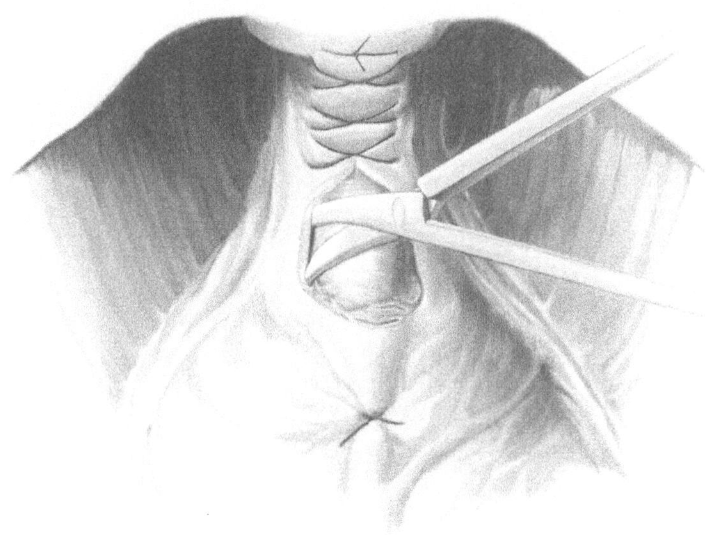

The dorsal vein complex is oversewn to provide stability for the anastomotic sutures and to control backbleeding.

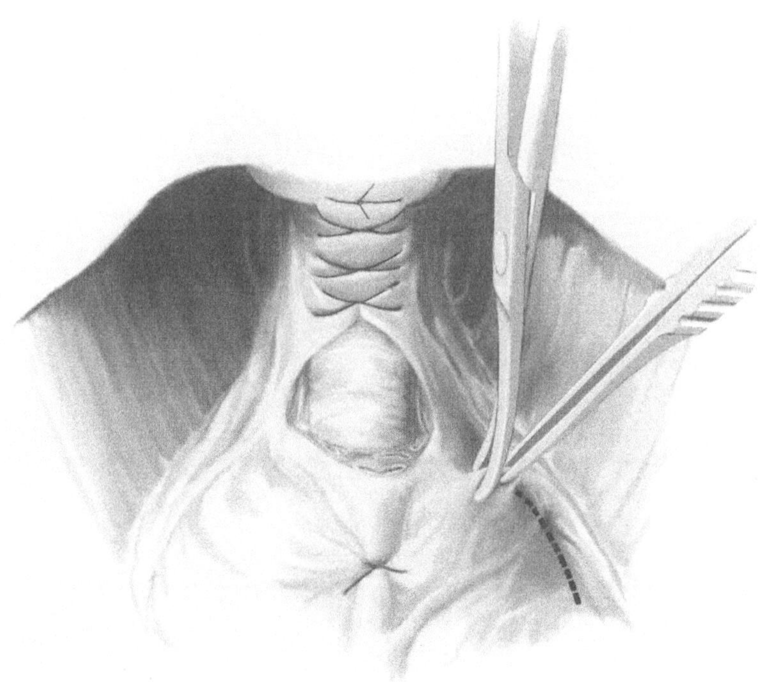

Nerve sparing technique requires that the medial fascia lateral to the apices be opened and a plane dissected close to Denonvilliers fascia. The neurovascular bundle is separated completely from the apex and the proximal 5 mm of the urethra before the urethra is divided from the apex.

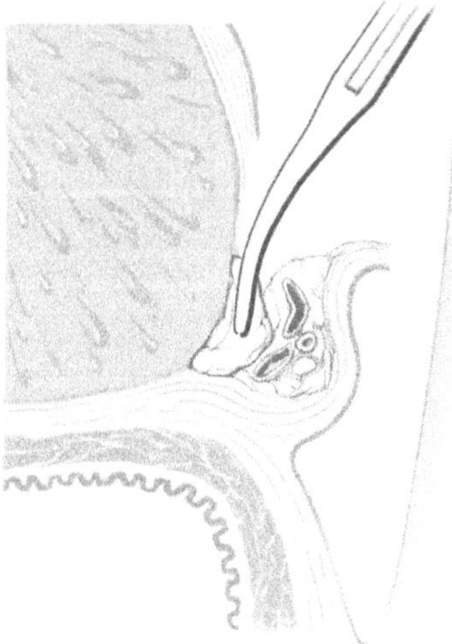

With a peanut dissector, the neurovascular bundle can be gently pushed downwards and laterally.

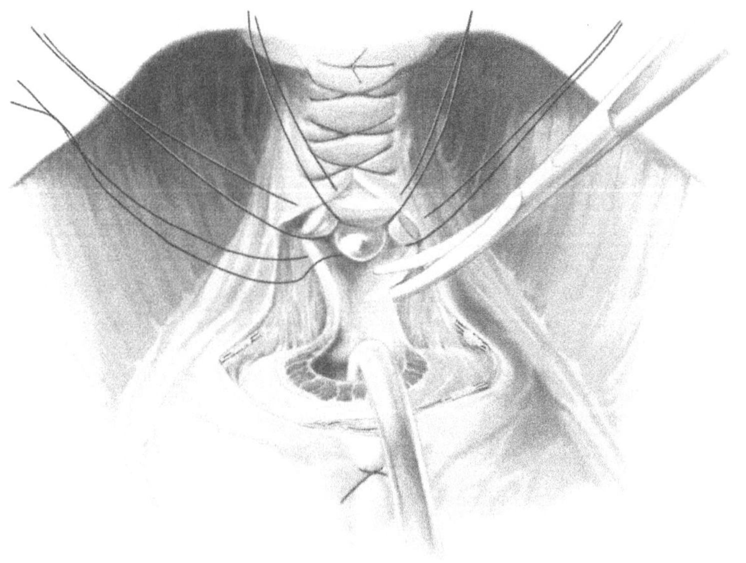

Five anastomotic sutures are placed before dividing the posterior aspect of the urethra.

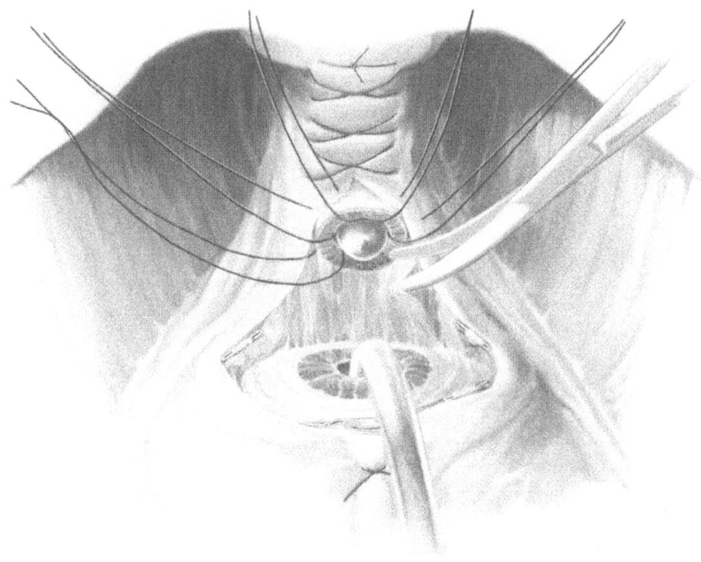

The two-layered character of Denonvillier's fascia being surgically insignificant, it is divided.

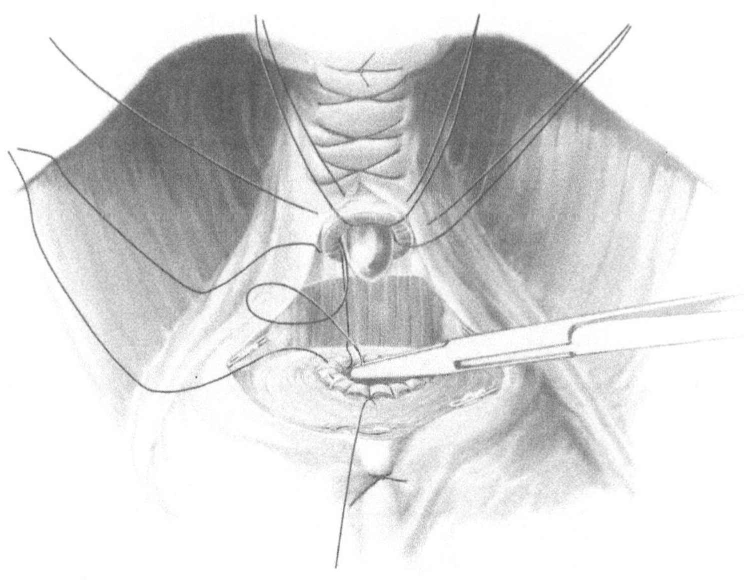

Bladder mucosa is everted by two running semicircular sutures. The five and seven o'clock anastomotic sutures in the urethra are placed appropriately in the everted bladder neck.

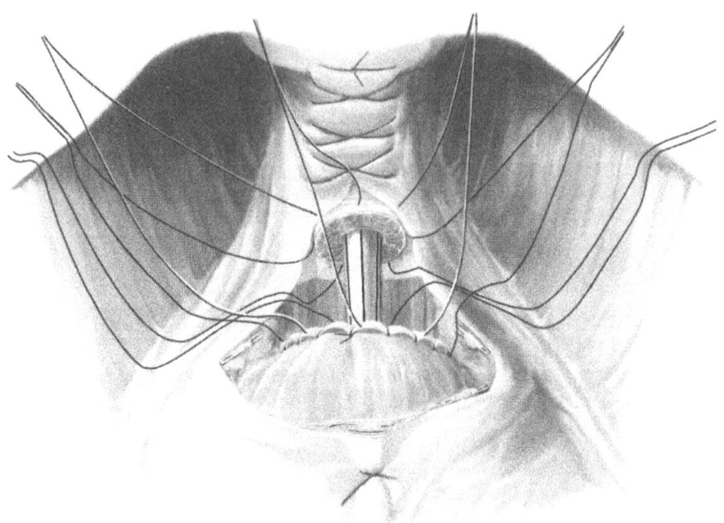

The urethral catheter is placed in the bladder, the ballon inflated and pulled cranially. Overall seven anastomotic sutures are placed.

17 Perineal Prostatectomy

D. Paulson, R. Hofmann

It is advisable to perform perineal prostatectomy only when the prostate weighs less than 40 g, intertuberosity distance is wide, and there has been no previous perineal surgery.

The sacrum is brought to the end of the table, the buttocks extending a bit beyond. The feet are elevated in stirrups and the patient moved into extended lithotomy position. The perineum should be parallel to the floor. Skin incision is performed in an inverted U-fashion.

After developing the ischiorectal fossa, the so-called central tendon, the fusion of the superficial anal sphincter with the raphe, is incised. The superficial part of the external anal sphincter is avoided and dissection begun anteriorly. Following transection of these fascial bands, the retrobulbar space is developed. Retracting the anus down leads to a plane beneath the deep external anal sphincter. Puborectalis and pubococcygeus muscles have to be retracted to find access to the prostate. Distal to the apex of the prostate the rectourethralis muscle reaches up from the rectum to the perineal body. In some patients it can be broad and pronounced, while in others very few fibers can be found.

The Lowsley retractor can help in finding the apex of the prostate and defining the plane for transecting the rectourethralis muscle. To avoid incising the rectum, which is in most danger at this point, the index finger is used to displace the rectum posteriorly and put tension on the rectourethralis muscle.

Following central incision of the rectourethralis, the muscle fibers of the levator are moved laterally away from the prostate. As a nerve sparing procedure, the slings of levator muscles and the neurovascular bundle can be dissected away from the prostate. With the use of the Lowsley retractor, the prostate is rotated in the direction of the surgeon. A plane is developed between Denonvilliers' fascia and the rectum to expose the posterior aspect of the prostate and the seminal vesicles. Once the midline space behind the prostate has been exposed, the lateral vascular pedicles are developed and ligated. To reach the apex, the fibers overlying the urethra are cut away and the urethra is isolated with a rectangle clamp. The space between the apical vascular pedicles and the prostate is developed and the dissection continued under the dorsal vein complex. Now the urethra can be cut and the ends secured with anastomotic sutures. With a Young retractor the prostate can be drawn into the wound and the anterior plane of dissection defined. The plane between the bladder and prostate is identified and the detrusor fibers moved away. The urethra at the bladder neck is cut anteriorly. A Foley catheter is inserted into the bladder, grabbed, and removed through the incision. With the catheter loop, the prostate can be further pulled down and out. When dissecting toward the rectum, fatty tissue is encountered and the seminal vesicles and vasa deferentia exposed. The prostate is fixed to the rectum only by Denonvilliers' fascia at this point in the operation. The prostate is lifted up anteriorly and the tissue transected sharply. The tips of the seminal vesicles and the vasa deferentia are clipped and divided. A racket-handle closure of the bladder neck is performed from the 6 and

12 o'clock positions using interrupted 0 monocryl sutures and the mucosa of the bladder everted outwards. Overall, six anastomotic sutures are placed and tied over a 20F Foley catheter.

A finger is placed in the rectum to ensure that no defect has been caused. In case of a rectal laceration, the defect is closed in two layers with imbricating 2–0 Vicryl sutures.

Wound closure is done by interrupted sutures, bringing the central tendon muscles to the perineal body. A Penrose drain is left in the prerectal space and the skin closed.

With the technique of extended perineal prostatectomy, the paraprostatic fascia or lateral pelvic fascia is also removed, in contrast to the conventional perineal prostatectomy, in which the prostate only is removed from within the paraprostatic fascia.

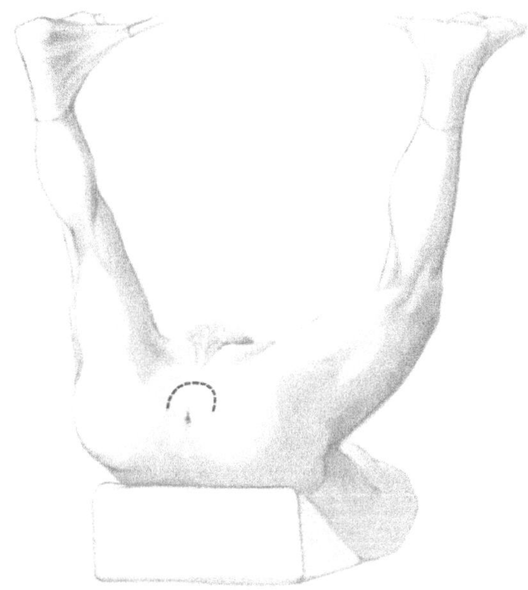

The patient is placed in an exaggerated lithotomy position and a broad U-shaped incision is made around the rectum.

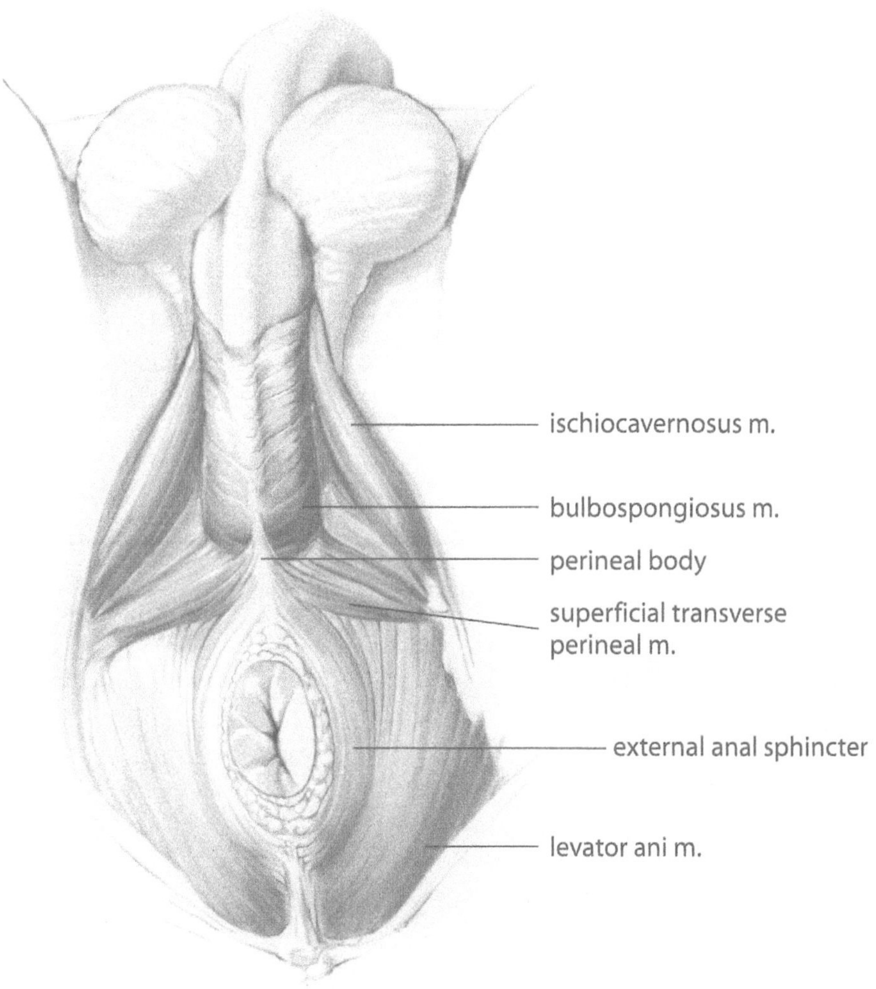

Superficial perineal space

The central tendon is divided at the level of its insertion on the perineal body.

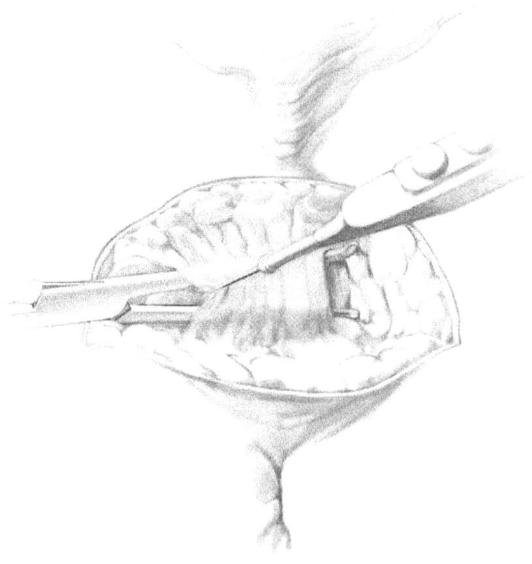

Division of the central tendon.

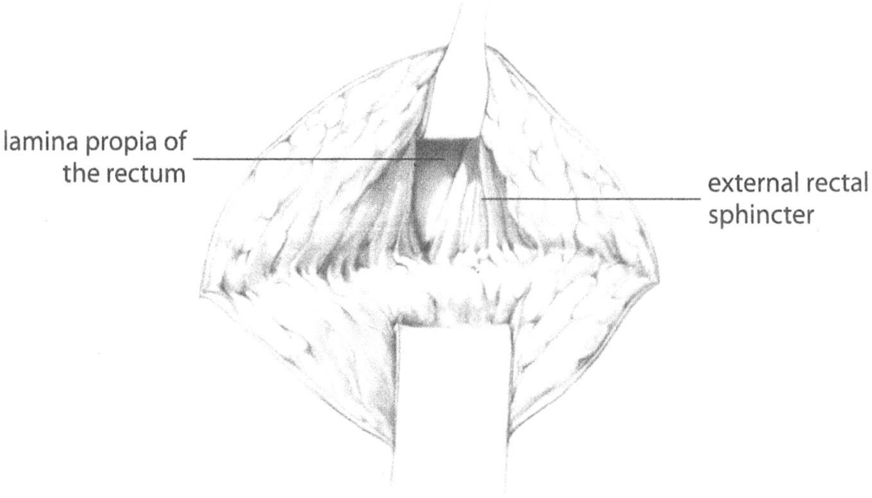

The external rectal sphincter is lifted away from the rectal lamina propria.

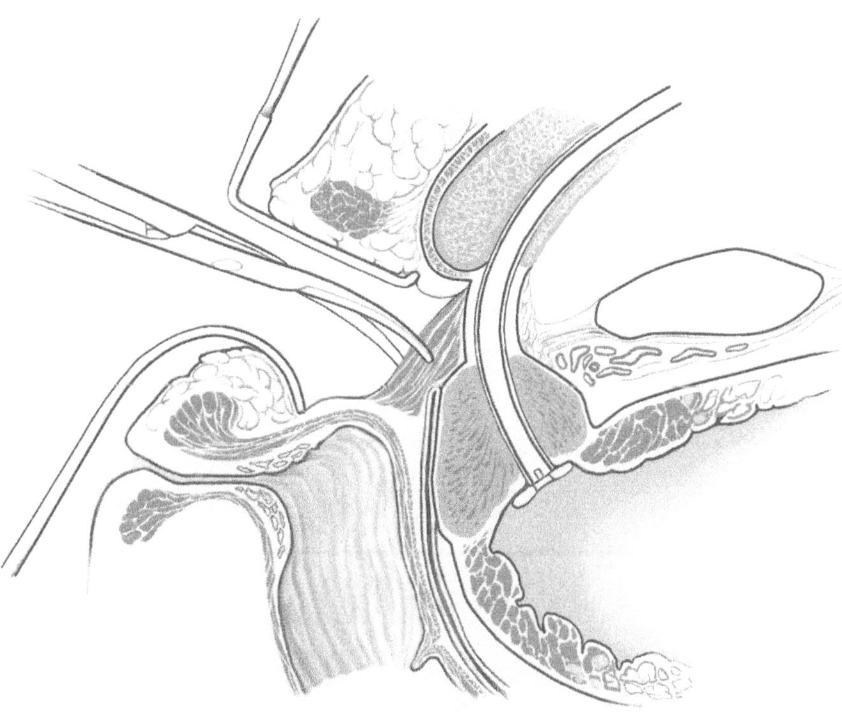

Division of the rectourethralis muscle in the midline.

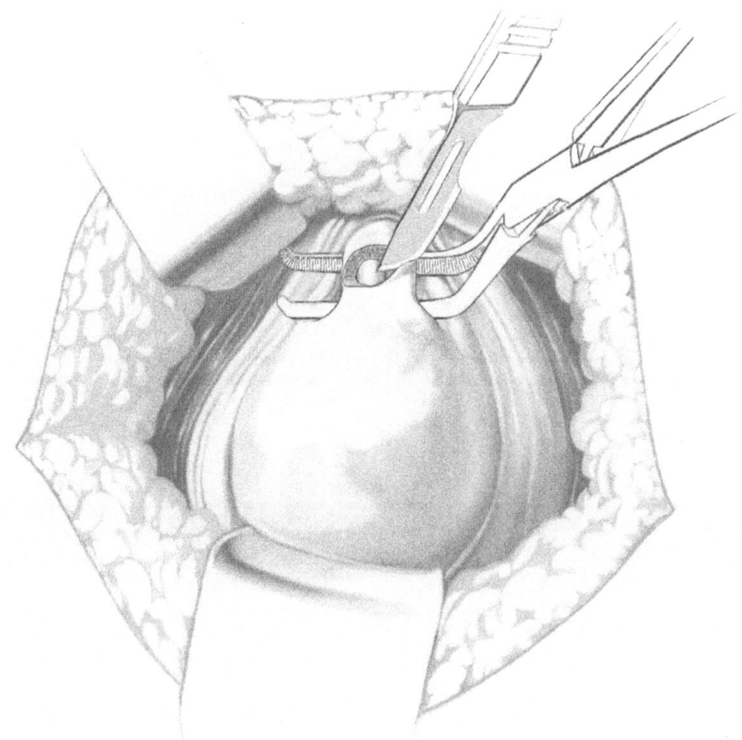

A right angle clamp is placed around the urethra and the urethra is partially divided.

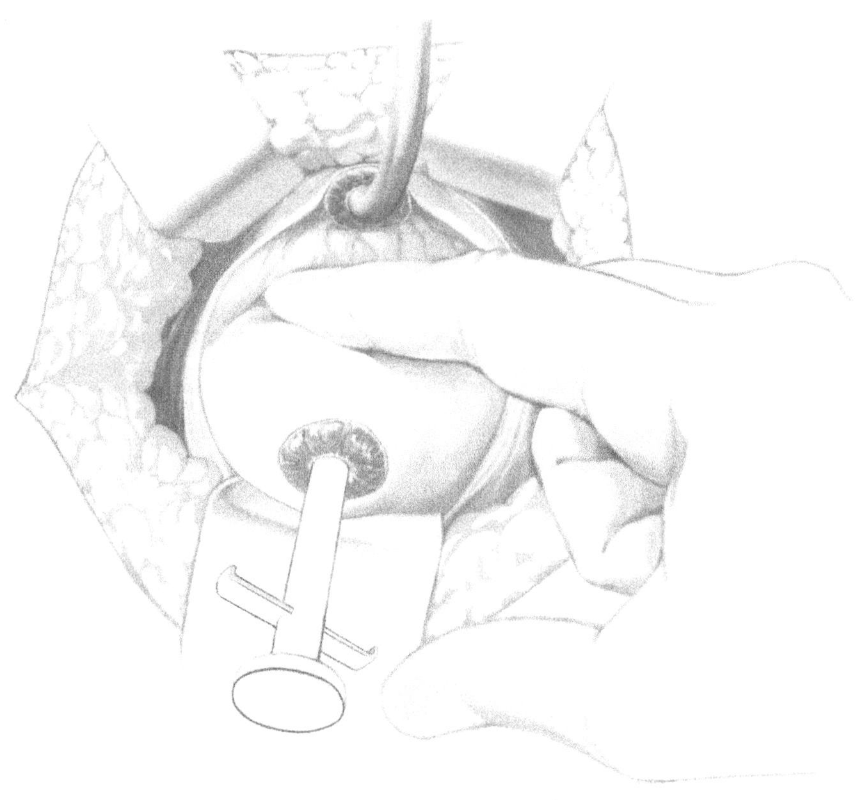

Blunt finger dissection at the anterior surface of the prostate is performed.

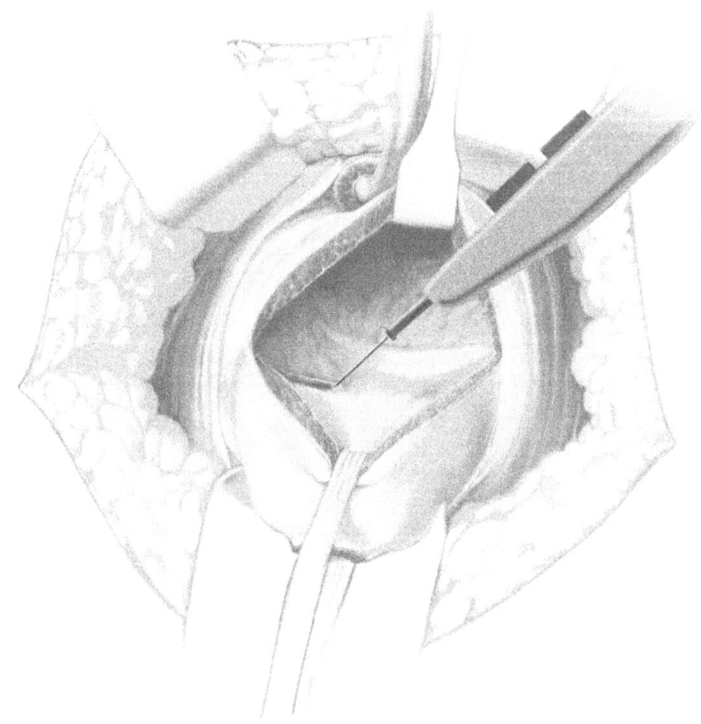

The anterior bladder wall is divided. The posterior bladder wall is cut by electrocautery.

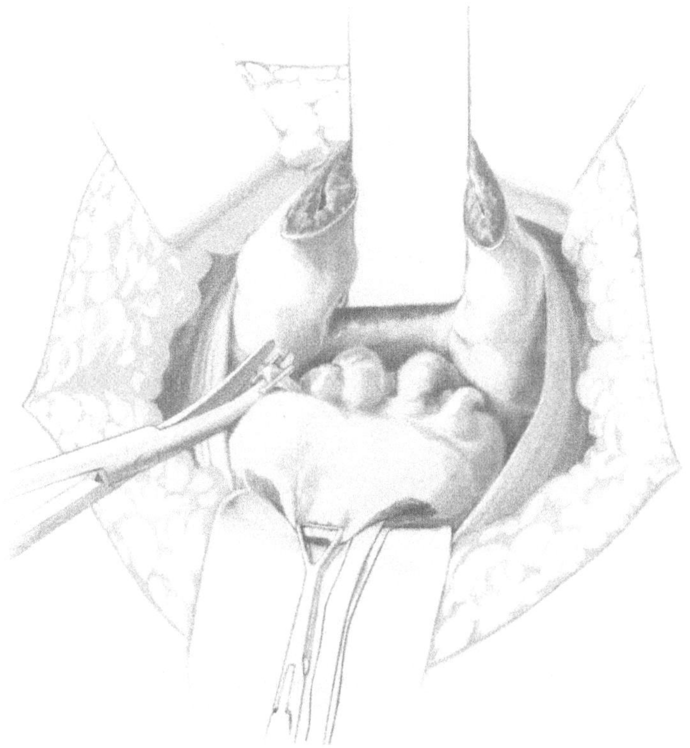

The seminal vesicles and the vas deferens are exposed.

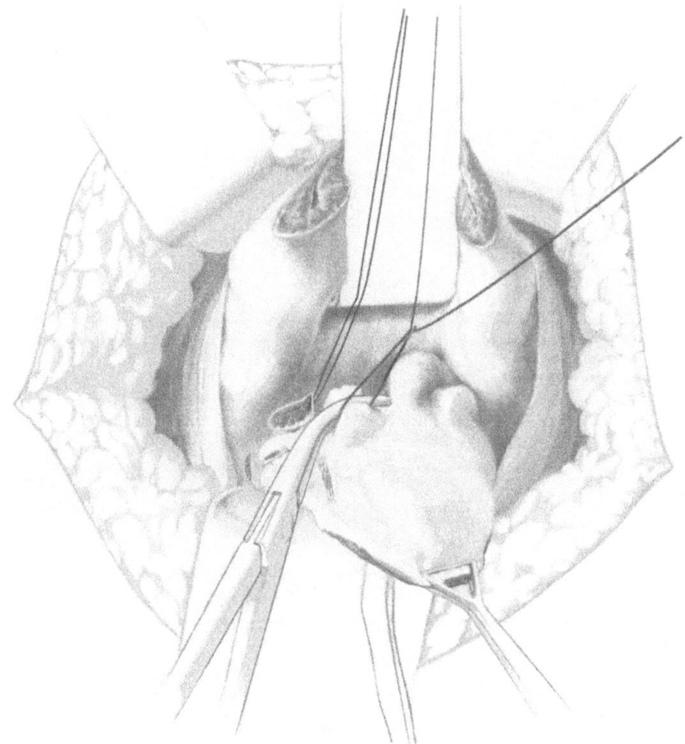

The artery to the seminal vesicles is controlled by ligation.

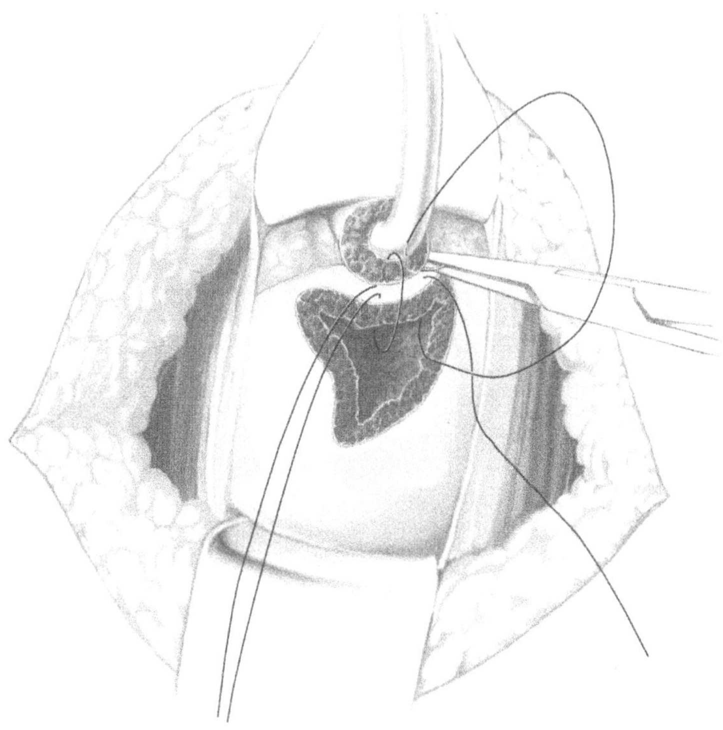

4-0 Monocryl sutures are placed between urethra and bladder neck.

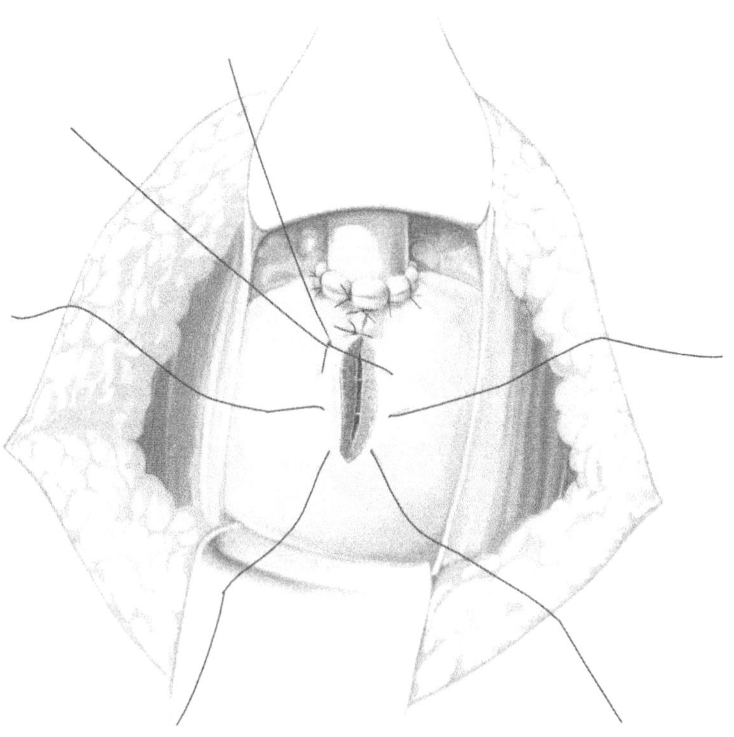

The bladder neck is closed with zero Monocryl sutures with a racket handle closure.

18 Penile Prosthesis Implantation

F. Schreiter, R. Hofmann

Broad spectrum antibiotics (cephalosporins) are given preoperatively and continued for 7 days. The patient is to take a povidine iodine shower before operation. Suprapubic and genital hair is removed in the OR, a 15-min scrub is done, and operating room traffic limited.

A transverse incision is made 1 cm above the symphysis.

The base of the penis is exposed and cleared from fat. A 2 cm incision in the corpus cavernosum is made between stay sutures. The corpus cavernosum is dilated distally and proximally by Hegar 9–13 bougies or Jarrett bougies to 43 F. The dilation should be completely distal to the corpus underneath the glans to avoid tilting the glans with inserted cylinders. Measurement of the penile length from the incision distally and from the incision proximally is done. Exact measurement for proper size is necessary; oversizing should be avoided. The total length minus 1 cm for the Ultrex AMS prosthesis is preferred. A needle is completely inserted into the Furlow inserter and passed to the distal end of the corpus cavernosum. Then the needle is advanced through the gland lateral and proximal to the urethral meatus. The needle is pulled out and the suture clamped and pulled.

The cylinder is held under traction while the proximal end is inserted into the crus. The tunica is closed with interrupted 2-0 absorbable sutures. The same procedure is commenced at the other side. Care has to be taken not to perforate the septum with the dilators or to cross the needle.

For pump insertion, a pocket is created with a slightly curved clamp beneath the dartos fascia lateral to the testicle. The opening is widened by a long nose speculum and the pump is placed at the most dependent portion of the hemiscrotum. The pump is held in place by a Babcock clamp when connecting the tubes. The reservoir is placed inside the peritoneum to avoid encasement in scar tissue, which may ensue if it is placed in an extraperitoneal area. Therefore the rectus abdominus muscle sheath is opened and the belly of the rectus divided bluntly to the transverse fascia and the peritoneum.

The reservoir is filled with 100 cc Ultravist 150 for penile prosthesis longer than 18 cm and with 65 cc for smaller ones. The prosthesis is half filled, and will be emptied on the second day and reactivated gradually over the course of 6 weeks. Thereafter full erection can be performed. A 14 F bladder catheter should be placed for 1 to 3 days.

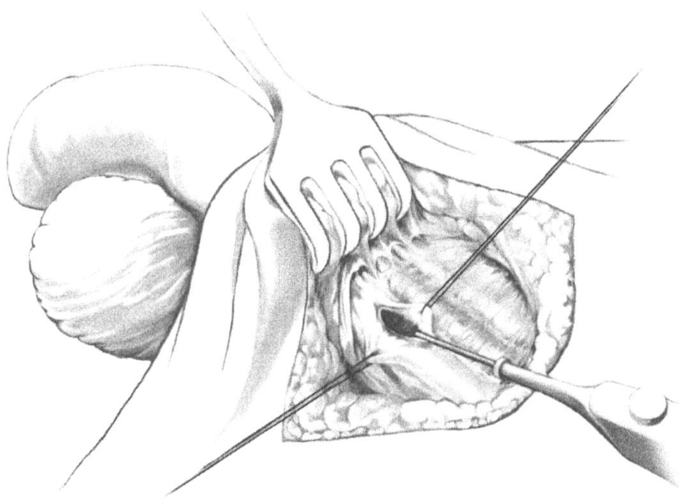

A 2 cm incision in the corpus cavernosum is made between stay sutures.

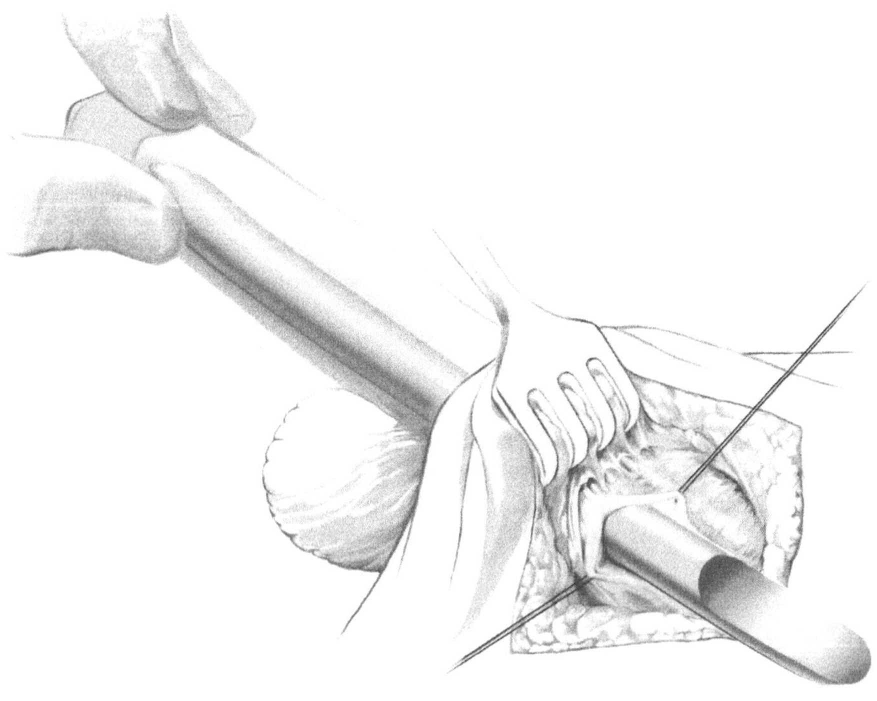

The corpus cavernosum is dilated distally. The dilation should be completely distal to the corpus underneath the glans to avoid tilting the glans with inserted cylinders.

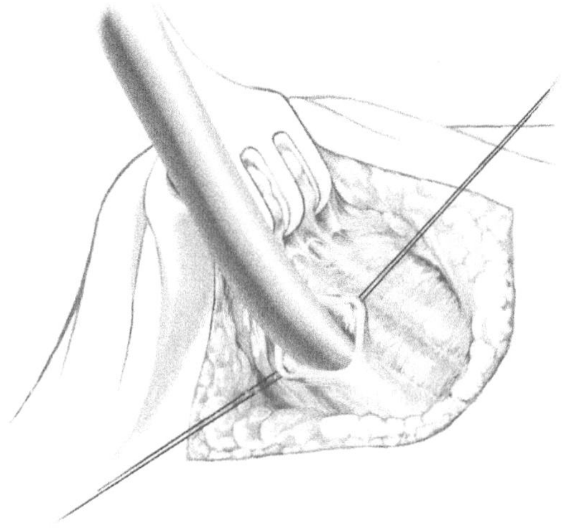

Dilation proximally by Hegar 9 to 13 bougies or Jarrett bougies to 43 F.

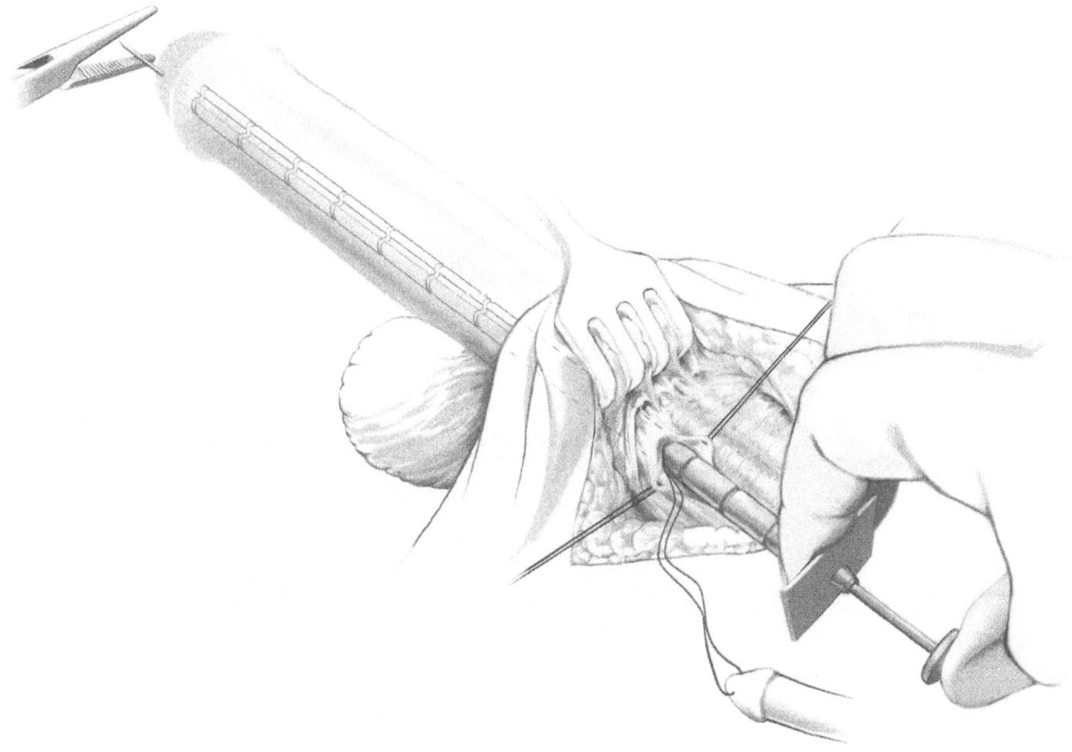

A needle is completely inserted into the Furlow inserter and passed to the distal end of the corpus and ejected to the glans lateral and proximal to the meatus.

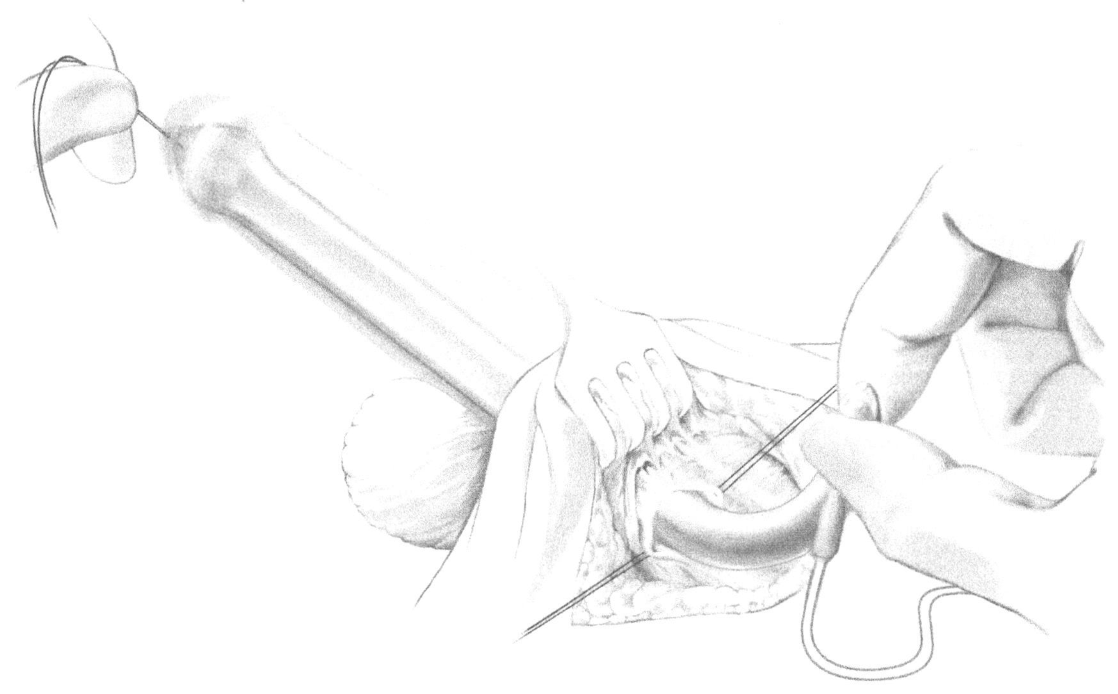

The cylinder is held under traction while the proximal end is inserted into the crus.

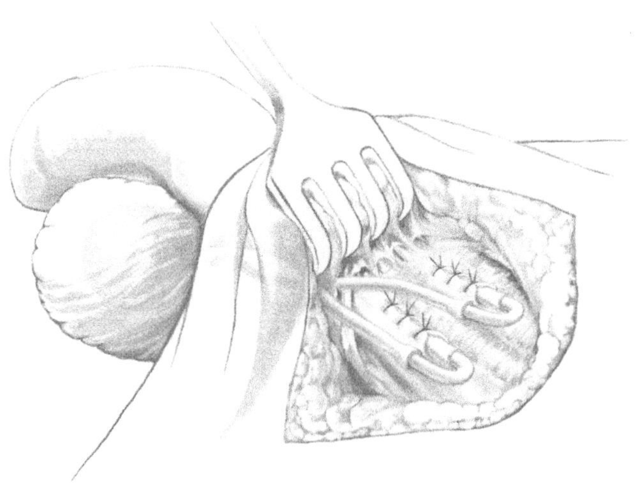

The tunica is closed with interrupted 2-0 absorbable sutures.

19 Artificial Urinary Sphincter Implantation

F. Schreiter, R. Hofmann

The artificial sphincter consists of three parts:

1. A pressure regulating reservoir with a pressure of 50–60, 60–70 and 70–80 cm H_2O
2. A cuff, which is placed around the urethra and can be filled and emptied
3. A control pump, which regulates fluid transport from the reservoir to the cuff

Normally the cuff is fluid filled and compresses the urethra circumferentially. The pressure in the cuff is determined by the pressure in the reservoir. Usually 60–70 cm H_2O is sufficient for continence. Pressing the pump empties the cuff and lets the urethra open. After 2 min fluid runs back to the cuff passively, impelled by the reservoir's elasticity. The whole sphincter system can also be completely deactivated.

In order to qualify for sphincter implantation, the patient should have a bladder capacity of at least 200 cc H2o, a normotonic or hypoactive detrusor, and no major urethral or bladder neck stricture. Following incision or resection of a bladder neck stenosis, a sphincter should be implanted no less than 3 months postoperatively. Patient motivation and normal intelligence and dexterity are prerequisites for implantation. Ureterorenal reflux higher than grade 2 should be corrected at the same time of sphincter implantation.

Urinary tract infection should be treated until a sterile urine is documented.

Preoperatively the patient is administered cephalosporin antibiotics for 3 days to cover for *Staphylococcus epidermidis*; he takes a sitz bath with betadine solution, and washes his genitals with betadine the evening before the operation. Shaving is done in the OR, immediately before a 15 min scrub of the operative field with betadine solution. Traffic in the OR should be restricted to a minimum. During the operation the wound is irrigated with Gentamicin solution.

The urethral sphincter cuff can be implated at the membranous urethra, which is our preferred placement in single cuff implantation, or at the bulbous urethra, where we nrmally implant the double cuff (tandem cuff).

For the membranous implantation of a single cuff the central tendon is cut and the triangular ligament is exposed and incised immediately below the bifurcatio of the crura and beside the urethra. With a right angle clamp the urethra is gently mobilized between the covering sheet of the triangular ligament and the symphysis. At the 12 o'clock position the corpus spongiosum of the urethra is thin, the covering part of the triangular ligament protects the urethra from erosion. For double cuff implantation the bulbous urethra is mobilized from the underlying corpora cavernosa after splitting the bulbo cavernous muscle. Two 4.5 cm or 4.0 cm long cuffs are implanted closed together. Care has to be taken not to enter the urethra or the surraounding thin fascia of the urethra. If the urethra is injured the implantation of the cuffs can only be continued, when the cuffs can be placed on a different, not injured segment of the urethra.

The catheter is removed and the size of the urethra with surrounding bulbospongiosus muscle measured. Usually a cuff size of 4.5 to 5.0 cm is appropriate. The cuff should fit exactly, but not so tight as to cause tissue atrophy underneath the cuff. Next the cuff is placed around the urethra, leaving the measuring band in place while pulling the cuff through. The centrum tendineum is reconstructed, thus moving the urethral cuff upward and horizontally. With this move, the cuff sits right under the pelvic floor and is covered by bulbospongiosus muscle tissue. Thus the patient does not sit on his sphincter and does not feel the device.

The cuff tube is advanced subcutaneously to an incision in the right groin. The pump is placed in the right hemiscrotum after gently opening a plane above Scarpa's fascia subcutaneously to the most dependent portion of the scrotum.

A pocket is dissected into the right scrotum with a long straight clamp and then a long nose speculum inserted. With this maneuver, postoperative scrotal edema is minimized. The reservoir is placed intraperitoneally to avoid scarring around the reservoir and consequent higher pressure than desired.

The tubes should be isolated from blood and from towel fibers, as blood and fiber may hamper the pump function. Mosquito clamps with a Silicone tubing are used and closed only to first click.

Drains are not necessary.

Pump and cuff tubing is brought to the side of hand dominance, usually to the patients right side.

From the same inguinal incision the peritoneum is opened through an incision in the rectus abdominus muscle, and a 60–70 cm H_2O reservoir is inserted intraperitoneally. The reservoir is filled with 22 cc of water and connected to the pump and the cuff. A right angle connector is used between the pump and the cuff tubing to prevent kinking, whereas connection between reservoir and pump is done by a straight connector.

The sphincter is deactivated for 6 weeks to allow healing, then activated by compressing the distal end of the pump and filling the cuff.

A 12-F transurethral catheter is inserted and left for 3 days. The pump has to be manually pulled down twice daily to prevent upwards movement.

The perineal wound is closed with running 3–0 SAS sutures. Care has to be taken, when adjusting the bulbar muscle and closing the central tendon not to puncture the cuff.

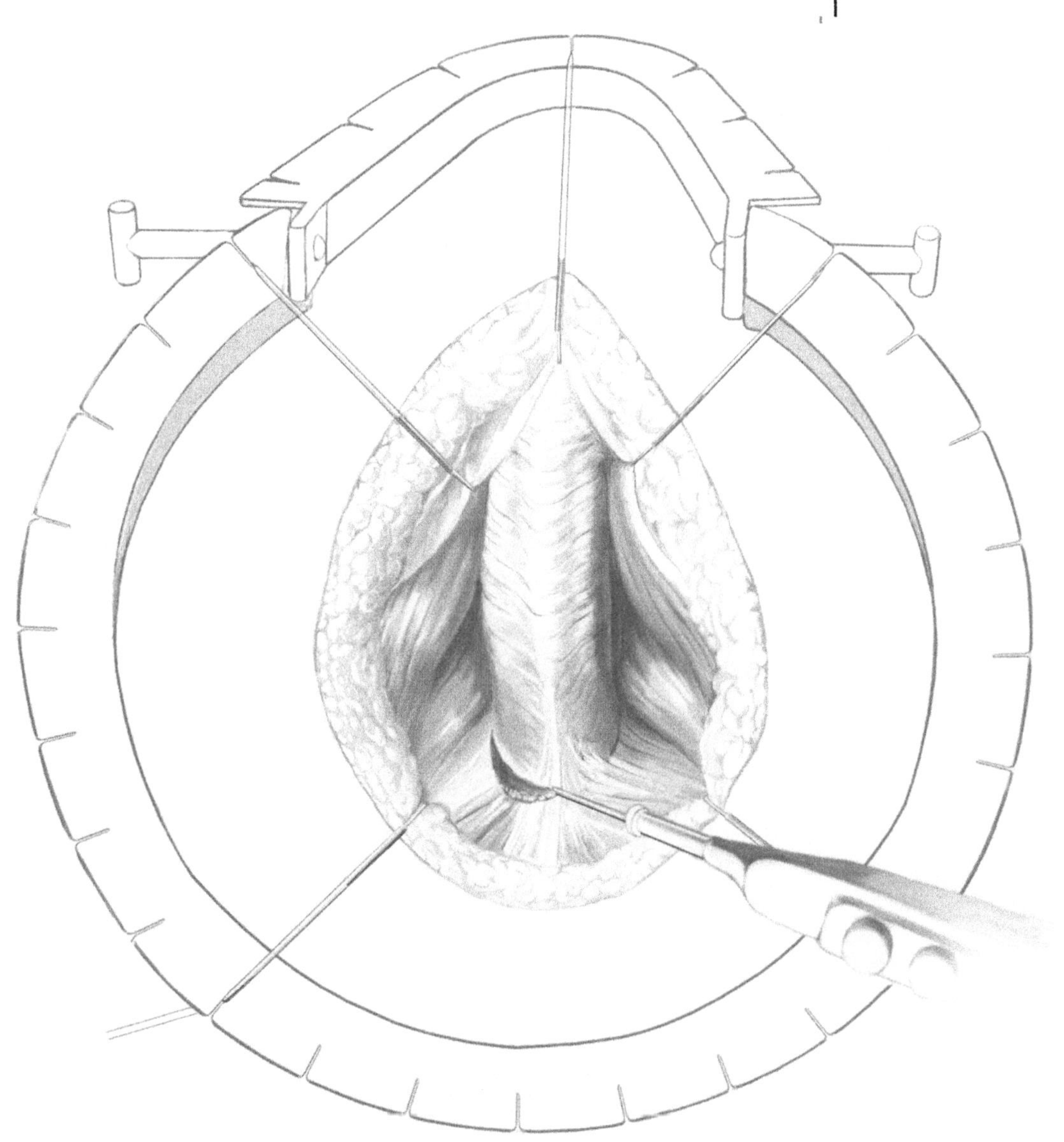

The perineal body (centrum tendineum) is exposed and cut by electrocautery.

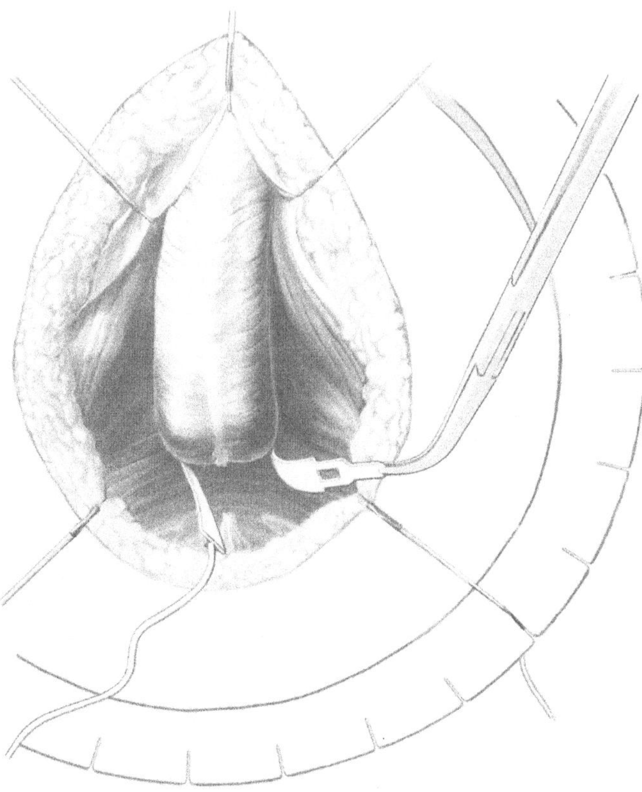

The cuff is placed around the urethra.

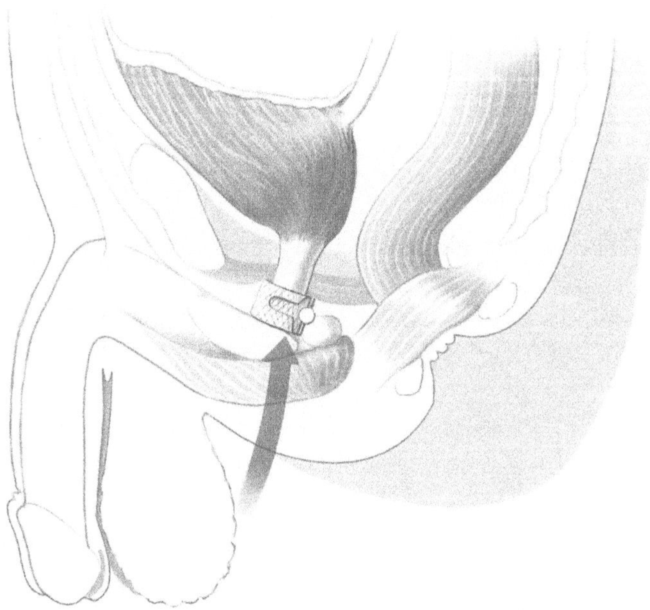

The cuff sits right under the pelvic floor and is covered by bulbospongiosus muscle tissue. The patient does not sit on his sphincter and does not feel the device.

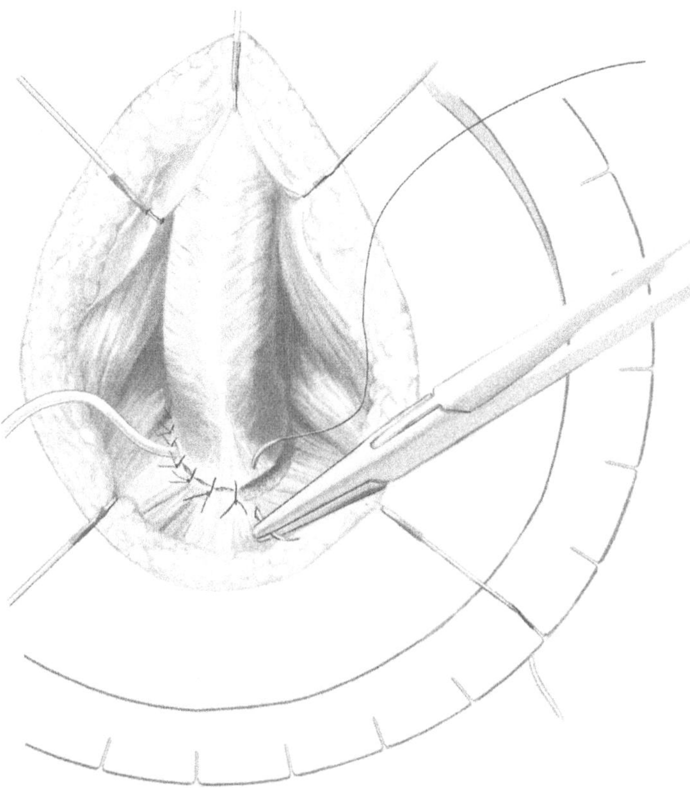

The perineal body (centrum tendineum) is reconstructed, thus moving the urethral cuff upward and horizontally.

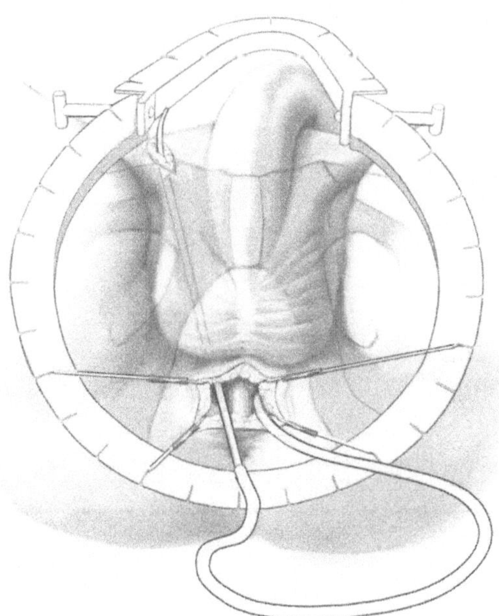

The cuff tube is advanced subcutaneously to an incision in the right groin.

Radiotherapy for Localized Prostate Cancer

20 Radiation Therapy of Prostate Cancer

P. Vacha, R. Engenhart-Cabillic

20.1 Introduction

Radiation therapy for nonmetastatic cancer of the prostate is a highly effective treatment modality. Local control and disease-free 10-year survival rates are equal to those of surgery. Despite the radiation doses of at least 70 Gy necessary for tumor control, the rate of radiation-related side effects can be clearly reduced by using computed tomography (CT)-based three dimensional conformal radiation therapy techniques.

20.2 Indications for Radiation Therapy

Definitive radiation therapy is indicated in tumor stage T1–3, N0, M0. Further, it should be employed after incomplete microscopic or macroscopic tumor resection. Because of the high risk of recurrence, pathologically staged T3 tumors are an indication for adjuvant radiation therapy, especially if unfavorable Gleason scores, high pretherapy prostate-specific antigen (PSA) levels, seminal vesicle involvement, or tumor growth within the proximal urethra has been a finding. Radiation therapy is indicated as well if increasing PSA levels suggest local recurrence, or if histologically proved local tumor recurrence has been found after surgery. If massive pelvic extension of the carcinoma or lymph node metastasis cause pelvic pain, hematuria, or urethral obstruction, palliative radiation therapy may be effective.

20.3 Irradiation

Definitive radiation therapy should be started immediately after the diagnostic examinations are finished. If the tumor is large, endocrine therapy before irradiation may be helpful since tumor reduction leaves a smaller target volume. After surgery at least 4 weeks should elapse before irradiation is started in order to decrease sequelae such as urinary incontinence or urethral stricture. If radiation therapy follows prostatectomy after a delay of 12–16 weeks no increase in side effects should be expected.

To minimize radiation-related side effects, irradiation should be performed only after therapy has been planned making use of CT-based three-dimensional techniques that conform with the anatomy and make use of linear accelerators with an energy of at least 6 MeV (Fig. 20.1). For best protection of organs at risk, individualized field shapes, realized by a multi-leaf-collimator or blocks that physically conform with the structures involved, are necessary.

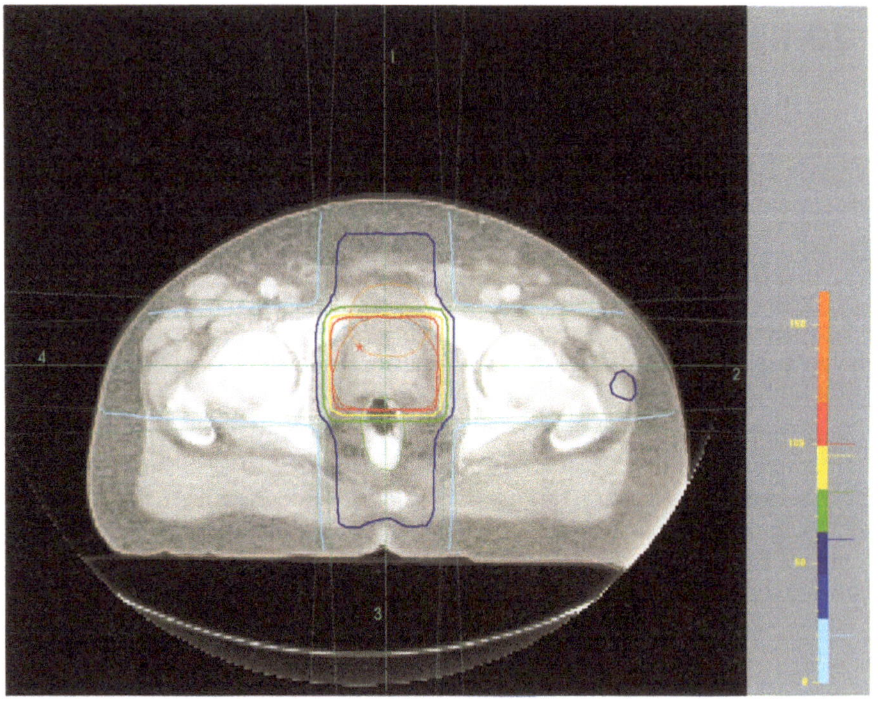

Fig. 20.1. Isodose curves with 18 MeV photons as a result of CT-based three-dimensional conformal therapy using four fields

20.3.1 The Volume To Be Treated

The planning target volume for stage T1–3 cancer encompasses the prostate and the seminal vesicles, with a small zone of 0.5–0.7 cm of surrounding tissue. Motion of organs and position variabilities must be considered. Only for stage T1a is the inclusion of the prostate without seminal vesicles sufficient. If possible, the planning target volume will be reduced after 50 Gy has been delivered, only the prostate itself remaining as the target for boost irradiation. No evidence has appeared to date that irradiation of pelvic lymph nodes has any effect on overall or disease-free survival rates. For that reason, irradiation of these nodes is only recommended if metastases are likely.

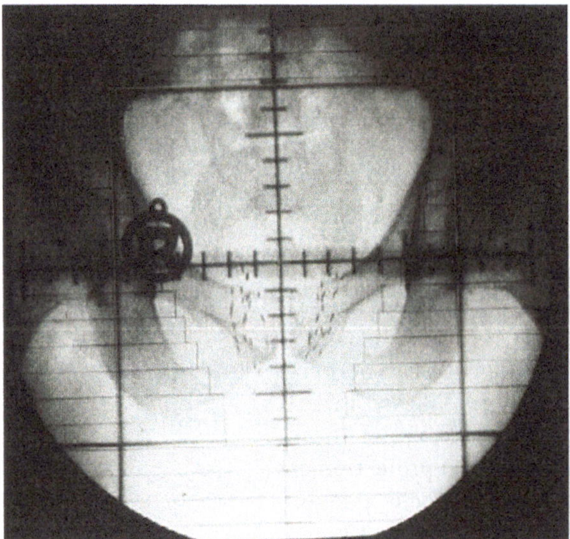

Fig. 20.2. Anterior-posterior three-dimensional, conformal, multileaf-collimator shaped portal for irradiation of prostate and seminal vesicles. Note: patient was treated with iodine-125 seeds before external beam irradiation

20.3.2 Radiation Therapy Techniques

As the result of CT-based three-dimensional conformal therapy planning, patients are treated via four, five, or six isocentric portals (Fig. 20.2). In the future, intensity modulated radiotherapy will be integrated in the treatment of prostate cancer. This technology promises to improve dose distribution, providing higher doses to the tumor without increasing tissue doses.

20.3.3 Treatment Doses

Minimum doses for long-term tumor control in patients with cancer of prostate are set forth in Table 20.1.

Table 20.1. Minimum tumor doses for adenocarcinoma of prostate depending on tumor stage

Tumor stage	Dose (Gy)
T1a	64–66
T1b,c–T2	66–70
T3	70–72
T1–3, irradiation following incomplete tumor resection (R1/2)	66/70
Recurrent tumor	70–72
T4; palliative irradiation	50–65

Because doses above 72 Gy may cause extensive reactions in normal tissue, higher tumor doses should not be applied except for clinical trials. At present, such trials are investigating whether doses up to 80 Gy improve treatment results. Conventional treatment is performed with administration of 1.8–2.0 Gy daily five times per week, to continue until the total dose has been given as outlined in Table 20.1. Dose prescription (Fig. 20.3) should follow the guidelines of International Commission on Radiation Units [9, 10].

20.4 Brachytherapy

20.4.1 Remote Afterloading Technique

Local dose escalation by interstitial radiation therapy, especially in T3 stage cancer of prostate, may improve local control and survival rates. At present the most used brachytherapeutic treatment modality is a temporary placement of a radioactive source such as iridium-192. Needles are introduced transperineally under ultrasound or CT guidance. With computerized treatment planning systems, dwell times, and positions are calculated for best dose distribution. Interstitial irradiation is performed in one to three courses with tumor doses of 18–30 Gy each. Additional conventional fractionated external beam irradiation is necessary before or after interstitial irradiation to a dose amount of 30–50 Gy. Unfortunately, long-term results of this combined treatment modality are not available at this time.

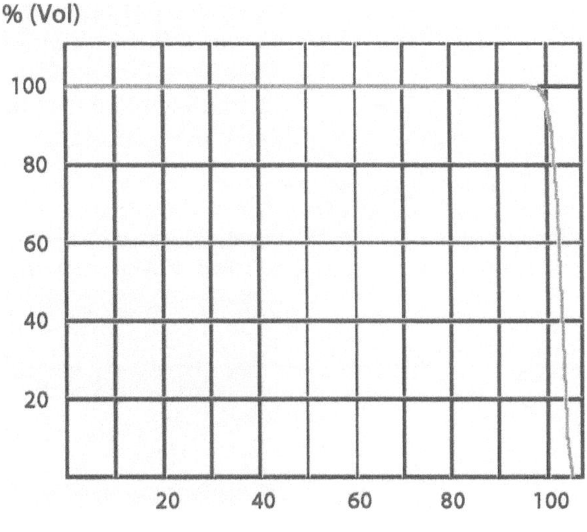

Fig. 20.3. Dose–volume histogram for a four-field three-dimensional conformal irradiation, demonstrating a homogeneous dose distribution according to ICRU report 50/62

20.4.2 Permanent Seed Implants

In contrast to temporary interstitial irradiation by remote afterloading, radioactive seeds with low energy and low specific dose rates (e.g., iodine-125, palladium-103) are implanted permanently in the prostate through an open retropubic laparatomy or by transperineal ultrasound-guided positioning.

This treatment modality should be restricted to T2 stage tumors because tumor doses in periprostatic tissue may be too low for cancers of higher stage. Despite the realization of radiation doses of at least 80 Gy obtainable by seed, external beam irradiation (30–50 Gy) is also necessary.

20.5 Results of Radiation Therapy

20.5.1 Definitive Radiation Therapy

The results obtained with radiation therapy in nonmetastatic carcinoma of the prostate are summarized in Table 20.2. Perez et al. [14], reported on data of 963 patients with cancer of the prostate that no survivors of stage T4 were found after 7 years. The same data showed a strong correlation between local tumor control, dose levels, and stage of the tumor. While in stage T1 5 years after radiation therapy, recurrent tumor was diagnosed in 8% of the patients, the rate was 21% in stage T3.

Pelvic failure after 10 years in patients with stage T3 occurred in 46% if irradiation dose levels were below 61 Gy. In patients treated with dose levels between 67 and 70 Gy, recurrent tumor was observed in 26%. Data published by Hanks et al. [8] and Pollack et al. [16] showed that radiation doses below 67 Gy are inadequate. They demonstrated the importance of sufficient tumor doses as a significant predictive factor for overall survival rate and disease-free survival.

20.5.2 Irradiation after Surgery

Irradiation after radical prostatectomy has been shown to be a clear benefit for the patients. Anscher et al. [1] described results of 159 patients treated with postoperative irradiation up to 65 Gy in pathologic T3/4 disease. The disease-free survival in the irradiated group after 10 years was 55% versus 37% for the group treated with radical prostatectomy alone. A significant reduction in local relapse rates was observerd after adjuvant radiation therapy (8%) compared with only prostatectomy (40%). Despite the improvement in local tumor control, there was no difference in the incidence of distant metastasis. The same

Table 20.2. Disease free survival-rate with 70 Gy external-beam irradiation in patients with stage T1-T3 carcinoma of the prostate

	No. of patients					
	T1	T2	T3	5 years	10 years	15 years
Bagshaw et al. 1990 [2]	308			90%	70%	
		218		87%	65%	
Bagshaw et al. 1993 [3]	335[a]					70%[a]
		242				50%
			409			35%
Perez et al. 1993 [13]			412	58%	38%	
Del Regato et al. 1993 [7]			372	77%	63	50%

[a] Disease-specific survival rate.

conclusion was reached by Valicenti et al. [19] after adjuvant postoperative irradiation in pT3 N0 M0 carcinoma of the prostate.

20.5.3 Irradiation and Endocrine Therapy

Further improvement in treatment results may be expected by combination of irradiation with endocrine therapy. Bolla et al. [5] found in a randomized study including 415 patients with nonmetastatic prostate cancer that disease survival after 5 years in a group treated with goserelin and radiation therapy was significantly better (85%) than in the group received radiotherapy alone (48%). Goserelin was administered at a dose of 3.6 mg subcutaneously every 4 weeks starting on the first day of irradiation and continuing for 3 years. Those patients also received 150 mg cyproterone acetate orally per day for 1 month starting 1 week before first dose of goserelin. Similar findings of a significant reduction in distant metastasis were reported by Pilipich et al. [15] as the result of Radio-Therapy Oncology Group (RTOG) trial, study number 86-10. In neither study was there a difference in morbidity between patients treated with endocrine therapy and irradiation or with irradiation alone. Despite these results, a meta-analysis published by Roach et al. [17] showed that further studies are necessary for the evaluation of criteria for long- versus short-term hormonal treatment.

20.6 Side Effects of Radiation Therapy

Tissue reaction due to radiation therapy depends on single and total dose, the fractionation regimen, and the irradiated volume. Despite the fact that patients undergoing treatment have become older over the last 40 years, the rate of side effects is getting lower [18]. As Hanks [8] pointed out, this reduction seems to be the result of using CT-based three-dimensional conformal therapy techniques, which allow application of high tumor doses while organs at risk are better protected (see Table 20.3). Similar results were reported by Dearnaley et al. [6] namely, a significant reduction in chronic radiation-induced proctitis and rectal bleeding when conformal radiation therapy was used. A further improvement is expected by using intensity-modulated radiation therapy. At this time the incidence of fatal complications due to radiation therapy is about 0.2%. Perez et al. [14] demonstrating the low risk to life of this treatment modality.

Acute gastrointestinal side effects are diarrhea, abdominal cramping, rectal discomfort, and rectal bleeding caused by transient enteroproctitis. Symptoms secondary to cystourethritis include dysuria, frequency, and nocturia. Urinary tract infections are also possible. Acute side effects of the

Table 20.3. Side effects correlated with the treatment modality [12]

	Standard radiation therapy (%)	Three-dimensional conformal therapy (%)
Dysuria/nocturia	25–36	27–33
Diarrhea	9–21	3–6
Proctitis/rectal bleeding	12	3
Difficulty in urinating	6–9	2–5

skin are erythema and dry or moist desquamation, mostly in the perineum and intergluteal fold.

The summarized incidence of late radiation-related urinary and rectosigmoid sequelae according to the RTOG scale is approximately 3%–5% for severe sequelae and 7%–10% for moderate sequelae [4, 12].

The most frequent urinary sequelae are uretheral stricture and cystitis with intermittent hematuria. The risk of severe side effects such as bladder fistula, hemorrhagic cystitis, uretheral stricture, pubic bone or soft tissue necrosis, and leg, scrotal, or penile edema is below 1%. Urinary incontinence occurs in 1% of patients after definitive radiation therapy. If postoperative radiation therapy is not started until 12–16 weeks after surgery, irradiation has not been found to cause urinary incontinence Van Cangh et al. [20], radiation-related sexual dysfunction is seen in 10%–15% after therapy.

The incidence of severe rectosigmoid and small bowel injury that needs surgery, such as perineal abscess, anal stricture, or chronic rectal bleeding is less than 1%. Most of RTOG grade 2 sequelae are proctitis with telangiectasia and occasionally bleeding ulcers. These side effects usually have been treated conservatively.

References

1. Anscher MS, Robertson CN, Prosnitz LR (1995) Adjuvant radiotherapy for pathologic stage T3/4 adenocarcinoma of the prostate: ten year update. Int J Radiat Oncol Biol Phys 33:37–43
2. Bagshaw MA, Cox RS, Ramback JE (1990) Radiation therapy fo localized prostate cancer: Justification by long-term follow-up. Urol Clin North Am 17:787-802
3. Bagshaw MA, Kaplan ID, Cox RC (1993) Radiation therapy for localized disease. Cancer 71:939–952
4. Boehmer D, Dinges S, Budach V (2000) Radiotherapie des Prostatakarzinoms Onkologe 6:130–136
5. Bolla M, Gonzalez D, Warde P, Dubois JB, Mirimanoff RO, Storme G, Bernier J, Kuten A, Sternberg C, Gil T, Collette L, Pierart M (1997) Improved survival in patients with locally advanced prostate cancer treated with radiotherapy and goserelin. N Engl J Med 337:295-300
6. Dearnaley DP, Khoo VS, Norman AR, Meyer L, Nahum A, Tait D, Yarnold J Horwich A (1999) Comparison of radiation side-effects of conformal and conventional radiotherapy in prostate cancer: a randomised trial. Lancet 9149:267–272
7. Del Regato JA, Trailing AH, Pittman DD (1993) Twenty years follow-up of patient with inoperable cancer of the prostate (stage C) treated by radiotherapy: report of a National Cooperative Study. Int J Radiat Oncol Biol Phys 26:197–201
8. Hanks GE, Hanlon AL, Pinover WH, et al (1999) Survival advantage for prostate cancer patients treated with high-dose three dimensional conformal therapy. Cancer J Sci Am 5:152–158
9. International Commission on Radiation Units and Measurements (1993) Report 50: prescribing, recording and reporting photon beam therapy. International Commission on Radiation Units and Measurements, Bethesda
10. International Commission on Radiation Units and Measurements (1999) Report 62: prescribing, recording and reporting photon beam therapy (supplement to ICRU report 50). International Commission on Radiation Units and Measurements, Bethesda
11. Perez CA (1995) Carcinoma of the prostate: a model for management under impending health care reform. Radiology 196:309–322
12. Perez CA, Brady LW (1998) Principles and practice of radiation oncology, 3rd edn. Lippincott-Raven, Philadelphia
13. Perez CA, Lee HK, Georgiou A, et al (1993) Technical and tumor-related factors affecting outcome of definitive irradiation for localized carcinoma of the prostate. Int J Radiat Oncol Biol Phys 26:565–581
14. Perez CA, Michalski J, Lockett MA (1995) Radiation therapy in the treatment of localized prostate cancer: an alternative to an emerging consensus Mol Med 82:696–704
15. Pilipich MV, Sause WT, Shipley WU, et al (1995) Androgen deprivation with radiation therapy compared with radiation therapy alone for locally advanced prostatic carcinoma: a randomised comparative trial of the Radiation Therapy Oncology Group. Urology 45:616–623
16. Pollack A, Smith LG, von Eschenbach AC (2000) External beam radiotherapy dose response characteristics of 1127 men with prostate cancer treated in the PSA era. Int J Radiat Oncol Biol Phys 48:507-512

17. Roach M 3RD, Lu J, Pilepich MV, Asbell SO, Mohiuddin M, Terry R, Grignon D,Lawton C, Shipley W, Cox J, Mohuidden M (2000) Predicting long-term survival, and the need for hormonal therapy: a meta-analysis of RTOG prostate cancer trials. Int J Radiat Oncol Biol Phys 47:617-627
18. Thompson IM, Middleton RG, Optenberg SA, Austenfeld MS, Smalley SR, Cooner WH, Correa RJ, Miller HC, Oesterling JE, Resnick MI, Wasson JH, Roehrborn C (1999) Have complication rates decreased after treatment for localized prostate cancer? J Urol 162:107-112
19. Valicenti RK, Gomella LG, Ismail M, Strup SE, Mulholland SG, Dicker AP, Petersen RO, Newschaffer CJ (1999) The efficacy of early adjuvant radiation therapy for pT3NO prostate cancer: a matched-pair analysis. Int J Radiat Oncol Biol Phys 45(1):53–58
20. Van Cangh PJ, Richard F, Lorge F, Castille Y, Moxhon A, Opsomer R, De Visscher L, Wese FX, Scaillet P (1998) Adjuvant radiation therapy does not cause urinary incontinence after radical prostatectomy: results of a prospective randomised study. J Urol 159:164–166

21 Brachytherapy of Localized Prostate Cancer

S. Deger, D. Böhmer, I. Türk, J. Roigas, S.A. Loening

21.1 Introduction

The Annual Report on the status of cancer in the USA 1973–1997 revealed that prostate cancer was the number one cancer site in men for each of the race/ethnic groups in the country. However, the rates showed a fourfold variation, from 49.6 per 100,000 for American Indian/Alaska Native men to 225.0 for Black men. Four trends in the incidence rates were identified: a steady increase from 1973 to 1988, an acceleration in the increase from 1988 to 1992, a substantial decline from 1992 to 1995, and approximately level rates thereafter. Over 50% of all cancer cases and cancer deaths were caused by cancers of the breast, prostate, lung and bronchus, and colon/rectum [63]. The increases seen in rate of incidence were clearly linked to the initiation of screening by means of prostate-specific antigen (PSA). The augmented incidence of prostate cancer was thus principally accounted for by earlier diagnosis, which in turn led to a stage migration to lower stages [43, 67].

PSA screening led to increased public awareness, and different treatment strategies began to compete. In 1997 Lu-Yao and Yao presented data on 59,876 cancer-registry patients aged 50–79. Ten-year prostate cancer-specific survival for grade 1 cancer after prostatectomy was 98% [95% confidence interval (CI) 97–99], 89% (87–92) after radiotherapy, and 93% (91–94) after conservative management [48].

Brachytherapy is a broad term referring to local application of any radioactive isotope. The idea of using a radioactive source locally to treat malignancies came from Pierre Curié's work in about 1901. Between 1910 and 1922 Paschkis, Pasteu, Degrais, and Denning pioneered the use of radium in the urethra [22, 55, 56]. Barringer inserted radium needles into the prostate in 1915 at New York's Memorial Sloan-Kettering Cancer Center (MSKCC). He used a perineal approach under digital rectal guidance [2].

There were almost no further developments over the next 40 years. In 1952 Flocks injected colloidal gold in to the prostate after open perineal exposure. Then in the mid 1950s radiation sources were developed which decreased the exposure of risk organs such as the rectum and urethra, and these low energy radioisotopes defined a new period of brachytherapy. Physicians at Sloan-Kettering started to test ^{125}I in 1970, using a retropubic approach for the treatment of prostate cancer. In early 1990s the current period of brachytherapy began with the introduction of three-dimensional (3D) computer planning systems, of transrectal ultrasound, and of additional low-energy sources. A change in patients' conception of treatment also helped make brachytherapy an attractive alternative to radical prostatectomy in the therapy of localized disease.

There are two defined brachytherapy categories: low dose rate (LDR) and high dose rate (HDR) brachytherapy. These two differ as to the dose rate of radioisotopes used as well as to overall treatment strategy.

Table 21.1. Radiobiological features of commonly used radionuclides

Source	Half-life (days)	Energy (kEV)	Initial dose rate (cGy/h)
Permanent			
^{125}I	60.2	28	5.8
^{103}Pd	17	21	15.3
^{198}Au	2.7	412	21.4–27
Temporary			
^{192}Ir	74.2	380	60–90

The most common radioisotopes used for LDR brachytherapy are ^{125}I) and ^{103}Pd. For HDR treatment, ^{198}Au and ^{192}Ir are most frequently used. Table 21.1 shows the radiobiological differences in these sources.

21.2 LDR Brachytherapy

21.2.1 ^{125}I and ^{103}Pd

^{125}I was introduced in 1970 at the Sloan-Kettering center by Hilaris and Whitmore using an open retropubic approach. Employment of a radioisotope with a long half-life of 60 days, which allowed a continuous irradiation for a slow growing cancer, at first evoked euphoria [76]. Unfortunately, data between mid 1970s and mid 1980s showed clearly that iodine was not suitable for patients who had a T3 lesion or an undifferentiated cancer.

Between 1970 and 1985, 1,013 patients with stage T2 and T3 lesions were treated with ^{125}I implantations and pelvic lymph node dissection at MSKCC. The approach was retropubic. After mobilization of the prostate from the surrounding tissues, hollow needles were inserted and used for implantation [30]. No severe complications were described due to iodine implantation. All rectal and urinary complications resolved spontaneously [66]. In patients with stage T2 and T3 tumors and negative nodes who received a peripheral dose of 140 Gy or more, the 15-year overall local disease-free survival rate was 60% [27].

Kuban et al. defined clinically progression free survival as no clinical evidence of disease (NED) (in the absence at that early time of PSA values). Their data in 120 patients is shown in Table 21.2 [40]. Findings of other study groups such as Peschel et al. and Rohloff et al. were similar [58, 64].

^{103}Pd was introduced in 1987. The characteristics of ^{103}Pd are similar to those of ^{125}I. It emits a low-energy photon with an average energy of 21 KeV. With a half-life of 17 days, it delivers an initial dose rate of 20–24 cGy/h for a typically prescribed dose [12, 45]. At many institutions, the choice between the ^{125}I and ^{103}Pd is based on the Gleason score. It has been generally accepted that patients with Gleason scores seven or higher benefit from the use of ^{103}Pd, while tumors with a lower Gleason score respond better to ^{125}I. It is thought that tumors with a high proliferative rate respond better to ^{103}Pd with a dose rate of 20 to 24 cGy/h, and tumors with low rate respond better to ^{125}I with a dose rate of 8 to 10 cGy/h. However, there have been no clinical trials to verify this belief [61].

A renaissance of LDR brachytherapy started in the early 1990s with technical improvements, including better visualization of the prostate, improved

Table 21.2. Progression-free survival using ^{125}I, the Eastern Virginia Medical School experience between 1974 and 1984 [40]

Stage	NED^{+} 5 years (%)	NED^{+} 10 years (%)	Grade	NED 5 years (%)	NED 10 years (%)
T1	100	90	G1	93	86
T2a	88	88	G2	67	30
T2b	77	50	G3	46	10[a]
T3	50	14			

NED, no evidence of disease.
[a] Nine-years follow-up.

computer planning systems, as well as the addition of ^{103}Pd as an effective radioisotope. The introduction of PSA led to the identification of prostate cancer in early stages, which was favorable for patient selection for LDR brachytherapy. Patients were selected in low-, intermediate-, and high-risk groups and dosages were tailored for each group.

In 1995 and 1998 the American Association of Physics and Medicine Task Group No. 43 (TG-43) recommended changing the algorithm used to calculate doses from ^{125}I and ^{103}Pd sources [54]. The American Brachytherapy Society (ABS) recommended adaptation of these changes for ^{103}Pd and revised the dose of ^{125}I to unify LDR dosimetry. ^{125}I implants were calculated to receive 144 Gy, and ^{103}Pd implants to receive 115–120 Gy using point source approximation [4, 47, 53].

The ABS further has recommended that patients whose cancer was stage T1 to T2a, whose Gleason score was 2 to 6, and whose PSA was less than 10 ng/ml should undergo LDR monotherapy. Patients with clinical stage T2b, T2c, *or* Gleason score 8–10, *or* PSA more than 20 ng/ml have been recommended to be considered as candidates for LDR brachytherapy as a boost to external beam radiation therapy. Relative contraindications for LDR brachytherapy based on ABS recommendations are patients with increased risk factors for developing complications. These factors include a large median lobe, previous pelvic irradiation, high American Urological Association (AUA) symptom score, history of multiple pelvic surgeries, severe diabetes with healing problems, technical difficulties which may result in inadequate dose coverage, previous transurethral resection of the prostate (TURP), gland size more than 60 cc at time of implantation, and tumor infiltration of seminal vesicles [53].

In 2000, using these criteria, Radge and Korb published data on 152 patients with stage T1–T3 using ^{125}I. Ninety-eight patients with low grade/low stage underwent ^{125}I implant alone. The observed 10-year disease free survival rate (PSA less than 0.5 ng/ml) was 60%. Another 54 patients received additional 45 Gy external radiation, and their 10-year disease free survival was 76% [61].

Beyer and Priestley reported on 489 T1–T2 patients with a median PSA value of 7.3 ng/ml who were treated with ^{125}I monotherapy [3]. The 4-year biochemically disease-free rate was 88% for patients with Gleason score ≤ 4, and 60% for those with Gleason score ≥ 5.

In 2000 the long awaited data of Blasko et al. [5] on the treatment of 230 patients with clinical stage T1–T2 with ^{103}Pd alone was also published. (56.1% of these patients had a T2a lesion, 28.3% a T1c lesion). In 75.7% the initial PSA level was less than 10 g/ml, and only 40% had a Gleason score ≥ 7. The overall biochemical control rate achieved at 9 years was 83.5%. Failures were local in 3.0%, distant in 6.1%. PSA progression was observed in 4.3%. These authors defined PSA progression as two consecutive rises in serum PSA, which differs from the American Society of Therapeutic Radiology and Oncology (ASTRO) Consensus Conference [1]requirement of three rises before failure is adjudged.

Dattoli et al. treated 124 patients with unfavorable risk factors, such as T3 tumor, Gleason score >6, PSA >15 ng/ml, using ^{103}Pd plus external irradiation of 41 Gy. Biochemical progression free survival was 79% at 3 years, preservation of potency 77% [18]. Wallner et al. reported a potency protection of 82% 6 years after treatment with ^{125}I [75]

Critz et al. combined external beam radiation with LDR treatment. Reporting on about 250 patients treated between 1984 and 1994 with a minimum follow-up of 5 years, they found that 98% of patients reached a PSA value less than 0.5 ng/ml, 87% below 0.2 ng/ml. In a later publication of this study group, it became clear that these patients had been highly selected, 93% with a tumor stage less than T2c [15, 16].

Looking at the literature, there are several studies published on LDR brachytherapy, differing definitions of patient risk and biochemical failure to be noted. Mostly, patients with a PSA ≤10 ng/ml, Gleason score less than 7, and stage ≤T2a were defined as low risk patients. For these populations, biochemical control values between 50 and 100% were achieved. Biochemical failure was variously defined as existing when PSA exceeded values between 0.4 and 1 ng/ml, or when its level increased twice consecutively [3, 19, 28, 62, 65, 69]. In moderate risk patients, defined as those with a PSA value between 10 and 20 ng/ml, biochemical survival ranged from 45% to 82% [3, 5, 28, 65, 68, 71, 75]. In high-risk patients characterized by PSA >20 ng/ml or Gleason score >7, unsatisfactory 5-year biochemical control rates of 30%–65% were reported [3, 5, 28, 68, 71, 75].Combining external beam irradiation with implants was reported to improve 10-year biochemical survival from 64% to 76% (PSA failure being defined as above 0.5 ng/ml) [14, 62].

An increasingly important aspect of LDR brachytherapy is preservation of sexual potency. Potency rates from 75% to 79% with a follow-up maximum of 3 years were reported after implants in two series [70, 75]. When this therapy was combined with external beam irradiation, the sexual potency rate dropped to 62% in 5 years [18].

The main problem in analyzing LDR data from the 1990s is the lack of prospective randomized trials in which the two isotopes are compared. Largely for the same reason, the impact of additional external beam radiation therapy or hormonal treatment remains unclear.

At last authors experienced in LDR brachytherapy could not demonstrate a difference in outcome between ^{125}I and ^{103}Pd [12, 28, 68].

21.3 HDR Brachytherapy

21.3.1 Gold-198

^{198}Au was introduced by Flocks for the treatment of prostate cancer in 1952. Doses of 3 mCi/cm^3 were injected into prostates smaller than 25 cm^3, and of 1 mCi/cm^3 into glands with a size over 150 cm^3, up to a maximum dose of 160 mCi [26]. Later, Flocks and associates injected colloidal ^{198}Au as an adjuvant therapy after radical prostatectomy for T3 disease. After removal of the prostate and seminal vesicles, colloidal ^{198}Au was injected in the pedicles with an activity of 100 mCi [25]. Because of the short half life (2.7 days) and penetration depth of 3 mm, gold 198 was ideal for an operative field.

In 1973 Flocks et al. published data from their neoadjuvant ^{198}Au injection of 345 patients. Complication rate was low and only 4.4% of the patients had local progression of disease. Progression-free survival in patients with no lymphatic involvement was 74% after 5 years, 66.7% after 10 years, and 27.5% 15 years after treatment [24]

Colloidal ^{198}Au was not available after the mid 1970s, and seed implantation was therefore introduced in the Urological Department at the University of Iowa. Gold seeds were implanted into the pedicles after radical prostatectomy. Between 1977 and 1988, 80 patients were treated with this adjuvant radiation therapy,73.8% of them with T3 disease. The 10-year progression-free survival for them was 84.4% for pT2 tumors and 79.1% for pT3 tumors [42]. This study group progressed in their work to the use of interstitial seed placement as primary therapy. In 1997, Loening published long-term data of the patient population thus treated between 1984 and 1995. With a median follow-up of 48 months, cancer-specific survival was 100% for T1 and T2a patients, 90% for T2b, and 76% for those with T3 tumors. The negative biopsy rate 5 years after treatment was 80% (n=77). Overall observed complications were minimal; two patients had mild radiation cystitis, treated with anticholinergic medications. However, two patients developed rectal ulceration, with one requiring a colostomy [46].

In 1997 a study group from Baylor University also reported on the use of ^{198}Au implantation. Butler et al. treated 510 patients between 1965 and 1980, employing ^{198}Au as boost to a delivery of external beam radiotherapy. Patients received their implantation via the open retropubic approach, the mean dose of ^{198}Au being 26 Gy (5–60 Gy). The mean dose of external beam was 43 Gy (30–50 Gy), resulting in a mean total dose of 69 Gy (45–105 Gy). Only 23% of the patients had T3 tumor, but 30% had lymph node metastasis. Actuarial survival rates for all stages were 83%±3% after 5 years, 53%±5% after 10 years, and 25%±10% after 15 years [10].

Table 21.3. The 5- and 10-year progression-free survival using ^{198}Au

Study	Progression-free survival according to tumor stage (%)			Follow-up (years)
	T1	T2	T3	
Carey [11]		73	74	5
Butler [10]	89±6	81±8[a] 78±10[b]	61±21	5 5
Loening [46]	100	90	76	
Gutierrez [29]		100	68	5
Carey [11]		60	63	7
Butler [10]	76±12	61±12[a] 53±16[b]	34±14	10
Lannon [44]	83	91.3[a] 64.4[b]	50.5	10
Gutierrez [29]		85	43	10

[a] T2a.
[b] T2b.

After introduction of transrectal ultrasound by Holm et al. [31], the Baylor group reported on the treatment of 54 patients between 1992 and 1996. Of these, 40.7% had a T1, 50% had a T2, and only 7.4% of them had a T3 lesion. Total delivered dose averaged 71 Gy (59–85 Gy). Pelvic lymph node dissection was performed in 30 patients, and additional external radiation was given in nine. Using this regime, no "acute toxicity" was seen in 11 patients (20.8%), single "acute toxicity" in 22 (41.5%), and multiple "acute toxicity" in 20 patients (40.7%). "Toxicity" according to Radiation Therapy Oncology Group (RTOG) criteria included proctitis in 50.9%, urethritis in 39.5%, and cystitis in 37.7%. Late rectal toxicity occurred in 6.3% and radiation cystitis in 16.7%. No grade III or IV acute or late toxicity was seen. The "PSA nadir" was defined as <1 ng/ml, and treatment was considered a success if reached. According to this definition, success was achieved in three of four patients with an initial PSA value between 0 and 4 ng/ml. Eighty-one percent of patients with an initial PSA level >4–10 ng/ml reached PSA nadir, while 65% patients with an initial PSA level >10 ng/ml achieved PSA nadir. Median follow-up was between 12.5 and 21.6 months [10]. Table 21.3 summarizes the 5-year and 10-year progression-free survival using ^{198}Au.

21.3.2 Iridium-192

Specific activity of ^{192}Ir is 60.3×10^{10} Bq/g, which is 16 times higher than that of ^{60}Co. The half-life is 74.4 days. Delivered electron energy is between 0.097 and 0.67 MeV, mean 0.59 MeV. Photon values measured at 0.3–0.6 MeV, mean 0.38 MeV. Because of the low gamma energy, radiation protection is much easier than with radium. For effective protection 5 cm of lead or 2.6 cm uranium are enough [9]. These considerations made iridium popular in the mid 1990s, especially in Europe.

Because of the high dose performance, iridium is used primarily as a temporary implant [50, 60]. ^{192}Ir offers the advantage of modifying dose distribution in case of suboptimal needle placement, which is the risk of a permanent implant.

^{192}Ir in a LDR technique has been used since 1977 [13]. Available data from different study groups of this era, with a follow-up of 1 to 60 months, showed a tumor control rate of 90%–95% using clinical criteria for failure [7, 8, 13, 34, 37, 52, 59, 72, 74]. Since these data lack PSA levels, they are difficult to analyze by today's standards.

Syed et al. reported on 200 patients, treated between 1977 and 1985. An open approach was used for delivering the treatment interstitially. Additional external irradiation of 30–40 Gy was applied. Local tumor control was 90%–95.5%, with complications such as proctitis and urethral strictures seen in 4%–11% of the patients. One patient required a colostomy. They found a significant correlation between complications and a previous transurethral resection of the prostate [73].

In 1986 Porter et al. described transperineal open surgical application of a device called a MicroSelectron [59]. This device opened the era of remote control afterloading technique. The advantage of this system is the maximum security of radiation exposure.

This system was adapted by different study groups. Khan et al. reported their experience with 321 patients. The total dose was 6500 cGy, with a 3100 cGy interstitial dose. Grade II complications, according the RTOG system, such as mild dysuria, diarrhea, and proctitis, were observed in 0.6% to 6.5% of cases. Grade III toxicity was seen in three patients. Five-year local tumor control was 95% for T1c, 93% for T2a, 83.6% for T2b and 73.1% for T3 disease [35].

Based on experiences such as these, transperineal, transrectal ultrasound-guided application using a high-dose source was established, and became the basis for modern HDR brachytherapy.

In summary HDR brachytherapy nowadays is an afterloading technique, based on a treatment plan adapted to actual geometry using computer algorithms to allow a more homogenous dose with better coverage within the implant volume.

The main goal of HDR brachytherapy is to deliver a high dose of radiation to the target while minimizing radiation to the surrounding normal tissue. In 2000 Hsu et al. published the critical volume-tolerance analysis using dose-volume information to estimate the possibility of further dose escalation using HDR brachytherapy boost. Seven-field conformal prostate-only external beam and HDR brachytherapy treatment plans were constructed for each patient. Dose-volume histograms were plotted for comparison of the two techniques, and doses to the normal structures were calculated. They found that the areas of bladder and rectum receiving a high dose were significantly reduced when using the implant, while higher doses were thereby delivered inside the prostate. On average, 47% of the prostate received >150% of the prescribed brachytherapy dose, and 0.19 cc of the bladder received 100% of such a dose. This compared with 5.1 cc of the bladder receiving 100% of the prescription dose in the seven-field conformal external beam radiotherapy boost. Similarly, 0.25 cc of the rectum received 100% of the dose with the implant boost, as compared to 2.9 cc in the conformal external beam treatment [32].

In the mid 1990s, using this basic information, different study groups had provided evidence that HDR brachytherapy might be an alternative to LDR implants [6, 23, 38, 49, 51, 57]. HDR brachytherapy has been performed by four study groups, namely, at Charité Hospital in Berlin, Germany [21], Christian Albert University in Kiel, Germany [39], Göteborg-Sahlgrenzka Universitätshospital in Göteborg, Sweden [6], and William Beaumont Hospital (WBH) in Royal Oak, Mich., USA [33]. Interstitial doses were between 8.25 and 15 Gy in all institutions. Follow-ups were between 30 and 47 months. Tumor stages were similar, with precentage of T3 disease between 13% and 26%, except at Charité where the precentage of T3 disease was 58%: Only the Charité group performed laparoscopic lymph node dissection for staging in all patients. Only 20 patients at Sahlgrenzka Universitätshospital had a staging lymphadenectomy. Five year biochemical survivals ranging from 67% to 84%. (according to ASTRO criteria [1], with three consecutive rises in PSA value, except at Sahlgrenzka Universitätshospital) are shown in Table 21.4.

HDR brachytherapy has also been used as monotherapy. In this technique, the template is fixed to the perineum and a fractioned interstitial dose of 6 Gy is delivered up to a total dose of 48 to 54 Gy [77].

Table 21.4. Patient characteristics of high dose rate groups

	Number	Age (years)	Initial PSA (ng/ml)	Single interstitial dose (Gy)	External dose (Gy)	Follow-up (months)	Five-year PFS (%)
WBH, Royal Oak, Mich.	161	69	9.9	8.25–10.5	46	30	67
Kiel, Germany	174	68.2	-	15	50	47.1	79
Göteborg, Sweden	50	63	-	10	50	45	84[a]
Charité, Berlin, Germany	230	67	12.8	9–10	45–50.4	40.2	69

PSA, prostate-specific antigen; PFS, progression-free survival.
[a] PSA value less than 1 ng/ml.

21.4 Summary

In summary, brachytherapy for prostate cancer is an alternative option to surgery and external beam radiation. Patient selection is important in choosing the appropriate technique. LDR monotherapy seems to be best for patients with low-risk disease (T1-T2a lesion, PSA less than 10 ng/ml, and Gleason less than 7).

Looking at advanced disease, dose escalation seems to be necessary. There is no doubt that patients receiving radiation doses exceeding 72 Gy have significantly better biochemical and clinical disease-free survival rates [41]. The best treatment for advanced disease may be dose escalation with or without synergistic treatment combinations such as antiandrogen therapy and interstitial hyperthermia [17, 20, 41].

References

1. American Society of Therapeutic Radiology and Oncology (1997) Consensus statement: guidelines for PSA following radiation therapy. Int J Radiat Oncol Biol Phys 37:1035–1041
2. Barringer BS (1917) Radium in the treatment of carcinoma of the bladder and prostate: review of one year's work. J Am Med Assoc 68:1227–1230
3. Beyer DC, Priestley JB Jr (1997) Biochemical disease-free survival following 125 I prostate implantation. Int J Radiat Oncol Biol Phys 37:559–563
4. Bice WS, Prestidge BR, Prete JJ, Dubois DF (1998) Clinical impact of implementing the recommendations of AAPM Task Group 43 on permanent prostate brachytherapy using 125 I. Int J Radiat Oncol Biol Phys 40:1237–1241
5. Blasko JC, Grimm PD, Sylvester JE, Badiozamani KR, Hoak D, Cavanagh W (2000) Palladium-103 brachytherapy for prostate carcinoma. Int J Radiat Oncol Biol Phys 46:839–850
6. Borghede G, Hedelin H, Holmäng S, Johanson KA, Aldenborg F, Pettersson S, Sernbo G, Wallgren A, Mercke C (1997) Combined treatment with temporary short-term HDR iridium-192 brachytherapy and external beam radiotherapy for irradiation of localized prostatic carcinoma. Radiother Oncol 44:237–244
7. Bosch PC, Forbes KA, Prassvinichai S, Miller BJ, Golji H, Martin D (1986) Preliminary observations on the results of combined temporary iridium 192 implantation and external beam irradiation for carcinoma of the prostate. J Urol 135:722–725
8. Brindle JS, Benson RC, Martinez A (1985) Acute toxity and preliminary therapeutic results of pelvic lymphadenectomy, combined with transperineal implantation of iridium 192 and external beam radiotherapy for locally advanced prostate cancer. Urology 25:23
9. Brix F, Bertermann H (1989) Interstitielle Strahlentherapie mit Iridium 192. In: Sommerkamp H, Altwein JE (eds) Prostatakarzinom, Spektrum der kurativen Therapie. Karger, München, pp 84–115
10. Butler EB, Scardino PT, Teh BS, Uhl BM, Guerriero WG, Carlton CE, Berner BM, Dennis WS, Carpenter LS, Lu HH, Chiu JK, Kent TS, Woo SY (1997) The Baylor College of Medicine experience with gold seed implantation. Semin Surg Oncol 13:406–418
11. Carey PO, Lippert MC, Constable WC, Jones D, Talton BM (1988) Combined gold seed implantation and external radiotherapy for stage B2 or C prostate cancer. J Urol 139:989–994
12. Cha CM, Potters L, Ashley R, Freeman K, Wang XH, Waldbaum R, Leibel S (1999) Isotope selection for patients undergoing prostate brachytherapy. Int J Radiat Oncol Biol Phys 45:391–395
13. Court B, Chassagne C, Savatovski I (1977) Irradiation interstitielle par fils d'iridium 192 des cancers de la prostate. J Urol Nephrol 83:113–115
14. Critz FA, Levinson Ak, Williams W, et al (1997) The PSA nadir that indicates potential cure after radiotherapy for prostate cancer. Urology 49:322–326
15. Critz FA, Levinson AK, Williams WH, Holladay CT, Griffen VD, Holladay DA (1999) Prostate specific antigen nadir achieved by men apparently cured of prostate cancer by radiotherapy. J Urol 161:1199–1203
16. Critz FA, Williams WH, Holladay CT, Levinson AK, Benton JB, Holladay DA, Schnell FJ Jr, Maxa LS, Shrake PD (1999) Post-treatment PSA ≤ 0,2 ng/ml defines disease freedom after radiotherapy for prostate cancer using modern techniques. Urology 54:968–971
17. D'Amico AV, Schultz D, Loffredo M, Dugal R, Hurwitz M, Kaplan I, Beard CJ, Renshaw AA, Kantoff PW (2000) Biochemical outcome following external beam radiation therapy with or without androgen suppression therapy for clinically localized prostate cancer. JAMA 284:1280–1283

18. Dattoli M, Wallner K, Sorace R, Koval J, Cash J, Acosta R, Brown C, Etheridge J, Binder M, Brunelle R, Kirwan N, Sanchez S, Stein D, Wasserman S (1996) 103Pd brachytherapy and external beam irradiation for clinically localized, high-risk prostatic carcinoma. Int J Radiat Oncol Biol Phys 35:875–879
19. Dattoli MJ, Wallner KE, Cash JC, Ross RE, Koval JM, Sorace RA (1997) Palladium 103 brachytherapy for clinical T1/T2 prostate carcinoma. Int J Radiat Oncol Biol Phys 39 [Suppl 1]: 221
20. Deger S, Böhmer D, Marlies Franke, Roigas J, Turk I, Schnorr D, Loening SA (2000) Interstitial hyperthermia with self regulating thermoseeds in combination with conformal radiotherapy for prostate cancer. Preliminary results of a phase II trial. J Urol 163:S4 (Abstract 1300)
21. Deger S, Böhmer D, Roigas J, Tuerk I, Schnorr D, Dinges S, Budach V, Loening SA (2000) Iridium 192 afterloading, high dose rate brachytherapy of prostate cancer. Radiother Oncol 55 [Suppl 1]:48
22. Denning DL (1922) Carcinoma of the prostate, seminal vesicles treated with radium. Surg Gynecol Obset 34:99–118
23. Dinges S, Deger S, Koswig S, Boehmer D, Schnorr D, Wiegel T, Loaning SA, Dietel M, Hinkelbein W, Budach V (1998) High-dose rate interstitial with external beam irradiation for localized prostate cancer: results of a prospective trial. Radiother Oncol 48:197–202
24. Flocks RH (1974) The treatment of stage C prostatic cancer with special reference to combined surgical and rediation therapy. J Urol 109:461
25. Flocks RH, Kerr D, Elkins HB, Culp D (1952) Treatment of carcinoma of the prostate by interstitial radiation with radioactive gold 198: a preliminary report. J Urol 68:510–522
26. Flocks RH, Kerr HD, Elkins HB, Mador D (1959) The treatment of carcinoma of the prostate by interstitial radiation with radioactive gold. J Urol 34:628–633
27. Fuks Z, Leibel SA, Wallner KE, Begg CB, Fair WR, Anderson LL, Hilaris BS, Whitmore WF, et al (1991) The effect of local control on metastatic dissemination in carcinoma of the prostate: long-term results in patients treated with 125 I implantation. Int J Radiat Oncol Biol Phys 21: 537–547
28. Grado GL, Larson TR, Balch CS, Grado MM, Collins JM, Kriegshauser JS, Swanson GP, Navickis RJ, Wilkes MM (1998) Actuarial disease-free survival after prostate cancer brachytherapy using interactive techniques with biplane ultrasound and fluoroscopic guidance. Int J Radiat Oncol Biol Phys 42:289 –298
29. Guitierrez AE, Merino OR (1988) Adenocarcinoma of the prostate: radioactive gold seed implantation plus external irradiation. Int J Radiat Oncol Biol Phys 15:1317–1322
30. Hilaris BS (1997) Brachytherapy in cancer of prostate: an historical perspective. Semin Surg Oncol 13:399–405
31. Holm HH, Juul N, Pedersen JF, Hansen H, Stroyer I (1983) Transperineal 125 iodine seed implantation in prostatic cancer guided by transrectal ultrasonography. J Urol 130:283–286
32. Hsu CJ, Pickett B, Shinohara K, Krieg R, Roach M, Philipps T (2000) Normal tissue dosimetric comparison between HDR prostate implant boost and conformal external beam radiotherapy boost: potential for dose escalation. Int J Radiat Oncol Biol Phys 46:851–858
33. Kestin LL, Martinez AA, Stromberg JS, Edmundson GK, Gustafson GS, Brabbins DS, Chen PY, Vicini FA (2000) Matched-pair analysis of conformal high-dose-rate brachytherapy boost versus external-beam radiation therapy alone for locally advanced prostate cancer. J Clin Oncol 18:2869–2880
34. Khan K, Crawford ED, Johnson EL (1983) Transperineal percutaneous iridium 192 implant of the prostate. Int J Rad Oncol Biol Phys 9:1391–1395
35. Khan K, Thompson W, Bush S, Stidley C (1992) Transperineal percutaneous iridium 192 interstitial template implant of the prostate: results and complications in 321 patients. Int J Rad Oncol Biol Phys 22:935–939
36. Klein K, Ali MM, Hackler RH (1986) Bilateral pelvic lymphadenectomy, transperineal interstitial implantation of ir 192 and external beam radiotherapy for advanced localized prostatic carcinoma: toxicity and early results. Endocuriether Hypertherm Oncol 2:23–27
37. Koren H, Dollezal P (1988) Interstitielle Iridium Therapie des lokoregionalen Prostatakarzinoms mittels maschinellem Afterloading. In: Hammer J, Kärcher H (eds) Fortschritte in der interstitiellen und intrakavitären Strahlentherapie. Zuckschwerdt, München, pp 167–68
38. Kovács G, Wirth B, Bertermann H, Galalae R, Kohr P, Wilhelm R, Kimmig B (1996) Prostate preservation by combined external beam and HDR brachytherapy at node negative prostate cancer patients – an intermediate analysis after 10 years experience. Int J Radiat Oncol Biol Phys 36:198
39. Kovács G, Galalae R, Loch T, Bertermann H, Kohr P, Schneider R, Kimming B (1999) Prostate preservation by combined external beam and HDR brachytherapy in nodal negative prostate cancer. Strahlenther Onkol 175 [Suppl 2]:87–88
40. Kuban DA, El-Mahdi AM, Schellhammer PF (1989) I 125 interstitial implantation for prostate cancer, what have we learned 10 years after? Cancer 63:2415 – 2420
41. Kupelian PA, Mohan DS, Lyons J, Klein EA, Reddy CA (2000) Higher than standard radiation doses (>or =72 Gy) with or without androgen deprivation in the treatment of localized prostate cancer. Int J Radiat Oncol Biol Phys 46:567–574

42. Kwon ED, Loening SA, Hawtrey CE (1991) Radical prostatectomy with adjuvant radioactive gold seed placement: results of treatment at 5 and 10 year for clinical stages A2, B1 and B2 cancer of the prostate. J Urol 145:524–531
43. Landis SH, Murray T, Bolden S (1999) Cancer statistics. Cancer J Clin 49:8–31
44. Lannon SG, el-Araby AA, Joseph PK, Eastwood BJ, Awad SA (1993) Long-term results of combined interstitial gold seed implantation plus external beam irradiation in localised carcinoma of the prostate. Br J Urol 72:782–791
45. Ling CC, Li WX, Anderson LL (1995) The relative biological effectiveness of I-125 and Pd-103. Int J Radiat Oncol Biol Phys 32:373–378
46. Loening SA (1997) Gold seed implantation in prostate brachytherapy. Semin Surg Oncol 13: 419–424
47. Luse RW, Blasko J, Grimm PA (1997) Method for implementing the American Association of Physicists in medicine task group 43 dosimetry recommendations for 125 I transperineal prostate seed implants on commercial treatment planning systems. Int J Radiat Oncol Biol Phys 37:737–741
48. Lu-Yao GL, Yao SL (1997) Population-based study of long-term survival in patients with clinically localized prostate cancer. Lancet 349:906–910
49. Martinez A, Gonzalez J, Stromberg J, Edmundson G, Plunkett M, Gustafson G, Brown D, Yan D, Vicini F, Brabbins D (1995) Conformal prostate brachytherapy: initial experience of a phase I/II dose-escalating trial. Int J Radiat Oncol Biol Phys 33:1019 –1127
50. Martinez AA, Edmundsen GK, Cox RS, et al (1985) Combination of external beam radiation and multi-site perineal applicator (MUPIT) for the treatment of locally advanced or recurrent prostatic, anorectal and gynecologic malignancies. Int J Radiat Oncol Biol Phys 11:391–398
51. Mate TP (1998) High dose-rate afterloading 192 Iridium prostate brachytherapy: feasibility report. Int J Radiat Oncol Biol Phys 41:525–533
52. Miller LS (1979) Afterloading transperineal iridium 192 wire implantation of the prostate. Radiology 131:527 - 528
53. Nag S, Beyer D, Friedland J, Grimm P, Nath R (1999) American Brachytherapy Society (ABS) recommendations for transperineal permanent brachytherapy of prostate cancer. Int J Radiat Oncol Biol Phys 44:789–799
54. Nath R, Anderson LL, Luxton G, Weaver KA, Williamson JF, Meigooni AS (1995) Dosimetry of interstitial brachytherapy sources: recommendations of the AAPM Radiation Therapy Committee Task Group No. 43. Med Phys 22:209–233
55. Pasteau O (1911) Traitment du cancer de la prostate par le Radium. Rev Mal Nutr 1911 363–367
56. Pasteau O, Degrais P (1914) The radium treatment of cancer of the prostate. Arch Roentgen Ray (London) 18:396–410
57. Paul R, Hofmann R, Schwarzer JU (1997) Iridium 192 high-dose-rate brachytherapy: a useful alternative for localized prostate cancer? World J Urol 15:252–256
58. Peschel RE, Fogel TD, Kacinski BM, Kelly K, Mate TP (1987) I 125 implants for carcinoma of the prostate. Prog Clin Biol Res 243:177–195
59. Porter AT, Scrimger JW, Pocha JS (1988) Remote interstitial afterloading in cancer of the prostate: preliminary experience with the MicroSelectron. Int J Radiol Oncol Biol Phys 14: 571–575
60. Puthawala AA, Syed AM, Tansey L (1985) Temporary iridium 192 implant in the management of carcinoma of prostate. Endocurietherap Hypertherm Oncol 1:25–33
61. Radge H, Korb L (2000) Brachytherapy for clinically prostate cancer. Semin Surg Oncol 18: 45–51
62. Radge H, Elgamal AA, Snow PB, Brandt J, Bartolucci AA, Nadir BS, Korb LJ (1998) Ten year disease free survival after transperineal ultasonography-guided iodine 125 brachytherapy with or without 45 Gy external beam irradiation in the treatment of patients with clinically localized, low to high Gleason grade prostate carcinoma. Cancer 83:989–1001
63. Ries LA, Wingo PA, Miller DS, Howe HL, Weir HK, Rosenberg HM, Vernon SW, Cronin K, Edwards BK (2000) The annual report to the nation on the status of cancer, 1973–1997, with a special section on colorectal cancer. Cancer 88:2398–2424
64. Rohloff R, Tauber R, Schätzl M, Wendt T, Willich N (1988) Ergebnisse nach interstitieller Strahlentherapie mit J-125 Seeds bei der Behandlung des Prostatakarzinoms. Strahlentherapie und Onkologie 164:195–201
65. Sharkey J, Chovnick SD, Behar RJ, Perez R, Otheguy J, Solc Z, Huff W, Cantor A (1998) Outpatient ultrasound-guided palladium 103 brachytherapy for localized adenocarcinoma of the prostate: a preliminary report of 434 patients. Urology 51:796–803
66. Sogani PC (1983) Pelvic lymphadenectomy: techniques and complications. In: Hilaris BS, Batata MA (eds) Brachytherapy oncology – advances in prostate and other cancers. Memorial Sloan-Kettering Cancer Center, New York, pp 79–82
67. Stephenson RA, Stanford JL (1997) Population-based prostate cancer trends in the United States: patterns of change in the era of prostate-specific antigen. World J Urol 15:331–335
68. Stock RG, Stone NN (1997) The effect of prognostic factors on therapeutic outcome following transperineal prostate brachytherapy. Semin Surg Oncol 13:454–460
69. Stock RG, Stone NN (1999) Permanent radioactive seed implantation in the treatment of prostate cancer. Hem Oncol Clin North Am 13:489–501

70. Stock RG, Stone NN, DeWyngaert JK, et al (1996) Prostate specific antigen findings and biopsy results following interactive ultrasound guided transperineal brachytherapy for early stage prostate cancer. Cancer 77:2386–2392
71. Stokes SH, Real JD, Adams PW, Clements JC, Wuertzer S, Kan W (1997) Tansperineal ultasound-guided radioactive seed implantation for organ-confined carcinoma of prostate. Int J Radiat Oncol Biol Phys 37:337–341
72. Syed AM, Puthwala A, Tansey LA (1983) Management of the prostatic carcinoma. Combination of pelvic lymphadenektomy, temporary Ir-192 implantation, and external irradiation. Radiology 149:829–833
73. Syed AM, Puthwala A, Tansey LA, Shanberg A, Sawyer D, Baghdassarian R, Wachs B, Tomasulo J, Rao J, Syed R (1992) Temporary irdium 192 implant in the management of carcinoma of the prostate. Cancer 69:2515–2524
74. Tansey LA, Shanberg AM, Syed AMN(1983) Treatment of prostatic carcinoma by pelvic lymphadenectomy, temporary iridium 192 implant and external irradiation. Urology 21:594
75. Wallner K, Roy J, Harrison L (1996) Tumor control and morbidity of following transperineal iodine 125 implantation for stage T1/T2 prostatic carcinoma. J Clin Oncol 14:449–453
76. Whitmore WF (1980) Interstitial radiation therapy for carcinoma of the prostate. Prostate 1:157–168
77. Yoshioka Y, Nose T, Yoshida K, Inoue T, Yamazaki H, Tanaka E, Shiomi H, Imai A, Nakamura S, Shimamoto S, Inoue T (2000) High-dose-rate interstitial brachytherapy as a monotherapy for localized prostate cancer: treatment description and preliminary results of a phase I/II clinical trial. Int J Radiat Oncol Biol Phys 48:675–681

Complications Following Radical Prostatectomy

22 Quality of Life Following Radical Prostatectomy

R.R. Berges, T. Senge

22.1 Introduction

One dilemma regarding therapy for localized prostate cancer is the lack of randomized clinical trials to prove the superiority of treatment with curative intent over watchful waiting. Even if several studies are under way, their results will not be available within the next 10–15 years [29, 36, 47, 48].

In the last decade, in the United States, and later also in Europe, incidence rates of prostate cancer have shown a substantial increase, mainly as a result of prostate-specific antigen (PSA) screening. With radical prostatectomy now regarded around the world as standard procedure offered to patients with reasonable life expectancy and low co-morbidity on a regular basis [41], urologists for the first time claim to detect a decline in prostate cancer mortality [6, 42]. However, true outcome regarding cancer control remains uncertain in many cases even in pathologically proven organ-confined disease.Furthermore, side effects of treatment (loss of erectile function, incontinence, urethral strictures), may reduce quality of life substantially. Also, radical prostatectomy must compete with other forms of treatment with curative intent, such as conformal radiation, brachytherapy, or a combination of both, treatment options for which many radiation oncologists claim fewer side effects and equal tumor control.

In this context it is widely considered important to assess the outcome of radical prostatectomy from the viewpoint of "health-related quality of life" (HRQOL), a term which has gained substantial weight in cancer therapy in general in recent years. However, it is still a matter of discussion how exactly HRQOL should be measured in cancer patients in general and prostate cancer patients in particular. Indeed, the definition of HRQOL itself is a matter of discussion.

The single assessment of physical performance through instruments like the WHO Karnowsky Index or others have quickly shown that these functional scores fail to correlate with overall HRQOL. It is widely accepted today that multidimensional approaches covering both physical and psychological health, along with social and cultural aspects of personal well being, are more suitable for assessing HRQOL [28]. In order to address treatment outcomes from the HRQOL point of view, studies should use only such multidimensional instruments that are capable of delivering comparable results [16]. Unfortunately, reliable validated instruments have only become available within the past couple of years; it is therefore understandable that evidence for comparison of the various prostate cancer treatments is only now emerging.

22.2 Instruments That Measure HRQOL in Prostate Cancer Patients

Instruments measuring HRQOL should be reliable, sensitive enough to pick up changes in well being, and easy to understand and interpret. They should address global issues such as pain, mobility, mental health, and social conditions common to all cancer patients as well as typical organ- and treatment-related issues. Instruments should also be designed to meet international and cross cultural criteria and be validated in different languages to insure comparability of results.

Many instruments have been developed within recent years to assess HRQOL in cancer patients, most of which are self administered questionnaires.

The European Organization for Research and Treatment of Cancer (EORTC) QLQ-C30 (see Appendix) [5, 17, 39], the Functional Assessment of Cancer Therapy (FACT) [2], the Functional Living Index Cancer (FLIC) [18, 27], the Quality of Life Index Cancer (CQOLC) [45, 46], and the SF36 [short form of 36 items of the Medical Outcomes Study (MOS)] questionnaires [10, 13] are among the accepted multidimensional instruments in this field. Most of these questionnaires have lacked a prostate cancer-specific module addressing urinary, sexual, and bowel function, the main adverse consequences of prostate cancer treatment such as radical prostatectomy, external beam or brachytherapy, or even of hormone ablation. Such modules, however, have become available recently with the appearance of the Litwin disease-targeted quality of life survey [23] and of EORTC's prostate cancer module QLQ-PR25 to accompany its QLQ-C30 questionnaire [3, 40]. QLQ-PR25 adds 25 items to the main document that assess urinary (nine items), bowel (four items), treatment-related (six items), and sexual symptoms (six items). Because of their emergence only recently, these instruments still have to be validated in different languages and cultural backgrounds to insure their applicability in HRQOL assessments around the world.

In summary, up to the present it has been rather difficult to compare treatment results among various treatment options, clinical trials, or even countries and socio cultural backgrounds with regard to HRQOL.

22.3 Studies Addressing HRQOL after Radical Prostatectomy

Despite the lack of the kind of solid evidence that may be derived from large-scale prospective clinical trials using validated instruments to assess HRQOL in prostate cancer patients, there is growing information from a variety of studies addressing this issue, many of which were performed retrospectively and for comparison of radical prostatectomy with radiation therapy [1, 4, 8, 9, 12, 14, 19, 20, 22, 23, 30, 31, 34, 35]. Results from these studies vary widely due to differences in types of institutions involved in study designs, in definitions of, for instance, incontinence and erectile dysfunction, in the nature of patients included, as well as in the instruments used to address HRQOL.

From the aspect of "multidimensionality" it appears that morbidity alone does not represent the whole of HRQOL. Unfortunately, prostate cancer-related issues aside, instruments that measure general HRQOL or cancer-related quality of life were not used in many trials. In a recent retrospective survey on

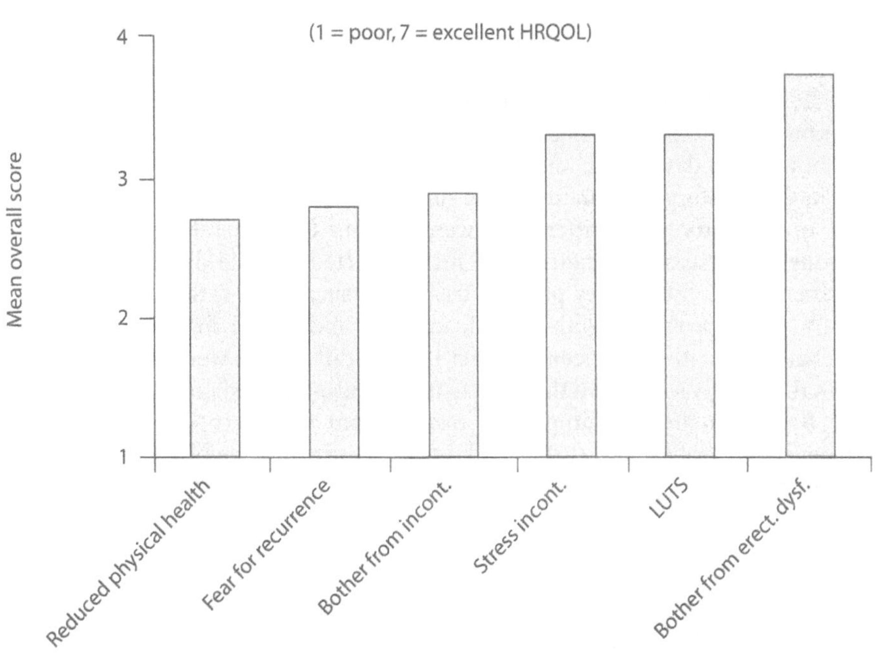

Fig. 22.1. Ranking of items to influence overall HRQOL in 430 patients after non-nerve-sparing radical prostatectomy performed in Herne, Germany, between 1986 and 1996, mean age 65 years. Instruments among others: QLQ-C30, IPSS, ICS-BPH incontinence including "bother," questions regarding pre- and post-operative erectile dysfunction and "bother", LUTS

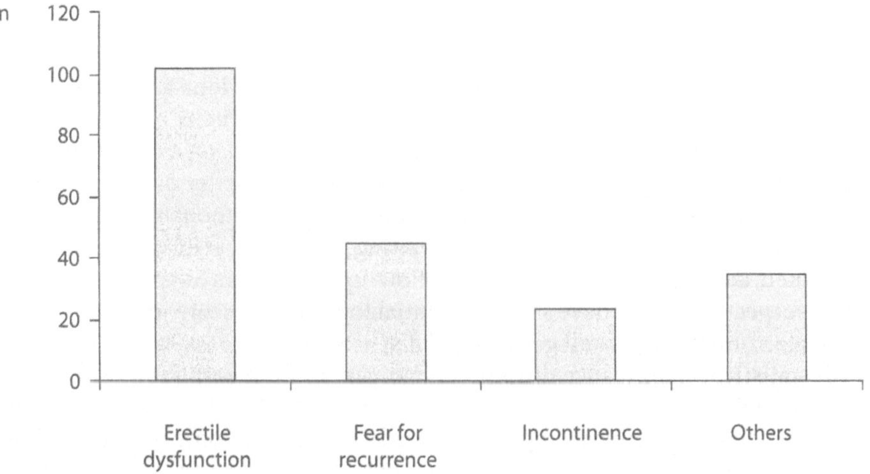

Fig. 22.2. Assessment of self-reported factors mostly imposing stress during cancer therapy in 430 patients after non-nerve-sparing radical prostatectomy performed in Herne, Germany, between 1986 and 1996 (in the order of items stated, multiple reasons possible)

HRQOL among 430 patients treated by radical prostatectomy during the years 1986 through 1996 in our institution, fear of tumor recurrence was cited by more patients as reducing the quality of life than was the "bother" from incontinence or erectile dysfunction, or indeed anything else except overall poor physical health (Fig. 22.1). Fear of recurrence was also given as the second most important cause of discomfort during follow-up (Fig. 22.2), a treatment aspect that would have been overlooked in conventional morbidity assessments.

One of the first clinical trials to assess overall HRQOL in men treated for clinically localized prostate cancer was a comparative cross-sectional analysis of men treated by radical prostatectomy (n=98), external beam radiation (56), or watchful waiting (60) with an age-matched population of 273 men without cancer living in California, USA [23]. In this survey, general health, cancer-related health, and prostate-specific treatment outcome were measured separately using different validated instruments. For cancer-specific HRQOL the Cancer Rehabilitation Evaluation System-Short Form and the Functional Assessment of Cancer Therapy (FACT) questionnaires were used.

To address disease-targeted HRQOL a specifically designed instrument assessing function and difficulty in three organ systems, namely sexual, urinary, and bowel, was developed; and it was later adopted by other investigators (e.g., Litwin disease-targeted quality of life survey).

In this survey no differences were seen in the general HRQOL factors. Although an occasional cancer-free man reported erectile dysfunction or incontinence, prostate cancer patients treated by surgery or radiation had significantly more problems with sexual, urinary, and bowel function than age-matched men without cancer. The fact that no differences were seen in general HRQOL strongly supported the need to use disease-targeted questionnaires [23].

Based on these findings and results from other cross-sectional, often retrospectively obtained, surveys a large-scale prospective observational trial was initiated using the same instruments to assess changes in HRQOL.

22.4 The Cancer of the Prostate Strategic Urologic Research Endeavor

The Cancer of the Prostate Strategic Urologic Research Endeavor (CaPSURE) is a database of patients with prostate cancer of any stage established through a number of academic as well as community-based urologists. There is no treatment protocol or recommendation; thus treatment decisions are made by the physician according to his or her clinical judgment. Patients enrolled in this database are assessed by self-administered questionnaires on a quarterly basis. From this database patients were evaluated immediately after diagnosis as well as 1 and 2 years after radical prostatectomy (with or without nerve sparing), external beam radiation, or watchful waiting. Trends in HRQOL scores were evaluated, adjusting for age, length of follow-up, and comorbidity. Results from this prospective survey have shown an initial low HRQOL score just after radical prostatectomy in almost all general and disease-specific areas, which improved with statistical significance during the first year of follow-up [26].

Sexual function and sexual problems were analyzed in 438 individuals treated with external beam radiation or radical prostatectomy with or without nerve sparing. Sexual function improved over time during the first year in all treatment groups. However, older patients who received external beam radiation showed substantial declines in sexual function after 2 years, a late aftermath not observed in the radical prostatectomy group. Also, sexual function was less often disturbed when nerve-sparing procedures were employed [24, 25].

22.5 The Prostate Cancer Outcomes Study

The Prostate Cancer Outcomes Study (PCOS) was initiated in 1994 by the National Cancer Institute (NCI) in the United States to look at the impact of treatments for primary prostate cancer on HRQOL. About 3500 men from six cancer registries are participating in this survey. Eighty-eight percent of the patients were diagnosed with clinically localized disease; 42% of these men were treated with radical prostatectomy, 24% with radiotherapy, 13% with hormonal therapy, and 22% were followed without treatment. This study is by far the largest survey, including now more than 1000 men treated by radical prostatectomy [32]. As in the CaPSURE database, men enrolled in POCS receive self-administered questionnaires, but on a yearly basis.

Of 1591 men with localized prostate cancer more than 2 years after treatment, those receiving radical prostatectomy (n=1156) reported more urinary incontinence (9.6% vs. 3.5%) and other urinary problems (11.2% vs. 2.3%) than men receiving radiotherapy (n=435). More men treated with prostatectomy also reported loss of erectile function (79.6% vs. 62.5%). However, only in younger men (ages 55 to 59) did more patients treated by radical prostatectomy report being bothered by loss of sexual function than did those receiving radiotherapy (59.4% vs. 25.3%). Again, men in the radical prostatectomy group recovered some urinary and sexual function during the second year after treatment, while men receiving radiotherapy worsened.

In general, prostatectomy had very little effect on bowel function while radiotherapy resulted in a decline in bowel function within the first 4 months of treatment. Two years after radiation 37.2% (vs. 20.9% in the radical prostatectomy group) reported suffering from diarrhea and 35.7% (vs. 14.5%) from bowel urgency.

No clear difference in emotional and mental health or overall physical health status was seen between the two groups [32].

At 18 months or more after surgery, 8.4% of the patients were incontinent and, at 24 months, 8.7% of men were bothered by the lack of urinary control. Regarding sexual function, 59.9% were unable to achieve an erection sufficient for sexual intercourse, of which number 41.9% reported to be bothered by it. Nevertheless, most men were satisfied with their treatment choice [38].

One of the unique features of both the CaPSURE and POCS trials is that the cohorts in these studies represent large community-based groups of patients from diverse racial and ethnic backgrounds treated in a broad range of health care settings. In contrast to the trials based on community settings, much better treatment outcomes have been reported in other studies where treatment was provided to a more selective patient cohort through a single institution.

This is clearly demonstrated when outcome data from the Johns Hopkins University, the state-of-the-art institution for radical prostatectomy, are compared to the outcome in the above-mentioned studies.

22.6 Johns Hopkins Outcomes of Radical Prostatectomy

To evaluate quality of life following radical retropubic prostatectomy using nerve-sparing techniques, self-reported outcomes of 62 men were recorded during 18 months of follow-up. The Litwin disease-targeted quality of life survey [23], assessing urinary, sexual, and bowel function and "bothersomeness," was used in this study for the large part, questions regarding bowel functions of the original questionnaire being eliminated in this study. The questionnaire was administered preoperatively as well as 3, 6, 12, and 18 months postoperatively.

By 18 months 93% of the patients were reported to have reached complete continence (e.g., wearing no pads). Ninety-three percent and 98% characterized urinary "bothersomeness" as none or minor, respectively.

Erectile dysfunction was rare in this study, with 86% of patients reporting achievement of unassisted intercourse with or without the use of sildenafil at 18 months. Eighty-four percent considered sexual "bothersomeness" as none or minor [43].

Self-reported treatment outcomes regarding erectile function and continence from these patients were also compared with data from patient charts

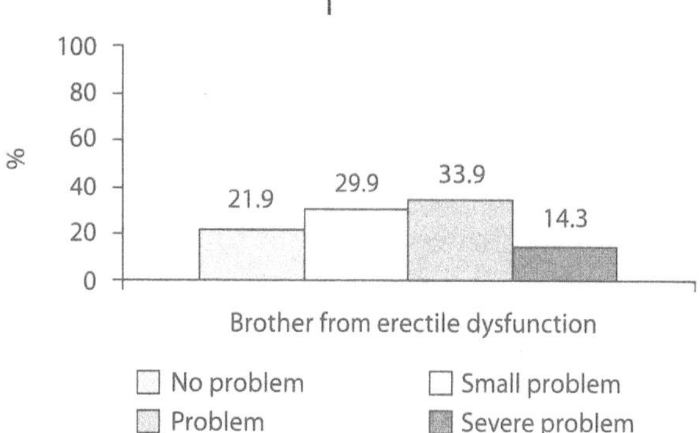

Fig. 22.3. Self-reported "bother" from loss of potency in 430 patients after non-nerve-sparing radical prostatectomy performed in Herne, Germany, between 1986 and 1996

and questionnaires administered to the patients' spouses. Remarkably, outcomes did not differ between the patients and spouses or from the physicians' evaluations. The author was prompted to question a widespread assumption that less favorable outcomes reported in clinical trials using self-administered instruments compared to in-office evaluations reflect patients' bias to inflate and investigators' to minimize adverse treatment outcomes [43].

As part of the extensively published data on long-term tumor control in more than 1500 men treated by this institution [33, 44], the report of this excellent outcome regarding adverse effects of radical prostatectomy gives a good idea of what may be achieved by this surgery,.

Other studies from single institutions have shown similar results in selected patient cohorts, showing that morbidity is low whenexperienced hands perform radical prostatectomy, and that excellent tumor control is provided as well. This latter is an important issue in terms of quality of life, since fear of tumor recurrence, as previously delineated, is substantial.

With regard to preservation of sexual function, it should be mentioned that many patients in that older age group already have erectile dysfunction from other causes, making nerve-sparing techniques irrelevant. In our patient population this was the fact in almost 30%. Also it should be pointed out that among those who lost their erection due to surgery, 50% were thereby bothered only mildly or not at all (Fig. 22.3). Comparable results have been published elsewhere [21]. These considerations should prompt discussion between patient and urologist as to whether nerves need be spared at surgery [11].

Patients in our institution were anonymously asked whether they would choose radical prostatectomy again for treatment, and whether they would suggest this form of treatment to a close relative or friend. These were patients who had had non-nerve-sparing radical prostatectomies, and whose postoperative rate of complete continence (defined as wearing no pads)was 76%. An answer of "Yes" was given by 97% to the first question and by 98% to the second. The same question (the first) was asked to more than 1300 patients receiving radical prostatectomy between the years 1962 and 1997 at various institutions (rate of complete continence defined as wearing no pads: 77%), Again the vast majority (77%) would choose radical prostatectomy again [15]. Both studies show, after all is said and done, a very high acceptance of this kind of therapy. They confirm that radical prostatectomy does preserve a reasonable good overall health-related quality of life.

Fig. 22.4. Self-reported acceptance of radical prostatectomy as cancer treatment: patients were anonymously asked whether or not they would retrospectively consider radical prostatectomy again as treatment (430 patients, non nerve sparing radical prostatectomy performed in Herne, Germany, between 1986 and 1996)

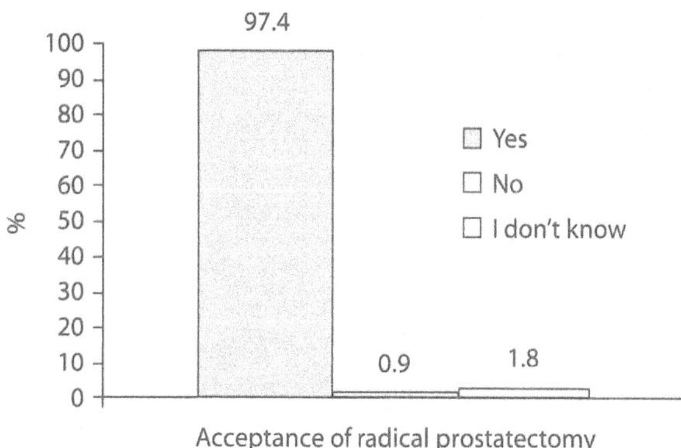

22.7 Summary

It can be stated that besides excellent tumor control, radical prostatectomy has an excellent overall outcome with regards to health-related quality of life. Overall health is only briefly affected and not altered in the long run. However, men with clinically localized prostate cancer who are treated with radical prostatectomy are more likely to experience urinary and sexual dysfunction than those treated with external beam radiation or watchful waiting. Bowel dysfunction, however, is uncommon in these patients, more commonly seen among men receiving external radiation therapy.

Stress incontinence reduces the quality of life in those affected; however, the vast majority of patients reach a stage of complete continence; and when minor urinary problems persist they do not influence well being at large. Those who are incontinent after surgery can be treated to gain HRQOL [7, 37], probably much more easily than those suffering from bowel urgency or bladder dysfunction resulting from radiation therapy.

Obviously, results are affected by training, but community studies have also demonstrated very good outcomes regarding continence. Again it should be emphasized that tumor control may be more important than possible morbidity in governing the choice of treatment.

Even nerve-sparing radical prostatectomy causes significant sexual dysfunction. The amount of "bother" resulting from this seems to vary and needs to be addressed before surgery. On the other hand, preservation of sexual function is certainly not guaranteed when the treatment is external beam radiation or brachytherapy, or a combination thereof. Once more, tumor control should be more important in the choice of therapy than erectile function.

Patient acceptance of radical prostatectomy is high, and so is fear of recurrence. As long as other forms of treatment have not shown at least the same long-term tumor control, radical prostatectomy for localized cancer of the prostate should be considered the gold standard in otherwise healthy males with a suitable life expectancy.

Appendix

ERTC QLQ-C30 (version 2.0.)

We are interested in some things about you and your health: Please answer all of the questions yourself by circling the number that best applies to you. There are no "right" or "wrong" answers. The information that you provide will remain strictly confidential.

Please fill in your initials:
Your birthdate (Day, Month, Year):
Today's date (Day, Month, Year):

	No	Yes
1. Do you have any trouble doin strenuous activities, like carrying a heavy shopping bag or a suitcase?	1	2
2. Do you have any trouble taking a long walk?	1	2
3. Do you have any trouble taking a short walk outside of the house?	1	2
4. Do you have to stay in a bed or a chair for most of the day?	1	2
5. Do you need help with eating, dressing, washing yourself or using the toilet?	1	2

During the past week:	**Not at All**	**A Little**	**Quite a Bit**	**Very much**
6. Were you limited in doing either your work or other daily activities?	1	2	3	4
7. Were you limited in pursuing your hobbies or other leisure time activities?	1	2	3	4
8. Were you short of breath?	1	2	3	4
9. Have your had pain?	1	2	3	4
10. Did you need to rest?	1	2	3	4
11. Have your had trouble sleeping?	1	2	3	4
12. Have you felt weak?	1	2	3	4
13. Have you lacked appetite?	1	2	3	4
14. Have you felt nauseated?	1	2	3	4
15. Have your vomited?	1	2	3	4

Please go on to the next page

During the past week:	Not at All	A Little	Quite a Bit	Very much
16. Have you been constipated?	1	2	3	4
17. Have you had diarrhea?	1	2	3	4
18. Were you tired?	1	2	3	4
19. Did pain interfere with your daily activities?	1	2	3	4
20. Have you had difficulty in concentrating on things, like reading a newspaper or watching television?	1	2	3	4
21. Did you feel tense?	1	2	3	4
22. Did you worry?	1	2	3	4
23. Did you fell irritable?	1	2	3	4
24. Did you feel depressed?	1	2	3	4
25. Have you had diffculty remembering things?	1	2	3	4
26. Has your physical condition or medial treatment interfered with your <u>family</u> life?	1	2	3	4
27. Has your physical condition or medical treatment interfered with your <u>social</u> activities?	1	2	3	4
28. Has your physical condition or medical treatment caused you financial difficulties?	1	2	3	4

For the following questions please circle the number between 1 and 7 that best applies to you

29. How would you rate your overall <u>health</u> during the past week?

1	2	3	4	5	6	7
Very poor						Excellent

30. How would you rate your overall <u>quality of life</u> during the past week?

1	2	3	4	5	6	7
Very poor						Excellent

Prostate Cancer module QLQ-RR25 in evaluation of EORTC.

References

1. Arai Y, Okubo K, Aoki Y, Maekawa S, Okada T, Maeda H, Ogawa O, Kato T (1999) Patient-reported quality of life after radical prostatectomy for prostate cancer. Int J Urol 6:78–86
2. Bonomi AE, Cella DF, Hahn EA, Bjordal K, Sperner-Unterweger B, Gangeri L, Bergman B, Willems-Groot J, Hanquet P, Zittoun R (1996) Multilingual translation of the Functional Assessment of Cancer Therapy (FACT) quality of life measurement system. Qual Life Res 5:309–320
3. Borghede G, Sullivan M (1996) Measurement of quality of life in localized prostatic cancer patients treated with radiotherapy. Development of a prostate cancer-specific module supplementing the EORTC QLQ-C30. Qual Life Res 5:212–222
4. Braslis KG, Santa-Cruz C, Brickman AL, Soloway MS (1995) Quality of life 12 months after radical prostatectomy. Br J Urol 75:48–53
5. Coates A, Porzsolt F, Osoba D (1997) Quality of life in oncology practice: prognostic value of EORTC QLQ-C30 scores in patients with advanced malignancy. Eur J Cancer 33:1025–1030
6. Feneley MRPartin AW (2000) Diagnosis of localized prostate cancer: 10 years of progress. Curr Opin Urol 10:319–327
7. Fleshner N, Herschorn S (1996) The artificial urinary sphincter for post-radical prostatectomy incontinence: impact on urinary symptoms and quality of life. J Urol 155:1260–1264
8. Fossa SD, Woehre H, Kurth KH, Hetherington J, Bakke H, Rustad DA, Skanvik R (1997) Influence of urological morbidity on quality of life in patients with prostate cancer. Eur Urol 31 [Suppl 3]:3–8
9. Fowler FJ Jr, Barry MJ, Lu-Yao G, Wasson J, Roman A, Wennberg J (1995) Effect of radical prostatectomy for prostate cancer on patient quality of life: results from a Medicare survey. Urology 45:1007–1013; discussion 1013–1005
10. Garratt AM, Ruta DA, Abdalla MI, Buckingham JK, Russell IT (1993) The SF36 health survey questionnaire: an outcome measure suitable for routine use within the NHS? BMJ 306: 1440–1444
11. Gralnek D, Wessells H, Cui H, Dalkin BL (2000) Differences in sexual function and quality of life after nerve sparing and nonnerve sparing radical retropubic prostatectomy. J Urol 163: 1166–1169; discussion 1169–1170
12. Heathcote PS, Mactaggart PN, Boston RJ, James AN, Thompson LC, Nicol DL (1998) Health-related quality of life in Australian men remaining disease-free after radical prostatectomy. Med J Aust 168:483–486
13. Jenkinson C, Coulter A, Wright L (1993) Short form 36 (SF36) health survey questionnaire: normative data for adults of working age. BMJ 306:1437–1440
14. Jonler M, Madsen FA, Rhodes PR, Sall M, Messing EM, Bruskewitz RC (1996) A prospective study of quantification of urinary incontinence and quality of life in patients undergoing radical retropubic prostatectomy. Urology 48:433–440
15. Kao TC, Cruess DF, Garner D, Foley J, Seay T, Friedrichs P, Thrasher JB, Mooneyhan RD, McLeod DG, Moul JW (2000) Multicenter patient self-reporting questionnaire on impotence, incontinence and stricture after radical prostatectomy. J Urol 163:858–864
16. Kempen GI (1992) The MOS Short-Form General Health Survey: single item vs. multiple measures of health-related quality of life: some nuances. Psychol Rep 70:608–610
17. King MT (1996) The interpretation of scores from the EORTC quality of life questionnaire QLQ-C30. Qual Life Res 5:555–567
18. King MT, Dobson AJ, Harnett PR (1996) A comparison of two quality-of-life questionnaires for cancer clinical trials: the functional living index-cancer (FLIC) and the quality of life questionnaire core module (QLQ-C30). J Clin Epidemiol 49:21–29
19. Kornblith AB, Herr HW, Ofman US, Scher HI, Holland JC (1994) Quality of life of patients with prostate cancer and their spouses. The value of a data base in clinical care. Cancer 73:2791–2802
20. Krupski T, Petroni GR, Bissonette EA, Theodorescu D (2000) Quality-of-life comparison of radical prostatectomy and interstitial brachytherapy in the treatment of clinically localized prostate cancer. Urology 55:736–742
21. Lerner SE, Richards SL, Benet AE, Kahan NZ, Fleischmann JD, Melman A (1996) [Detailed evaluation of sexual function after radical prostatectomy: is patient satisfaction correlated with the quality of erections?] Prog Urol 6:552–557
22. Lim AJ, Brandon AH, Fiedler J, Brickman AL, Boyer CI, Raub WA Jr, Soloway MS (1995) Quality of life: radical prostatectomy versus radiation therapy for prostate cancer. J Urol 154:1420–1425
23. Litwin MS, Hays RD, Fink A, Ganz PA, Leake B, Leach GE, Brook RH (1995) Quality-of-life outcomes in men treated for localized prostate cancer. JAMA 273:129–135
24. Litwin MS, Flanders SC, Pasta DJ, Stoddard ML, Lubeck DP, Henning JM (1999) Sexual function and bother after radical prostatectomy or radiation for prostate cancer: multivariate quality-of-life analysis from CaPSURE. Cancer of the Prostate Strategic Urologic Research Endeavor. Urology 54:503–508
25. Litwin MS, Pasta DJ, Yu J, Stoddard ML, Flanders SC (2000) Urinary function and bother after radical prostatectomy or radiation for prostate cancer: a longitudinal, multivariate quality of life analysis from the Cancer of the Prostate Strategic Urologic Research Endeavor. J Urol 164: 1973–1977

26. Lubeck DP, Litwin MS, Henning JM, Stoddard ML, Flanders SC, Carroll PR (1999) Changes in health-related quality of life in the first year after treatment for prostate cancer: results from CaPSURE. Urology 53:180–186
27. Morrow GR, Lindke J, Black P (1992) Measurement of quality of life in patients: psychometric analyses of the Functional Living Index-Cancer (FLIC). Qual Life Res 1:287–296
28. Nease RF Jr (2000) Challenges in the validation of preference-based measures of health-related quality of life. Med Care 38 [Suppl 9]:155–159
29. Norlen BJ (1994) Swedish randomized trial of radical prostatectomy versus watchful waiting. Can J Oncol 4 [Suppl 1]:38–40; discussion 41–42
30. Pedersen KV, Carlsson P, Rahmquist M, Varenhorst E (1993) Quality of life after radical retropubic prostatectomy for carcinoma of the prostate. Eur Urol 24:7–11
31. Perez MA, Meyerowitz BE, Lieskovsky G, Skinner DG, Reynolds B, Skinner EC (1997) Quality of life and sexuality following radical prostatectomy in patients with prostate cancer who use or do not use erectile aids. Urology 50:740–746
32. Potosky AL, Legler J, Albertsen PC, Stanford JL, Gilliland FD, Hamilton AS, Eley JW, Stephenson RA, Harlan LC (2000) Health outcomes after prostatectomy or radiotherapy for prostate cancer: results from the Prostate Cancer Outcomes Study. J Natl Cancer Inst 92:1582–1592
33. Pound CR, Partin AW, Eisenberger MA, Chan DW, Pearson JD, Walsh PC (1999) Natural history of progression after PSA elevation following radical prostatectomy. JAMA 281:1591–1597
34. Rossetti SR, Terrone C (1996) Quality of life in prostate cancer patients. Eur Urol 30 [Suppl 1]: 44–48; discussion 49
35. Schwartz EJ, Lepor H (1999) Radical retropubic prostatectomy reduces symptom scores and improves quality of life in men with moderate and severe lower urinary tract symptoms. J Urol 161:1185–1188
36. Schwartz JS (1995) Prostate Cancer Intervention Versus Observation Trial: economic analysis in study design and conditions of uncertainty. J Natl Cancer Inst Monogr 19:73–75
37. Smith DN, Appell RA, Rackley RR, Winters JC (1998) Collagen injection therapy for post-prostatectomy incontinence. J Urol 160:364–367
38. Stanford JL, Ziding F, Hamilton AS (2000) Urinary and sexual function after radical prostatectomy for clinically localized prostate cancer. JAMA 283:354–360
39. Stockler MR, Osoba D, Goodwin P, Corey P, Tannock IF (1998) Responsiveness to change in health-related quality of life in a randomized clinical trial: a comparison of the Prostate Cancer Specific Quality of Life Instrument (PROSQOLI) with analogous scales from the EORTC QLQ-C30 and a trial specific module. European Organization for Research and Treatment of Cancer. J Clin Epidemiol 51:137–145
40. Stockler MR, Osoba D, Corey P, Goodwin PJ, Tannock IF (1999) Convergent discriminitive, and predictive validity of the Prostate Cancer Specific Quality of Life Instrument (PROSQOLI) assessment and comparison with analogous scales from the EORTC QLQ-C30 and a trial-specific module. European Organisation for Research and Treatment of Cancer. Core Quality of Life Questionnaire. J Clin Epidemiol 52:653–666
41. Walsh PC (1998) Anatomic radical prostatectomy: evolution of the surgical technique. J Urol 160:2418–2424
42. Walsh PC (2000) Cancer surveillance series: interpreting trends in prostate cancer. I. Evidence of the effects of screening in recent prostate cancer incidence, mortality, and survival rates. J Urol 163:364–365
43. Walsh PC (2000) Radical prostatectomy for localized prostate cancer provides durable cancer control with excellent quality of life: a structured debate. J Urol 163:1802–1807
44. Walsh PC, Partin AW, Epstein JI (1994) Cancer control and quality of life following anatomical radical retropubic prostatectomy: results at 10 years. J Urol 152:1831–1836
45. Weitzner MA, McMillan SC (1999) The Caregiver Quality of Life Index-Cancer (CQOLC) Scale: revalidation in a home hospice setting. J Palliat Care 15:13–20
46. Weitzner MA, Jacobsen PB, Wagner H Jr, Friedland J, Cox C (1999) The Caregiver Quality of Life Index-Cancer (CQOLC) scale: development and validation of an instrument to measure quality of life of the family caregiver of patients with cancer. Qual Life Res 8:55–63
47. Wilt TJ, Brawer MK (1994) The Prostate Cancer Intervention Versus Observation Trial: a randomized trial comparing radical prostatectomy versus expectant management for the treatment of clinically localized prostate cancer. J Urol 152:1910–1914
48. Wilt TJ, Brawer MK (1997) The Prostate Cancer Intervention Versus Observation Trial (PIVOT). Oncology (Huntingt) 11:1133–1139; discussion 1139–1140, 1143

23 Diagnosis and Therapy of Erectile Dysfunction Following Radical Prostatectomy

A. Heidenreich, P. Olbert, R. Hofmann

23.1 Introduction

Radical prostatectomy has been the standard approach for the treatment of clinically organ-confined prostate cancer. The result has been long term cancer-specific survival and progression-free rates of more than 80% in specimen-confined disease [2, 42, 45]. Although the surgical technique in radical retropubic prostatectomy (RRP), radical perineal prostatectomy (and, recently, radical laproscopic prostatectomy) has seen dramatic improvement over the last decade, incontinence and impotence still persist as the most serious morbidities resulting from surgery [2, 42]. In classical RRP with no attempt to save the neurovascular bundles, impotence rates were as high as 100%; but even with nerve-sparing techniques designed to maintain potency, approximately 40%–70% of patients have been rendered impotent [7, 30, 42, 43, 45]. The Prostate Cancer Outcome Study demonstrated recently that 60% of men who had undergone RRP 24 months earlier reported erections not firm enough for sexual intercourse, and 44% were unable to achieve any erection [42]. Although retention of potency correlated with nerve-sparing approaches, no great difference existed among the different surgical strategies: 66% of non-nerve-sparing techniques, 59% of unilateral nerve-sparing procedures, and 56% of bilateral nerve-sparing techniques were associated with erectile dysfunction 24 months after therapy. Sexual dysfunction was reported by 42% of all men as a moderate to big problem in their life after surgery. Since sexual function is a significant patient/partner concern and significantly contributes to quality of life, many men diagnosed with prostate cancer search for alternative therapeutic options that may offer a lower risk of impotence despite the good disease control associated with radical prostatectomy [2].

It is the task of this chapter to briefly review the physiology of erection and the pathophysiology of erectile dysfunction following RRP, as well as to report on the different therapeutic strategies once impotence has developed.

23.2 Physiology of Erection

Penile erection is a neurovascular event modulated by psychological factors and hormonal status (Fig. 23.1). Each of the four columns depicted is important for normal erections, and disturbances in any one of these parameters will cause an imbalance in the physiologic situation and result in erectile dysfunction. The penis and the corpora cavernosaare innervated by somatic (pudendal) and autonomic nerves; sympathetic and parasympathetic nerves merge in the pelvis and form the cavernous nerves regulating blood flow during tumescence and rigidity.

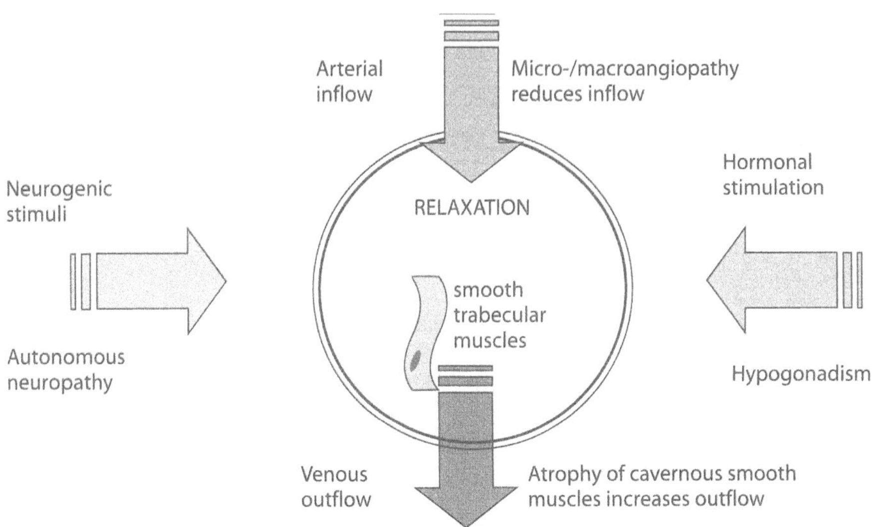

Fig. 23.1. Schematic and simplified model of the physiologic and pathophysiologic events involved in penile erections and erectile dysfunction

Sexual stimulation with consecutive release of neurotransmitters from the cavernous nerve terminals and of relaxing factors from the endothelial cells results in relaxation of the smooth muscles in the arteries and arterioles of the corpora cavernosa and in a significant dilatation of cavernosal and helical arteries. Parallel relaxation of the trabecular smooth muscles increases the compliance of the sinusoids. These rapidly fill, and their expansion results in an elongation and compression of the venules against the tunica albuginea. Blood is trapped within the corporal bodies and the penis widens and elongates to its full capacity. During sexual intercourse the base of the penis and the corporal bodies are compressed by the ischiocavernous muscles, leading to a significant rise of intracavernous pressure and an even harder erection. Nitric oxide (NO) released from the endothelium has been identified as the main neurotransmitter mediating penile erection [21, 38]. NO activates the enzyme guanylate cyclase which increases the intracellular concentration of cyclic guanosine monophosphate (cGMP) by transformation of guanosine triphosphate (GTP) (Figs. 23.1 and 23.2). By inhibiting calcium channels, cGMP causes the efflux of calcium and potassium and the influx of calcium, the result being a decrease in intracellular calcium concentration, which reduction initiates erection by trig-

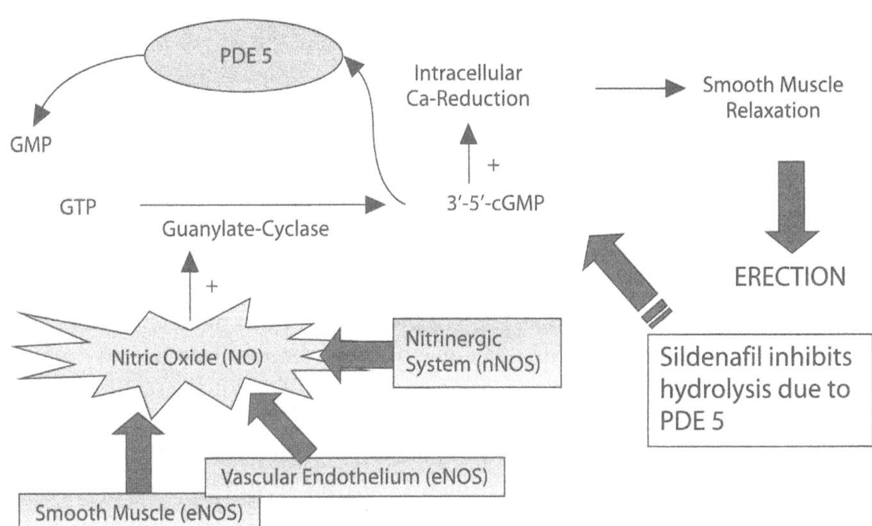

Fig. 23.2. Nitric oxide and GMP mechanisms involved in erections

gering a step-wise relaxation of the smooth muscles of the endothelium of the corpora cavernosa. A return to the flaccid state is introduced by the hydrolysis of cGMP to GMP by the specific phosphodiesterase type 5 (PDE5).

23.3 Pathophysiology of Erectile Dysfunction Following RRP

Impotence can be the result of various psychogenic, neurogenic, hormonal, arterial, cavernosal, drug-induced effects, or of a combination of these. Erectile dysfunction following RRP is potentially the result of neural and vascular injury during surgery. It has been hypothesized that damage to the neurovascular bundles leads to poor oxygenation of the smooth muscles of the corpus cavernosum, resulting in poor or absent erections, and eventually perhaps to corporeal fibrosis and veno-occlusive failure [8, 29, 31].

23.3.1 Injury to Cavernous Nerves

Injury to the cavernous nerves during RRP most commonly is caused by lateral dissection near the prostatic apex and around the prostatic capsule. According to an anatomic study of Paick et al. [34], the cavernous nerves run between the prostatic capsule and the endopelvic fascia. They travel beneath the posterolateral aspect of the prostate until reaching the prostatic apex some 9–12 mm cranial to the urogenital diaphragm. According to that study, the cavernous nerves divide into several branches and spread out anterolaterally, with the most medial branches lying in close proximity to the membranous urethra, and the most lateral branches piercing the urogenital diaphragm close to the external sphincter. The lateral branches might survive apical dissection, thereby explaining reports on potency following non-nerve-sparing RRP. The classical dissection techniques, however, will injure all medial and lateral branches and result in the high impotence rate of close to 100%. Although the nerve-sparing technique described by Walsh [44, 45] preserves the cavernous nerves, it has been reported to take 6–18 months before 41% to 69% of the patients recover erectile function [13, 20, 36] – a phenomenon not well understood.

Recently, Carrier et al. [5] presented a potential explanation with regard to this phenomenon in an experimental animal model. After uni- and bilateral cavernous nerve transsection in rats, the number, distribution, and regeneration of NO syntase-containing nerves in the corpus cavernous and dorsal nerves were studied by immunohistochemistry and electrostimulation. As compared to a control group, a significant increase in the number of NOS-containing nerves was observed in the unilateral ablation group 6 months after surgery – which still was lower than in the control group – but no regeneration was identified in the bilateral ablation group. After electrostimulation there was no increase in intracavernous pressure in the bilateral ablation group, whereas there was no significant difference between the unilateral ablation group and the control group. These data demonstrate that nerve regeneration even after unilateral dissection can take place and result in a normal response to stimuli. The calculated time required for nerve regeneration correlates well with clinical observation. These experimental findings are further corroborated by the clinical observation that the response to sildenafil – a drug requiring an intact NO pathway – for the treatment of erectile dysfunction is best in patients with bilateral nerve-sparing RRP. However, it may take 18–24 months until peak treatment satisfaction rate is reached by patients with unilateral nerve-sparing RRP [20].

Therefore, since cavernous nerve regeneration also might take place at some time following RRP, a bilateral nerve-sparing procedure should be performed whenever possible.

23.3.2 Vascular Injury

It has long been hypothesized that a significant number of patients suffer from erectile dysfunction, despite nerve-sparing surgery, because of injury to penile arterial system or to that providing veno-occlusive function.

Breza et al. [3] described the detailed anatomy of the penile neurovascular structures. In addition to the normal arterial blood supply by the pudendal artery, they found an accessory pudendal artery traveling along the lower part of the bladder and the anterolateral surface of the prostate in seven of ten cadavers; in one the accessory pudendal artery alone provided blood to the corpus cavernosum and the erectile tissue. The authors pointed out that, due to their closeness to the bladder and prostate, the accessory pudendal arteries might be easily dissected during RRP. This loss might contribute to the development of erectile dysfunction, especially in older patients with an already diminished penile blood flow. In their clinical series, however, Polascik et al. [35] identified accessory pudendal arteries in only 4% of the patients undergoing RRP. The arteries were preserved in 19/33 (57.6%) and dissected in 14/33 (42.4%), and the authors could not identify a significant difference between the two groups with regard to the recovery of sexual function, 67% versus 50%, respectively. The interval to recovery of sexual function was 7.9±3.2 months versus 15.6±18.4 months. The role of dissected accessory pudendal arteries in the pathogenesis of postsurgical impotence after RRP is still unclear, but if the incidence is only 4%, it certainly is not a major contributor to erectile dysfunction.

A number of studies have assessed the role of penile vascular injury in erectile dysfunction after radical prostatectomy by the use of intracavernosal injection of vasoactive agents and pulsed Doppler ultrasonography. Kim et al. [22] did not demonstrate any significant differences with regard to cavernous artery diameter, peak systolic flow velocity, penile blood flow, end diastolic flow, and resistance index regardless of the type of radical prostatectomy performed. All findings were similar to those in the unilateral nerve sparing analysis. On the other hand, Aboseif et al. [1] and DeLuca et al. [11] demonstrated a significant decrease in peak flow velocity and in diameter of the cavernosal arteries after intracavernosal injection of vasoactive agents, in 40% [1] and 16% [11] of the patients, respectively. Based on these results, it has to be concluded that post-prostatectomy impotence is a multifactorial problem, with neurogenic and vascular injury playing substantial roles.

Table 23.1. Therapeutic options for the management of impotence following radical prostatectomy

Therapeutic options
Oral pharmacologic therapy
Vacuum constriction devices
Intraurethral application of vasoactive agents
Intracavernous injections of vasoactive agents
Penile prosthesis

23.4 Therapy of Erectile Dysfunction Following RRP

As outlined, pathogenesis of post-prostatectomy impotence is the result of combined vascular and neurogenic injury so that no specific diagnostic approach is necessary prior to initiation of therapy. With regard to treatment, there are a variety of therapeutic options which have to be discussed extensively with the patient and his female partner [25] (Table 23.1). We also have to respect that not all patients are bothered by postoperative erectile dysfunction (Fig. 23.3): basically all young patients are significantly bothered by their impotence whereas less than a majority (45%) of patients older than 70 years experience impotence as a significant problem.

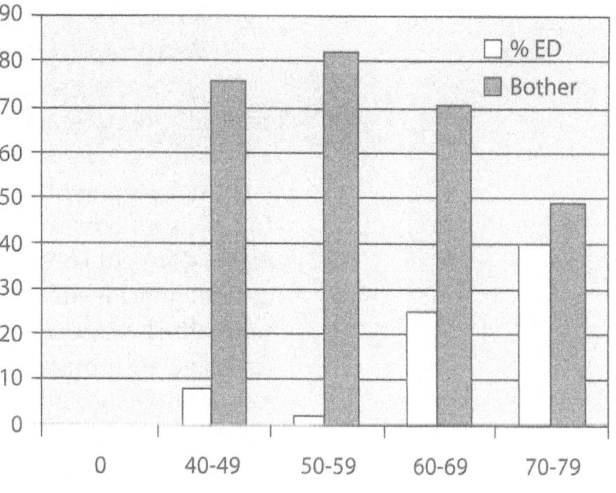

Fig. 23.3. Percentage of patients experiencing erectile dyfunction (*ED*) due to various etiologies and being bothered by impotence

23.4.1 Oral Pharmacologic Therapy

Sildenafil citrate (Viagra) has revolutionized the therapy for erectile dysfunction that is independent of pathophysiology [26]. As previously discussed (Sect. 23.2, Figs. 23.1, 23.2), hydrolysis of cyclic GMP to GMP by phosphodiesterase type 5 (PDE5) terminates erection and results in the return to the flaccid state. Sildenafil citrate is a selective inhibitor of PDE5, and thus produces a marked elevation of intracellular cyclic GMP concentrations in the glans penis, corpora cavernosa, and corpus spongiosum, leading to an increased smooth muscle relaxation and better erection [21, 38]. To be effective, sildenafil citrate requires both sexual stimulation and intact NO-generating pathways.

With regard to the treatment of post-prostatectomy impotence, a number of studies have been performed with divergent results [13, 20, 24, 33, 47, 48]. Zippe et al. [48] treated 28 patients after a mean interval after surgery of 12.8 months with a starting dose of 50 mg sildenafil citrate. A positive response with the ability to penetrate was observed in 80% of patients having undergone bilateral nerve-sparing RRP; in unilateral nsRRP and in classic RRP, none of the patients achieved adequate erections. Similar results were reported by Lowentritt et al. [24], who observed an improvement of erections in 58% of men with both sides, 57% with one side, and 20% with no nerves spared in RRP; sexual ability improved in 46%, 39%, and 10%, respectively. The most important predicitve factor for a positive response to sildenafil was the degree of nerve sparing during the surgical procedure. Other significant predictive factors included patient age (<55 years), time since surgery (<6 months), and preoperative potency status [36]. In another study, Hong et al. [20] demonstrated a 60% satisfaction rate which was found to peak between 18 months and 2 years following RRP, indicating that early nonresponders should not be discouraged as they might do so later. An update of their initial study including 91 patients confirmed the high satisfaction rate of sildenafil following bilateral nsRRP; however, with a longer mean interval from surgery even 50% of the unilateral nsRRP group and 15% of the non-nsRRP group responded to sildenafil, findings in accord with experimental studies suggesting a spontaneous regeneration of the cavernosal nerves with time [5]. Similar results were reported by Feng et al. [13] who observed 71%, 80%, and 5.9% response rates following bilateral, unilateral, and non- nsRRP, respectively, in 53 consecutive patients.

In conclusion, 80% of patients with post-prostatectomy impotence respond well to sildenafil citrate if both neurovascular bundles are preserved during surgery. Preservation of only one bundle reduces the chance of recovery to 25% and in patients with a non-nerve-sparing RRP the chance for erectile recovery is basically nonexistent. Therefore, nerve-sparing procedures performed by experienced urologists should be the surgical treatment of choice for clinically localized prostate cancer.

23.4.2
Vacuum Constriction Devices

Basically all patients suffering from impotence are candidates for vacuum therapy. Patients with severe scarring of the corpora cavernosa may not get a sufficient engorgement, and some patients with Peyronie's disease are unable to use the vacuum device because of the degree of deviation; however, other absolute or relative contraindications are few. Patients with bleeding disorders or on anticoaguation therapy should not use a vacuum device. Among 161 patients with short-term use (average 3 months) and 115 patients with long-term use (average 29 months) patient and partner satisfaction were 82% and 87% and 84% and 89%, respectively [9]. "Quality of erection" with regard to hardness, length, and circumference of the penis was greater than 90% of perfect satisfaction in both groups. Moreover, the adequate erection achieved in about 90% is accompanied by low morbidity and low cost. Still, only 50%–60% of patients and their partners accept vacuum devices permanently as treatment for erection problems. This low acceptance rate compared to other treatment modalities is mainly due to the "technical" induction of erections, the dribbling ejaculation, penile coldness, livid change in penile color, all three the result of the penile shaft ring, and finally because of diminishing erection during intercourse. A recent study [41] found the acceptance rate lowest among young men, men with a short duration of erectile dysfunction, and among men with impotence due to classic RRP.

Although a noninvasive treatment option, complications and side effects such as penile skin necrosis, urethral bleeding, Peyronie's disease, and testicular migration are potential problems after long-term use of vacuum devices [14].

23.4.3
Intraurethral Application of Vasoactive Agents

Efficacy and safety of intraurethral alprostadil (MUSE) in patients with erectile dysfunction following RRP have only been evaluated in one study [10] composed of 384 patients. This was a multicenter double-blind, parallel-placebo-controlled trial consisting of a clinical titration phase to assess the adequate dose required to achieve erections sufficient for sexual intercourse and a home treatment phase. During the clinical phase 270 patients (70.3%) achieved adequate erections for sexual intercourse with 66.3% of the patients requiring a dose of 500 or 1000 µg alprostadil, but in the home treatment phase only 57.1% of the patients had sucessful sexual intercourse. Combining the clinical with the home success rate yields an overall response rate of 40.1%, which appears to be the realistic likelihood of successful use of alprostadil at home. The most common side effects were penile pain in 39.9%, urethral/meatal burning in 18.3%, and dizziness in 2.4%.

In conclusion, MUSE appear to be a treatment option for post-prostatectomy impotence with similar response rates to sildenafil in patients with unilateral or non-nsRRP.

23.4.4
Intracavernous Injections of Vasoactive Agents

Prostaglandin E_1 (PGE_1) is the most commonly used intracavernous drug for the treatment of organic erectile dysfunction and achieves success rates of approximately 90%. This substance directly relaxes the the trabecular smooth muscle (with or without sexual stimulation), acts independently of endogenous vasoactive substances such as NO production, and has the further benefit of inhibiting connective tissue synthesis [31]. Treatment-related side effects are priapism in 3%, cavernosal fibrosis in about 10%, and pain at injection in some 17%–34% of men. The dropout rate from penile self-injection therapy is reported at about 30% due to cost, problems with the concept of self injection, and spontaneous improvement of erections [32].

Studies with regard to efficacy, safety and patient acceptance of intracavernous injections for management of post-prostatectomy impotence are rare although the first experiences were reported as early as 1988 [15]. A success rate of 95% adequate penile stiffness resulted in a patient acceptance of 82% in the study by Rodriguez Vela et al. [37]; furthermore, the authors observed a decrease of the minimally effective dose if active treatment had been started within 6 months after nsRRP in men younger than 60. Soderdahl et al. [41] compared the acceptance of intracavernosal self-injections versus external vacuum devices in the treatment of erectile dysfunction of various etiologies in 45 patients. The authors found a similar acceptance rate of 80% for injection therapy and the use of vacuum devices; however, patients younger than 60 years, those with a shorter duration of impotence, and those impotent after radical prostatectomy strongly favored injection therapy.

Intracavernosal injections of PGE_1 have been demonstrated to be more effective in achieving good erections than MUSE (90% vs 60%) as well as in ability to have intercourse (85% vs 55%) [41]. Nevertheless, MUSE was accepted by 90% of the patients due to its easy application as compared to intracavernosal PGE_1.

Switching from intracavernosal PGE_1 injections to oral sildenafil citrate appears to be an attractive concept which, however, has been found to be successful in only two thirds of trial patients [19]. The problem herecan probably be explained by the different pharmacologic mechanisms of the two drugs. On the other hand, PGE_1 has been found to be effective in 90% of those failing sildenafil therapy [39]. Accounting for this is quite likely the fact that PGE_1 acts directly on the trabecular smooth muscles of the corpus cavernosum without the need of an intact NO pathway.

23.4.5 Pharmacologic Agents and Spontaneous Return of Potency

Besides providing their own specific activity, it has been demonstrated that early use of pharmacologic agents enhances the recovery of spontaneous potency in patients following RRP [4, 27]. Three months after nsRRP 30 patients were randomized to receive intracavernous injections of alprostadil three times a week for 12 consecutive weeks (group 1), or to be observed for 12 weeks without active treatment (group 2). Of the 12 patients in group 1 who could be evaluated for response, 67% demonstrated recovery of spontaneous erections sufficient for intercourse, and 33% experienced at least some degree of spontaneous recovery of potency. In group 2, however, spontaneous recovery of sufficient erections was only observed in 20%, while recovery of some type of erections was described in 67% of the patients. These data would appear to suggest that the early use of intracavernous injections of PGE_1 should be offered to all patients having undergone nsRRP to facilitate spontaneous recovery of potency.

These results were substantiated by Brock et al. [4], who observed a return of spontaneous erections in 26/70 men (37%) during long-term intracavernous alprostadil treatment for erectile dysfunction of various etiology.

23.4.6 Penile Prosthesis

A penile prothesis is currently implanted in about 3% of all men suffering from erectile dysfunction following RRP [2]. The majority of these implantations have taken place within the first 2 years following RRP, only 8% after that.

Implantation of penile prosthesis is indicated in all patients who have failed or who do not accept other kinds of medical or surgical therapy. Currently, two-piece and three-piece inflatable penile prostheses, such as the Mentor Alpha-1 or the AMS 700CX, are the models most commonly used, whereas semirigid rods rarely are implanted in non-disabled patients.

Patient acceptance of both models is excellent, with 89% and 90% of couples reporting satisfaction with, respectively, the quality of erections and intercourse [6, 16, 17]. Both men with a penile prosthesis and their female partners have the highest satisfaction rates of all treatment options in the management of erectile dysfunction. However, a recent study published by Montorsi et al. [28] indicated that 30% and 20% of men complain about penile shortening and poor glandular engorgement, respectively; partners complained of the unnaturalness of the prosthetic erection.

With regard to long term survival 93% of the Menor Alpha-1 devices were not found to need replacement or revision over a mean follow-up period of 22 months [16]. The most common complications necessitating Alpha-1 device replacement were infection in 2.8%, and device malfunction and fluid loss in 2.1% each. In a study of 372 patients using the AMS 700CX, with a mean follow-up time of 57 months [6], device malfunction complications occurred in 17.5%, surgical revision was necessary in 13.7%, and 28 devices (7.5%) were explanted. These two studies demonstrate that the reliability of the devices is very high, especially when the length of follow-up is considered; postoperative complication and morbidity rates are low while the satisfaction rates of patients and partners is very high (Tables 23.2, 23.3).

In confirmation of the results described above, other investigators have found that the most common complication in the use of a penile prosthesis is infection at the site of the implant; rates have been reported from 2% to 16% [6, 12, 17]. Infection ususally results in explantation of the infected part of the prosthesis, wound irrigation with antibiotics, and insertion of a new prosthesis followed by intravenous antibiotic therapy. This salvage procedure has been said to result in eradication of the infection in 85% of the cases. Another option is to remove all parts of the prothesis, drain the wound, and implant a complete, new device after 3 to 6 months. This procedure has, however, been reported to

Table 23.2. Complications of penile implants with regard to infection and total revision rates including revision for infections and technical malfunction

Author	*n*	Implant	Infection	Revision	Median
Kabalin et al. [?]	62	AMS Dynaflex	4.8%	32%	no data
Holloway et al. [?]	45	AMS 700	2.7%	??%	no data
Wilson et al. [46]	253	Hydroflex	2.4%	33%	4.53 J.
	42	Dynaflex	2.4%	55%	2.61 J.
	306	AMS 700CX	6.9%	17%	6.65 J.
	720	Mentor α-1	2.3%	9.3%	>8.0 J.
Goldstein et al. [16]	434	Mentor α-1	2.8%	6.9%	>8.0
J. Montorsi et al. [?]	200	AMS 700	6.0%	10%	>5.0 J.

Table 23.3. Patient's and partner's satisfaction with penile implants

Expectations fulfilled	89%
Satisfaction with sexual activity	83%
Sexual self-esteem ↑	80%
Satisfaction with function	84%
Partner's satisfaction	68%

result in fibrosis and contraction of the corpora cavernosa. Erosion and migration most commonly are associated with semirigid prostheses. Glandular ischemia and penile necrosis are disastrous but very rare complications developing in severe diabetes, extensive vascular disease, and in severe edema with tissue dissection. Perineal pain existing longer than 1–2 months may reflect a periprosthetic infection or a too large prosthesis. Besides these medical problems, mechanical problems such as fluid leakage, auto-inflation, and cylinder aneurysm and/or rupture have been known to occur.

References

1. Aboseif S, Shinohara K, Breza J, et al (1994) Role of penile vascular injury in erectile dysfunction after radical prostatectomy. Br J Urol 73:75–82
2. Benoit RM, Naslund MJ, Cohen JK (2000) Complications after radical retropubic prostatectomy in the medicare population. Urology 56:116–120
3. Breza J, Aboseif SR, Orvis BR, et al (1989) Detailed anatomy of penile neurovascular structures: surgical significance. J Urol 141:437–443
4. Brock G, Tu LM, Linet OI (2000) Return of spontaneous erection during long-term intracavernous alprostadil (Caverject) treatment. Urology 57:536–541
5. Carrier S, Zvara P, Nunes L, et al (1995) Regeneration of nitric oxide synthase-containing nerves after cavernous nerve neurotomy in the rat. J Urol 153:1722–1727
6. Carson CC, Mulcahy JJ, Govier FE (2000) Efficacy, safety and patient satisfaction outcomes of the AMS 700CX inflatable penile prosthesis: results of a long-term muticenter study. AMS 700CX Study Group. J Urol 164:376–380
7. Catalona WP, Basler JW (1993) Return of erections and urinary continence following nerve-sparing radical retropubic prostatectomy. J Urol 150:905–907
8. Ciancio SJ, Kim ED (2000) Penile fibrotic changes after radical retropubic prostatectomy. Br J Urol 85:101–106
9. Cookson MS, Nadig PW (1993) Long-term results with vacuum constriction device. J Urol 149:290–294
10. Costabile RA, Spevak M, Fishman I, et al (1998) Efficacy and safety of transurethral alprostadil in patients with erectile dysfunction following radical prostatectomy. J Urol 160:1325–1328
11. DeLuca V, Pescatori ES, Taher B, et al (1996) Damage to the erectile function following radical pelvic surgery: prevalence of veno-occlusive disease. Eur Urol 29:36–40
12. Evans C (1998) The use of penile prostheses in the treatment of impotence. Br J Urol 81:591–598
13. Feng MI, Huang S, Kaptein J, et al (2000) Effect of sildenafil citrate on post-radical prostatectomy erectile dysfunction. J Urol 164:1935–1938
14. Ganem JP, Lucey DT, Janosco EO, Carson CC (1998) Unusual complications of the vacuum erection device. Urology 51:627–631
15. Goldstein M (1988) Intracavernous injection of vasoactive drugs after radical prostatectomy. J Urol 139:800
16. Goldstein M, Newman L, Baum N, et al (1997) Safety and efficacy outcome of Mentor Alpha-1 inflatable penile prosthesis implantation for impotence treatment. J Urol 157:833–839
17. Govier FE, Gibbons RP, Correa RJ, et al (1998) Mechanical reliability, surgical complications and patient and partner satisfaction of the modern three-piece inflatable penile prosthesis. Urology 52:282–286
18. Gralnek D, Wessells H, Cui H, Dalkin BL (2000) Differences in sexual function and quality of life after nerve-sparing and nonnerve sparing radical retropubic prostatectomy. J Urol 163: 1166–1169
19. Guiliano F, Montorsi F, Mirone V, et al (2000) Switiching from intracavernous prostaglandin E1 injections to sildenafil citrate in patients with erectile dysfunction: results of a multicenter European study. The Sildenafil Multicenter Study Group. J Urol 164:708–711

20. Hong EK, Lepor H, McCullough AR (1999) Time dependent patient satisfaction with sildenafil for erectile dysfunction after nerve-sparing radical retropubic prostatectomy. Int J Impot Res 11 [Suppl 1]:15–22
21. Ignarro LJ, Bush PA, Buga GM, et al (1990) Nitric oxide and cyclic GMP formation upon electrical field stimulation cause relaxation of the corpus cavernosum smooth muscle. Biochem Biophys Res Commun 170:843–850
22. Kim ED, Blackburn D, McVary KT (1994) Post-prostatectomy penile blood flow: assessment with color flow doppler ultrasound. J Urol 152:2276–2279
23. Lebret T, Herve JM, Yonneau L, et al (1999) Erectile dysfunction after radical prostatectomy: value of preoperative programming of intracavernous injections. Prog Urol 9:483–488
24. Lowentritt BH, Scardino PT, Miles BJ, et al (1999) Sildenafil citrate after radical retropubic prostatectomy. J Urol 162:1614–1617
25. Lue T (2000) Erectile dysfunction. N Engl J Med 342:1802–1813
26. McMahon CG, Samali R, Johnson H (2000) Efficacy, safety and patient acceptance of sildenafil citrate as treatment for erectile dysfunction. J Urol 164:1192–1196
27. Montorsi F, Guazzoni G, Strambi LF, et al (1997) Recovery of spontaneous erectile function after nerve-sparing radical retropubic prostatectomy with and without early intracavernous injections of alprostadil: results of a prospective randomized trial. J Urol 158:1408–1410
28. Montorsi F, Rigatti P, Carmignani G, et al (2000) AMS three piece inflatable implants for erectile dysfunction: a long-term multi-institutional study in 200 consecutive cases. Eur Urol 37: 50–55
29. Moreland RB (1998) Is there a role of hypoxemia in penile fibrosis? Int J Impot Res 10:113–120
30. Mulcahy JJ (2000) Erectile dysfunction after radical prostatectomy. Semin Urol Oncol 18:71–75
31. Mulhall JP, Graydon RJ (1996) The hemodynamics of erectile dysfunction following nerve-sparing radical retropubic prostatectomy. Int J Impot Res 8:91–94
32. Mulhall JP, Jahoda AE, Cairney M, et al (1999) The causes of patient drop out from penile self-injection therapy impotence. J Urol 162:1291–1294
33. Nehra A, Goldstein I (1999) Sildenafil citrate (Viagra) after radical retropubic prostatectomy: con. Urology 54:587–589
34. Paick JS, Donatucci CF, Lue TF (1993) Anatomy of cavernous nerves distal to prostate: microdissection study in adult male cadavers. Urology 42:145–149
35. Polascik TJ, Walsh PC (1995) Radical retropubic prostatectomy: the influence of accessory pudendal arteries on the recovery of sexual function. J Urol 153:150–152
36. Rabbani F, Stapletin AM, Kattan AW, et al (2000) Factors predicting recovery of erections after radical prostatectomy. J Urol 164:1929–1934
37. Rodriguez Vela L, Gonzales Ibarra A, Bono Arino A, et al (1997) Erectile dysfunction after radical prostatectomy. Etiopathology and treatment. Actas Urol Esp 21:909–921
38. Saenz de Tejada I, Goldstein I, Azadzoi K, et al (1989) Impaired neurogenic and and endothelium mediated relaxation of penile smooth muscle from diabetic men with impotence. N Engl J Med 320:1025–1030
39. Shabsigh R, Padma-Nathan H, Gittleman M, et al (2000) Intracavernous alprostadil alfadex (EDEX/VIRIDAL) is effective and safe in patients with erectile dysfunction after failing sildenafil (Viagra). Urology 55:477–480
40. Shokeir AA, Alserafi MA, Mutabagani H (1999) Intracavernosal versus intraurethral alprostadil: a prospective randomized trial. Br J Urol 83:812–815
41. Soderdahl DW, Thrasher JB, Hansberry KL (1997) Intracavernosal drug-induced erection therapy versus external vacuum devices in the treatment of erectile dysfunction. Br J Urol 79:952–957
42. Stanford JL, Feng Z, Hamilton AS, et al (2000) Urinary and sexual function after radical prostatectomy for clinically localized prostate cancer. JAMA 283:354–360
43. Talcott JA, Riecker P, Propert KJ, et al (1997) Patient-reported impotence and incontinence after nerve-sparing radical prostatectomy. J Natl Cancer Int 89:1117–1123
44. Walsh PC (1987) Radical prostatectomy, preservation of sexual function, cancer control: controversy. Urol Clin North Am 14:663–673
45. Walsh PC (2000) Radical prostatectomy for localized prostate cancer provides durable cancer control with excellent quality of life: a structured debate. J Urol 163:1802–1807
46. Wilson SK, Cleves M, Delk II JR (1996) Long-term results with hydroflex and dynaflex penile prostheses: device survival comparison to multicomponent inflatables. J Urol 155:1621–1623
47. Zippe CD, Kedia S, Kedia AW, et al (1999) Sildenafil citrate (Viagra) after radical retropubic prostatectomy: pro. Urology 54:583–586
48. Zippe CD, Jhaveri FM, Klein EA, et al (2000) Role of Viagra after radial prostatectomy. Urology 55:241–245

24 Diagnosis and Therapy of Urinary Stress Incontinence Following Radical Prostatectomy

R. Hofmann, F. Schreiter

24.1 Introduction

Postoperative urinary incontinence can be encountered after radical retropubic or perineal prostatectomy, transurethral surgery, or open adenomectomy. With refined techniques in prostatic surgery and better endoscopic equipment for transurethral surgery, the rate of incontinence should be reduced.

Radical prostatectomy is the therapy of choice for localized prostatic carcinoma. Postoperative incontinence can vary from 0.5%–40%. Twelve months after radical retropubic prostatectomy 80% of the patients required no pads, 8% one or two pads/day, 7% three to five pads/day and 5% more than five pads/day. Only 2% of all patients were completely incontinent [6]. In the patient group of Schreiter, 8.6% of the total required therapy for postradical incontinence.

Continence usually returns in 66% of the patients within 3 months, 20% within 6 months, and 5% after 6 months. Continence can continue to improve in some patients for up to a year postoperatively.

Postprostatectomy continence relies on the function and integrity of the striated urethral sphincter in the pelvic floor musculature. The striated sphincter consists of three layers in this area: an outer layer of striated muscle, a middle layer of elastic tissue and smooth muscle, and an inner mucosal lining. This inner urothelium is important for tissue adaptation and sealing.

Postprostatectomy incontinence should be fully evaluated 6 months after surgery and an artificial genito-urinary sphincter (AGUS) implantation considered. This time should be allowed for continence to return after radical prostatectomy, with a focus on ascertaining if the patient can stop his urinary stream during voiding.

Postprostatectomy incontinence is not only due to sphincter damage, but also to detrusor instability, decreased bladder compliance, chronic infection, or a bladder neck stenosis that mimics surgical incontinence. Chronic infection, sometimes due to a relative urethral or bladder neck stenosis, requires appropriate antibiotic therapy. If infection is recurrent, incision or repeated dilatation of the relative outlet obstruction may be required.

24.2 Diagnosis

Evaluation of the postoperative incontinent patient should include a careful history, physical examination, ultrasound of the bladder and residual urine, urinalysis, urethro- and cystoscopy, and urodynamics. If there is an improvement of continence over time following radical retropubic prostatectomy (RRP) only ultrasound evaluation and urinalysis is warranted within the first 3–6 months. Only if loss of urine is complete and the patient cannot hold any urine back in the bladder is evaluation with cystoscopy and urodynamic testing advised; such patients usually want early therapy.

Physical examination should include a gross neurological examination with determination of sensitivity of the genital and anal region, anal sphicteric tonus, and bulbocavernosus reflex.

Digital rectal examination is mandatory to rule out scar formation or early recurrent disease.

If there is residual urine, cystoscopy is necessary to verify meatal, urethral or bladder neck stenosis.

Diagnosis and therapy of postoperative incontinence should be tailored to the patient, depending on the psychosocial impact of incontinence and quality of life. During follow-up, patients improving with their incontinence and those who have only mild to moderate incontinence need reassurance and instructions for pelvic floor exercises.

An incontinence work-up should be instituted with urethrocystoscopy and urodynamics, evaluating bladder wall compliance and detrusor activity as well as response to the Valsalva maneuver and straining, and to coughing and standing up.

If clinical and urodynamic evaluation of the incontinent patient leads to the diagnosis of detrusor instability, pharmacologic therapy is indicated. Anticholinergics (propantheline bromide), musculotropic relaxants (oxybutynin chloride), or tricyclic antidepressants (imipramine) are used. Combination therapy of these agents may lead to improvement; however, side effects like dry mouth, drowsiness, tachycardia, and decreased intestinal motility can ensue.

Not uncommonly, detrusor instability or reduced bladder wall compliance is connected with true sphincteric insufficiency or weakneess. Thus it does not necessarily mean that medical treatment has failed if the patient is still incontinent during anticholinergic treatment. Urodynamic testing can evaluate the effects of medical treatment at this point.

24.3 Surgical Treatment

Many options for postoperative incontinence surgery are available, either endoscopic or open surgery. Bladder neck reconstruction is not advised following radical prostatectomy. Procedures that increase urethral resistance such as ischial or bulbocavernosus muscle plication, transposition of the gracilis muscle around the urethra (unstimulated or with neurostimulation), embedding the urethra between the corpora cavernosa, or a fascial sling around the urethra can improve incontinence, but these only work when there is residual sphincteric function and incontinence is mild.

Endoscopic periurethral injection of bulking agents such as polytetrafluorethylene, carbon particles, or cross-linked collagen have limited success and are reserved for patients with residual sphincteric function.

The cornerstone of treatment of complete post radical urinary incontinence is the implantation of an artificial genitourinary sphincter, pioneered by Brandly Scott and American Medical Systems [7, 11, 12].

24.3.1 Artificial Sphincter System

The artificial sphincter consists of three parts:

1. A pressure regulating reservoir with a pressure of 50–60, 60–70, and 70–80 cm H_2O
2. A cuff, which is placed around the urethra and can be filled and emptied
3. A control pump, which regulates fluid transport from the reservoir to the cuff

Bulbar or membranous urethral cuff placement is necessary for postradical prostatectomy incontinence. Normally the cuff is filled with fluid that compresses the urethra circumferentially. The pressure in the cuff is determined by the pressure in the reservoir. Usually 60–70 cm H_2O is sufficient for continence. Pressing the pump empties the cuff and lets the urethra open. After 2 min fluid runs back to the cuff passively, impelled by the reservoir's elasticity. The sphincter system can also be completely deactivated [1, 9].

In order to qualify for sphincter implantation, the patient should have a bladder capacity of at least 200 cc H_2o, a normotonic or hypoactive detrusor, and no major urethral or bladder neck strictures. Following incision or resection of a bladder neck stenosis, a sphincter should be implanted in no less than 3 months postoperatively.

Bladder augmentation may be necessary for low compliant, low capacity bladders prior to sphincter implantation or at the same operative session.

Patient motivation and normal intelligence and dexterity are prerequisites for implantaion. Ureterorenal reflux higher than grade 2 should be corrected at the time of sphincter implantation.

Urinary tract infection should be treated until sterile urine is documented [2].

24.3.2 Operative Technique According to Schreiter

Preoperatively the patient is administered cephalosporin antibiotics, to be continued for 5 days perioperatively, principally to cover for *Staphylococcus epidermidis*. The evening before surgery the patient washes his genitals with Betadine. In the morning before surgery the patient should be disinfected with Betadine solution and covered by sterile drapes on the ward. The patient is then transferred to the OR, and shaving is done in the OR immediately before a 15-min scrub of the operative field with Betadine solution. The final skin disinfection is with a 70% alcoholic solution. Traffic in the OR should be restricted to a minimum. During the operation the wound is irrigated with gentamicin solution.

The urethral sphincter is implanted via a longitudinal incision in the perineum. A Scott retractor with large stays is used.

An indwelling catheter is placed and the bulbocavernosus muscle is exposed. The insertions of the crura above the bone are exposed beside the bulbocavernosus muscle on both sides as first landmarks in finding the exact place for the insertion of the cuff. The central tendon and the urethral rectal musculature are dissected and the membranous urethra exposed. Directly beneath the bifurcation of the crura of the corpora cavernosa, the triangular ligament is incised to a 2-cm width on both sides. A right angle clamp is moved on the posterior surface of the pubic bone (between that boneand the triangular ligament) so as to surround the urethra. The length of the cuff (4.5–6.0 cm) is chosen by measuring with a measuring tape. The cuff is then inserted, making use of the clamp placed as described above. Thus, the very thin posterior wall of the urethra is covered by a small piece of triangular ligament that serves to protect the urethra against pressure.

The catheter is removed and the appropriate cuff exactly placed around the membranous urethra. The cuff should fit exactly, but not be so tight as to cause tissue atrophy. The procedure is easier if the measuring tape remains in place during the cuff's insertion, to be removed after closure of the cuff. The central tendon is reconstructed, a process that moves the urethral cuff upward and horizontally to the membranous urethra. The cuff now sits right under the pelvic floor and the urethra is covered by muscle tissue. The patient does not sit on his cuff, which might empty when sitting down.

The cuff tube is advanced subcutaneously via an incision in the right groin. This tube and that between pump and reservoir should be isolated from blood and from towel fibers, as blood and fiber may hamper the pump function. Mosquito clamps with a Silicone tubing are used and closed only to first click The pump is placed in the right hemiscrotum after gently opening a plane between tunica dartos and tunica vaginalis with a long nose speculum or a long clamp. Preparation of this space, where no blood vessels occur prevents hematomas and edema. The reservoir is placed inside the peritoneum in order to avoid scarring around the reservoir and consequent higher pressure than desired.

Using the same inguinal incision used for passing the tube from the cuff, the peritoneum is opened and a 61–70 cm H_2O reservoir is inserted. The reservoir is filled with 22 cc of a mixture of 0.9% saline and contrast medium and connected to the pump. A right angle connector is used between the pump and the cuff tubing to prevent kinking, whereas connection between reservoir and pump is accomplished by a straight connector.

The perineal wound is closed with running 3–0 SAS sutures. Care has to be taken, when adjusting the bulbar muscle and closing the central tendon, not to puncture the cuff. Drains are not necessary.

A 12-F transurethral catheter is inserted and left for 3 days. The pump has to be manually pulled down twice daily to prevent upward movement.

The sphincter is not used for 6 weeks to allow healing, then activated by compressing the distal end of the pump and filling the cuff.

Urinary incontinence and erectile dysfunction ususally coexist following radical prostatectomy. A urinary sphincter and a penile prosthesis can be inserted at the same time or at staged procedures usually starting with implantation of the AGUS. The two pumps used in such cases have to be placed in either hemiscrotum and the reservoirs on either side of the abdomen in the peritoneal cavity.

24.3.3 Implantation of a Double Cuff

Implantation of a double cuff becomes necessary if the membranous urethra placement is not possible. Indications are irradiation of the anastomosis after radical prostatectomy, a defect of the membranous urethra caused by dissection failures or previous surgery, or erosion of the membranous urethra following primary surgery. Double cuff implantation also may become necessary because of tissue atrophy and recurrent incontinence after membranous urethral implantation.

Via a perineal longitudinal incision the distal bulbar urethra is exposed, splitting the bulbocavernosus muscle. The urethra is then carefully dissected free and two cuffs are wrapped one after the other around the distal bulbar urethra. Tubes from each cuff are passed into the inguinal incision and connected via a y-connector to the tube coming from the pump. The bulbocavernosus muscle is sutured over the two cuffs to cover them and the perineal wound is closed.

24.4 Patients

Between 1973 and 4/2001 a total of 1574 operations with implantation of an artificial urinary sphincter AMS 800 was performed by Schreiter and associates. Eight hundred and fifty-seven cases (54%) were primary implantations; 336 operations (21.3%) were performed after operations done outside had failed, and 381 were own revision operations (24.2%).

Of 1254 patients receiving AGUS, cuff location was at the bladder neck in 596 (47.5%) and membranous urethra in 658 (52.5%).

Up to 4/2001, 612 male patients received a bulbar urethral cuff for post-prostatectomy incontinence. Data and files of 396 of these, operated between 1983 to 4/1999, were fully evaluated and are reported here.

Patients ages varied from 54 to 81 years, with a mean age of 65 years. A total of 36,7% had previous anti-incontinence measures such as placement of older sphincteric devices (n=33), periurethral Teflon injection (n=93), and sling procedures (n=19). Forty-two patients had a postoperative bladder neck contracture and needed transurethral resection prior to AGUS implantation. Fifteen patients had prior irradiation before or after prostatectomy.

All patients received a bulbar urethral cuff implantation. Thirty percent received a 4.5-cm, 28% a 5.0-cm, 23.7% a 5.5-cm, and 17.7% a 6.0-cm cuff around the urethra.

Ninety-nine patients(25%) received a double cuff implantation, with 24 patients having a second cuff placed after primarily implanting a single cuff, while 75 patients had a double cuff at the first operative intervention.

Fifty-two patients received a pressure regulation balloon with 51–60 cm H_2O, 333 patients a balloon with 61–70 cm, 10 patients a balloon with 71–80 cm, and one patient a 81–90 cm H_2O reservoir balloon.

Ninety-seven of these 396 patients (24.5%) underwent revision with a total of 131 revisions (33%). Revisions were necessary for various reasons, including sphincter malfunction, pump displacement, leakage of the hydraulic system, and misplacement of the cuff.

Overall, 299/396 patients (75.5%) did not need any revision.

24.5 Results

Follow-up of 396 patients was available between 1 week and 76.8 months (average 6.4 years).

Of 396 patients 334 were fully continent (84.3%), needing no or at most one pad/day, 27 were improved (two or three pads/day), 24 were unsatisfied as they needed more than four pads/day, and 11 patients failed and had their device removed (Table 24.1).

Tissue-related complications were infection, cuff erosion, atrophy, and hematoma (n=66, 16.7%) (Table 24.2). Device-related complications included cuff or balloon leak, pump malfunction, connector leak, and tube kink (n=60, 15.1%) (Table 24.3).

Table 24.1. Continence rates of AMS 800 post radical prostatectomy implantation in 396 patients from 1/1983–4/1999

Continence	Maximum 1 pad/d	334 (84.3%)
Improved	2–3 pads	27 (6.5%)
Unsatisfied	4 or more pads	24 (6.1%)
Failed (device removed)	–	11 (2.5%)

Table 24.2. Complications of AMS 800 post radical prostatectomy implantation in 396 patients from January 1983 to April 1999

Tissue related complications	Number	Percentage
Infection	15	3.8
Cuff erosion	13	3.3
Tissue atrophy	33	8.3
Hematoma	5	1.3
Total	66	16.7

Table 24.3. Complications of AMS 800 post radical prostatectomy implantation in 396 patients from 1/1983–4/1999

Device-related complications	Number	Percentage
Cuff leak	40	10.3
Balloon leak	4	1.0
Pump malfunction	5	1.3
Connector leak	6	1.5
Tube kink	5	1.3
Total	60	15.4

Double cuff implantation was done in our series in 99/396 patients either as primary procedure in 75 patients or after insufficient continence with one cuff in 24 patients. The continence rate of 84% with a single cuff was increased to 94.8% using a double cuff.

24.6 Discussion

Urinary stress incontinence following radical prostatectomy is a distressing complication, tremendously impairing a patient's quality of life. Reported continence results following prostatectomy surgery vary over a wide range according to the definition of continence ("number of pads," "totally continent," "social continence"). The number of patients being completely incontinent and having the desire for treatment ranges between 2% and 5%. Excellent operative skills, knowledge of the important anatomical structures, and high-quality experience are prerequisites for a successful outcome of radical prostatectomy [5, 8].

Bulbar cuff placement is a straightforward procedure and needs only limited urethral exposure. Disadvantages of this technique are possible emptying of the cuff when sitting down and incomplete continence, as no abdominal pressure is directly transmitted to the cuff. Possibly a higher risk of erosion through the friable and thin bulbar urethra can occur. Thus, Schreiter devised an operative modification for the cuff site by placing the cuff around the membranous urethra directly below the pelvic floor [10]. With this technique, the bulbocavernous muscle is exposed, the central tendon incised horizontally, and the space exposed up to the diaphragm of the pelvis. Just below the bifurcation of the corpora cavernosa and above the membranous urethra, the diaphragm is split below the posterior rim of the pubic bone. The cuff is closed deeply around the proximal bulb of the urethra immediately below the pelvic floor musculature. Ample muscle and connective tissue lie around the urethra in this location. Care has to be taken not to enter the urethra ventrally as in this area between urethra and pubic symphysis, periurethral tissue is diminished.

By suturing the central tendon back, and thus mobilizing the cuff up to the pelvic floor, the cuff moves in a space located outside the compression zone while sitting. After this maneuver, the cuff is located in a horizontal position, to be comparedwith bulbar implantation where the cuff is in a vertical position.

The membranous implantation technique has advantages in that emptying of the cuff while sitting is unlikely, abdominal pressure transmission while straining is improved, and a lower risk for erosion exists due to better tissue quality around this portion of the urethra.

About 15% of all patients with a urethral cuff do not become completely dry due to incomplete closure of the cuff. Urethral resistance results from the balloon pressure x the compressing surface of the cuff. Urethral resistance can thus be increased either by increasing the pressure of the regulating balloon or by increasing the compressing surface of the cuff. Increasing the balloon pressure results in an increased risk of tissue atrophy under the cuff or early erosion through the urethra. Indications for double cuff implantation are recurrence after primary single cuff implantation, postirradiation of the bladder neck, or previous surgery at the bladder neck or posterior urethra [3].

A periprosthetic infection can occur at any time after surgery. An acute infection presents with swelling, redness, fever, induration, skin erosion, or abscess formation; evacuation and removal of the artificial system are necessary. Chronic infection usually is gradual and can be realized by slight induration at the pump site or along the tubes. Cuff erosion into the urethra will follow. An acute or chronic infection postoperatively is likely to be due to contamination during surgery [4]. Late infection, however, can be due to hematogenous seeding from dental or surgical procedures. Prophylactic antibiotics are advised as in all other prosthetic implantations. Our results with an overall 3.8% infection rate seems to be reasonably low. This is a result of a number of precautions undertaken, such as use of perioperative antibiotics, meticulous cleaning and scrubbing of the genital skin area, preoperative shaving of the genital hair in the OR, and careful surgical technique to prevent hematomas and wound drainage.

In conclusion, operative results with the implantation of an artificial urinary sphincter system are very encouraging for patients in the treatment of incontinence after radical prostatectomy [13]. A 95% overall improvement in continence is to be expected. Meticulous surgery and the experience of the surgeon provide the basis for a fully satisfactory therapy for patients with distressing and socially unacceptable urinary incontinence.

References

1. Barrett DM, Goldwasser B (1986) The artificial urinary sphincter: current management philosophy. AUA Update SeriesLesson 32, vol 5, American Urologic Association, Houston, Texas.
2. Blum MD (1989) Infections of genitourinary prostheses. Infect Dis Clin North Am 3:259–274
3. Britto CG, Mulcahy JJ, Mitchel ME, Adams MC (1993) Use of a double cuff AMS 800 artificial sphincter for severe stress incontinence. J Urol 149:283–285
4. Carson CC III (1989) Infections in genitourinary prostheses. Urol Clin North Am 16:139–147
5. Fowler FJ Jr, Barry MJ, Lu-Yao G, Wasson J, Roman A, Wenneberg J (1995) Effect of radical prostatectomy for prostate cancer on patient quality of life: results from a Medicare survey. Urology 45:1007–1015
6. Geary ES, Dendinger TE, Freiha FS, Stamey TA (1995) Incontinence and vesical neck strictures following radical retropubic prostatectomy. Urology 45:1000–1006
7. Gundian JC, Barrett DM, Parulkar BC (1989) Mayo clinic experience with use of the AMS 800 artificial urinary sphincter for urinary incontinence following radical prostatectomy. J Urol 142:1459–1461
8. Igel TC, Barrett DM, Segura JW, et al (1987) Perioperative and postoperative complications from bilateral pelvic lymphadenectomy and radical retropuic prostatectomy. J Urol 137:1189
9. Schreiter F, Noll F (1993) The artificial sphincter AS 800. In: Steg A (ed) Urinary incontinence. Churchill Livingstone, London, pp 241–257
10. Schreiter P (1985) Bulbar artificial sphincter. Eur Urol 11:294–299
11. Scott FB, Bradley WE, Timm GW (1973) Treatment of urinary incontinence by an implantable prosthetic sphincter. Urology 1:252–254
12. Scott FB, Bradley WE, Timm GW (1974) Treatment of urinary incontinence by an implantable prosthetic urinary sphincter. J Urol 112:74
13. Wein AJ, Barrett DM (1988) Voiding function and dysfunction: a logical and practical approach. Year Book, Chicago

Therapy of Advanced Prostate Cancer

25 Is Radical Lymphadenectomy Indicated in Lymph Node-Positive Disease?

R.S. Foster

Several alternative treatments exist for patients with clinically localized prostate cancer who have Gleason grades equal to or less than 7. Though an adequate randomized prospective study comparing these various treatment modalities has not been performed, many series of outcomes of treatment of patients with clinically localized prostate cancer exist. If in fact one of these treatments is more effective than the other, the difference is likely very small and could only be delineated in a very large randomized prospective trial. As is well recognized, these treatments include radical prostatectomy, external beam radiation therapy, and brachytherapy. Fortunately, because of the well-recognized stage migration of prostate cancer associated with the widespread use of prostate-specific antigen (PSA) testing, most patients diagnosed with prostate cancer are in this so-called "good risk" category.

Several studies, however, have shown that patients with higher risk disease may be managed best surgically. These higher risk patients are those with higher Gleason scores, higher PSAs, and higher volumes of cancer. Lu-Yao performed an analysis of a group of patients managed with either radical prostatectomy, radiation therapy, or observation [6]. This was a Cancer Registry-based series that included almost 60,000 patients from 1983 to 1992. Intent-to-treat analysis was performed. In low grade (Gleason 2 to 4) patients 10-year disease-specific survivals were essentially the same if treated with radical prostatectomy, radiation, or observation. In the Gleason 5 to 7 category an improved disease-specific survival for surgery as compared to radiation and observation was noted, and in the Gleason 8 to 10 category the incremental benefit on disease-specific survival of radical prostatectomy compared to the other two treatments was still greater.

Similarly, in a series of patients from the Cleveland Clinic treated with radical prostatectomy or radiation therapy from 1987 to 1993, it was found that radical prostatectomy appeared to have the greatest incremental impact in the high risk group [5]. This analysis of 551 patients with clinical T1 or T2 disease was well defined and reported. All patients had PSA and Gleason scores, and all pathology was reviewed at the Cleveland Clinic, including whole mounts on radical prostatectomies. There was a minimum 2-year follow-up. Two hundred and fifty three patients had radiotherapy, 298 radical prostatectomy. The biochemical relapse-free survival for the radical prostatectomy group was 57% against 43% for radiotherapy. In multivariable analysis, grade and PSA were predictors of relapse, but type of treatment was not. If this large group of patients was further divided into a low-risk group (defined as a PSA less than 10 and a Gleason score <6) and a high-risk group (PSA greater than 10 or Gleason >7), interesting trends emerge. In the low-risk group the biochemical relapse-free survival was 81% for radiotherapy and 80% for radical prostatectomy. However, in the high-risk group the biochemical relapse-free survival rate was 26% for radiotherapy and 37% for radical prostatectomy. In this high-risk group of radical prostatectomy patients, when surgical margins were negative, the biochemical relapse-free survival was 62%.

Therefore, these two studies (and others in the literature) lend credence to the concept that even though fewer patients with high-risk disease are cured of their cancer, the incremental benefit of surgery versus another treatment strategy is greatest in the high-risk group. Though patients in this high-risk group are considered to be the poorest candidates for radical prostatectomy, the benefit from surgery in this group may be the greatest.

In a series of radical prostatectomy patients from Baylor University in Texas who had Gleason scores of 7 or greater, an 85% non-progression rate was found in patients with organ confined disease and high-grade tumor [8]. In multivariable analysis neither grade nor volume of tumor influenced progression when the tumor was organ confined. Focusing on PSA alone, a study from Indiana University considered 79 radical prostatectomy patients who underwent radical prostatectomy with PSA values 20–100 at the time of prostatectomy. Fifteen patients had lymphatic metastases, 11 of whom did not undergo radical prostatectomy. At a median follow-up of 30 months with a mean PSA of 34.6 in these patients, the biochemical disease-free rate was 42% at 3 years and 31% at 5 years. In multivariate analysis Gleason score did not predict biochemical freedom of disease [4].

These studies would thus suggest that higher risk disease may be best managed with radical prostatectomy. A logical extension of this concept would be to ask whether radical prostatectomy in conjunction with extended lymphadenectomy is indicated in patients who have lymphatic metastases.

Of all the urological cancers, the cancer most curable surgically when lymphatic metastases have occurred is undoubtedly testis cancer. Roughly 50%–75% of patients who are not treated with chemotherapy and have low volume lymphatic metastases are cured with surgery alone. Surgery alone similarly cures approximately 50% of patients with penile cancer and low volume metastases. Smaller numbers of patients with bladder cancer (10%–35%) and renal cancer (5%–20%) plus lymphatic metastases are cured by surgery alone. Historically, prior to the PSA era the probability of systemic disease was very high in patients found to have lymphatic metastases of prostate cancer, and therefore surgical therapy was not indicated. However, in the modern era of PSA-driven diagnosis, nodal metastases that are found are usually part of overall low volume metastasis. Are pelvic lymphadenectomy and radical prostatectomy indicated in this group of patients? The answer lies in randomized prospective studies. Such studies will likely never be done, however, mainly due to the difficulty in finding adequate numbers of patients in this category. Therefore, the answer to this question will probably never be known. A review of the literature still allows us to make some interesting speculations.

The standard node dissection for radical prostatectomy as currently practiced involves resection of only the obturator nodes. Yet historical information, based on patients identified in the pre-PSA era, suggests that 7%–14% have metastases to the presacral nodes and 10%–17% to the external iliac nodes. In a series of patients treated with delayed hormonal therapy alone, the median time to therapy in patients with D1 prostate cancer was 12.2 months [9]. Fifty percent of these patients were dead at 34 months; however, in 15% disease had not advanced at 5 years. Clearly, at least some patients in this particular circumstance progress in a very indolent fashion. This is well recognized in all patients with prostate cancer.

A series of papers from the Mayo Clinic published in the late 1980s and early 1990s suggested that radical prostatectomy patients with low volume lymphatic metastases should be treated with immediate hormonal therapy. As the series matured it became clear that overall survival was improved only in those patients who had early hormonal therapy and who had diploid tumors [12].

The advantage of early hormonal therapy was to delay progression. As it turned out only a very small number of patients benefitted when considering the total number of patients in the entire series. DeKernion et al. published a series of 56 patients who underwent radical prostatectomy and who had nodal metastases [2]. Twenty-one underwent immediate hormonal therapy, based on the discretion of the treating physician; 35 did not. These two groups were similar for age, Gleason score, pathologic stage, volume, and aneuploidy. At a mean follow-up of 72 months for the early hormonal therapy group and 62 months for the observation group, two deaths from prostate cancer had occurred in the hormonal therapy group, seven in the observation group. The survival in the overall group was 84% at 60 months, 78% at 98 months. Control of progression and survival free of disease were significantly better in the endocrine group. Using the Cox proportional hazards model correcting for Gleason score and percentage of positive nodes, it was shown that those who did not undergo early hormonal therapy had a 3.1 times greater risk of progression or death ($P<0.032$). Interestingly, surgical therapy alone yielded a 5-year overall survival of 80%. This well-documented series showed that if patients are selected appropriately, some do extremely well with pelvic lymph node dissection and radical prostatectomy.

In a series from Johns Hopkins University published in 1997, 168 men were examined [1]; 127 had radical prostatectomy and 41 had pelvic lymph node dissection alone. All of these patients were classified as T1 to T3 and M0. Thirty-three percent of patients who underwent pelvic node dissection and radical prostatectomy had endocrine therapy. Seventy-one percent of those who had pelvic lymph node dissection alone had endocrine therapy. The only significant difference in the two groups was that the pelvic lymph node dissection group had higher volumes of metastases. The 5- and 10-year actuarial survival in the radical prostatectomy versus pelvic lymph node dissection group was 91% versus 63% and 61% versus 45% ($P=0.006$). Nineteen patients in each group were matched for age, PSA, stage, length of follow-up, volume of metastasis, and percentage of positive nodes. In comparing these two latter subgroups of patients there was no statistically significant difference in survival. Nonetheless, as was seen in the study of DeKernion, if patients are well selected, many do extremely well with pelvic lymph node dissection and radical prostatectomy alone. Another study from Hopkins was published in 1994 on prognostic factors in D1 disease [10]. A retrospective analysis of 113 men who had had radical prostatectomy and nodal metastases was performed. It was found that the only predictor of progression after surgery was the Gleason score of the preoperative biopsy. Patients with low Gleason scores did better than those with high scores.

Finally, in a study from Duke University published in 1994, 156 patients with D1 prostate cancer were examined. Forty two of them had radical prostatectomy, the remainder only pelvic node removal [3]. The cancer-specific survival was 11.2 years in the radical prostatectomy group and 5.9 years in the pelvic lymph node dissection alone group. The groups were well matched, but the benefit of surgery was seen only if fewer than three nodes were involved with metastatic tumor.

Recently a randomized study was published on the benefit of immediate hormonal therapy in patients undergoing radical prostatectomy with low volume lymphatic metastasis [7]. Of 98 patients, 47 had immediate hormonal therapy, 51 did not. At 7.1 years of follow-up, 7 of 47 had died in the hormonal group and 18 of 51 in the observation group. There were three prostate cancer deaths in the hormonal group and sixteen in the observation group. In multivariate analysis only the treatment type was predictive of outcome. It should be recognized, however, that this investigation was originally planned for 220 patients. The study was prematurely closed due to poor accrual. Hence, though the differences were statistically significant ($P<0.01$) the possibility of the difference being solely due to chance is increased. Nonetheless, this study adds to the growing body of literature suggesting that early hormonal therapy is beneficial.

Considered together, these studies suggest that properly selected patients who have very low volume lymphatic metastasis will do well in the short and moderate term with radical prostatectomy and lymphadenectomy alone. Because of the varied natural history of prostate cancer, the absolute answer to this question is only to be found in a properly performed prospective randomized study and, as discussed above, this will likely never happen. Another pertinent issue concerns the type of lymphadenectomy to perform. A recent study from Germany used lymphoscintigraphy in 11 patients with prostate cancer [11]. The goal was to determine the sites of lymphatic spread. Four patients indeed had micrometastasis and in three of these patients the lymphoscintigraphy accurately identified the involved nodes. Interestingly, in two cases the nodes with metastasis were outside the standard boundary of an obturator node dissection. Therefore, further study of the boundaries of the node dissection should be performed if the surgeon is considering surgical treatment in such high-risk patients.

In summary, if lymph nodes are palpably and visually normal at the time of exploration for radical prostatectomy, frozen section analysis is probably not necessary, since many of these patients who indeed have micrometastases will do well with lymphadenectomy and surgery alone. Based on the data discussed, there remains no justification for proceeding with radical prostatectomy in the face of high volume metastasis since high volume lymphatic metastasis has a strong correlation with distant micrometastatic disease. Finally, based upon the randomized prospective study discussed above, patients who undergo radical prostatectomy and are found to have low volume lymphatic metastasis should be considered strong candidates for early hormonal therapy.

References

1. Cadeddu JA, Partin AW, Epstein JI, et al (1997) Stage D1 (T1–3, N1–3, MO) prostate cancer: a case controlled comparison of conservative treatment versus radical prostatectomy. Urology 50: 251
2. DeKernion JB, Neuwirth H, Stein A, et al (1990) Prognosis of patients with stage D1 prostate carcinoma following radical prostatectomy with and without early endocrine therapy. J Urol 144:700
3. Frazier HA, Robertson JE, Paulson DF (1994) Does radical prostatectomy in the presence of positive pelvic lymph nodes enhance survival? World J Urol 12:308
4. Koch MO, Foster RS, Brandli DW, et al (2000) Biochemical disease free survival in patients with high PSA (20–100 ng/ml), stage TxNo prostate cancer after radical prostatectomy. J Urol 163:284
5. Kupelian P, Katcher J, Levin H, et al (1997) External beam radiotherapy versus radical prostatectomy for clinical stage T1–2 prostate cancer: therapeutic implications of stratification by pretreatment PSA levels and biopsy Gleason scores. Cancer J Sci Am 3:78
6. Lu-Yao GL and Yao SL (1997) Population-based study of long term survival in patients with clinically localized prostate cancer. Lancet 349:906
7. Messing EM, Manola J, Sarosdy M, et al (1999) Immediate hormonal therapy compared with observation after radical prostatectomy and pelvic lymphadenectomy in men with node positive prostate cancer. N Engl J Med 341:1781
8. Ohori M, Goad JR, Wheeler TM, et al (1994) Can radical prostatectomy alter the progression of poorly differentiated prostate cancer? J Urol 152:1843
9. Paulson DF, Cline WA, Koefoot, RB, et al (1982) Extended field radiation therapy versus delayed hormonal therapy in node positive prostate adenocarcinoma. J Urol 127:935

10. Sgrignol AR, Walsh PC, Steinberg GD, et al (1994) Prognostic factors in men with stage D1 prostate cancer: identification of patients less likely to have prolonged survival after radical prostatectomy. J Urol 152:1077
11. Wawroschek F, Vogt H, Weckermann D, et al (1999) The sentinel lymph node concept in prostate cancer – first results of gamma probe-guided sentinel lymph node identification. Eur Urol 36:595
12. Zincke H, Bergstralh EJ, Larson-Keller JJ, et al (1992) Stage D1 prostate cancer treated by radical prostatectomy and adjuvant hormonal treatment. Cancer 70:311

26 Hormone Therapy for Prostate Cancer

D. Raghavan

26.1 Introduction

It has been known for more than two centuries that the growth of the normal prostate and its malignancies is dependent upon hormonal function [9, 26, 68]. More recently, the application of this knowledge to the management of advanced prostate cancer has been rationalized, building upon the Nobel prize winning observation that castration or the administration of estrogens causes regression of advanced prostate cancer in dogs [25]. The physiology of prostatic growth is summarized in Fig. 26.1 [50].

Testosterone, the dominant stimulus for prostatic growth, is bound to two major proteins in the blood – sex hormone binding globulin (SHBG) and albumin. It is in dynamic equilibrium with the unbound or "free" fraction. Levels of SHBG decline with advancing age [66], which may explain the apparent decline in total testosterone with age that has been reported in some series. Free testosterone is converted to dihydrotestosterone (DHT) by 5α-reductase. There are at least two isoenzymes 5α-reductase, type I and type II, and the expression of this enzyme is controlled by the SRD 5A2 gene [37, 64]. Testosterone and DHT bind to the androgen receptor and, in turn, this complex interacts with DNA, leading to increased protein synthesis. Adrenal androgens are also converted to testosterone and DHT in the prostate, and it is believed that they also may contribute to the stimulation of growth of prostatic tissues. However, there is also evidence against the importance of adrenal androgens in this context – for example, patients with hypogonadotrophic hypogonadism do not have normal prostate development, despite the presence of adrenal androgens. Notwithstanding this observation, castration (medical or surgical) results in reduction of circulating androgens, and this leads to regression of normal or neoplastic prostatic tissue. One dominating mechanism of this process is apoptosis, or programmed cell death, which appears to be initiated by withdrawal of androgens [32].

Our knowledge of the role of androgen receptors in the response and resistance to hormonal therapy is still evolving. The androgen receptor is a ligand-activated nuclear transcription factor that mediates the cellular effects of androgens. As noted above, testosterone and DHT bind to this receptor. It appears that androgen receptor gene amplification and over-expression occur in association with the development of resistance to hormone therapy [36, 67]. In addition, it has been demonstrated that the androgen receptor may undergo mutation in patients with hormone-refractory disease [63].

In addition to the effects of testosterone in the prostate, estrogens and progestins interact with this gland. Estrogens compete for binding sites on SHBG, although testosterone has a greater avidity for this protein. Because of these interactions, there is a 40% rise in the ratio of free estradiol/free testosterone in males over 50–60 years of age. The major effect of estrogens on the prostate gland may be mediated via the hypothalmo-pituitary-end organ axis, with inhibition of testicular synthesis of testosterone. If estrogens and testosterone are administered jointly to castrate animals, normal growth of the prostate gland occurs – i.e. estrogens do not appear to block the replacement effects of the administered testosterone.

Prolactin may also have a function in the growth and metabolism of the prostate gland. In hypophysectomized rats, exogenous androgens are unable to restore full prostatic growth unless supplemented by prolactin [22], and the interaction of testosterone and prolactin has been confirmed in vitro in fragments of human prostatic tissue [19]. Prolactin receptors have been demonstrated in prostate gland and testis [1] and may mediate the interaction of prolactin in testosterone uptake and metabolism by the prostate.

26.2 Impact of Hormone Therapy

In advanced or metastatic disease, depending upon the criteria of assessment of outcome [17, 48, 62], tumor shrinkage can be achieved in 50–70 percent of cases in response to hormone therapy. This includes bilateral orchiectomy, the administration of systemic estrogens, the use of analogs of luteinizing hormone releasing hormone (LHRH), or by combinations of some of these approaches (combined androgenic blockade) [13, 21, 35] (Table 26.1). As discussed elsewhere, response can be defined by objective tumor reduction, reductions in levels of circulating prostate-specific antigen (PSA), or simply by improvements in indices of quality of life, such as pain, appetite, weight gain, or performance status [17, 48, 62].

The rationale for bilateral orchiectomy in the management of prostate cancer was determined by Huggins et al. [25]. The procedure results in a substantial decrease in plasma testosterone, usually from an initial range of 500–600 ng/ml down to less than 50 ng/ml [60], thus suppressing the growth of normal and cancerous prostatic tissue. This approach yields long-term suppression of testosterone production [60] that is demonstrable even after relapse.

In the past, systemic estrogens were widely used as a nonsurgical alternative for the management of newly diagnosed metastatic prostate cancer. The

Table 26.1. Options for primary hormone therapy of prostate cancer

Treatment option	Benefits	Drawbacks
Bilateral orchiectomy	Effective; usually no compliance problems; no need for repeated medical visits	Permanency if considering intermittent hormone Rx; psychological factors; side effects
Estrogens	Can be discontinued; effective	Gynecomastia; nausea; vascular problems; impotence
PC-SPES (phytoestrogens)	Can be discontinued; may have less estrogenic toxic effects	Some estrogenic toxic effects; unproven in long-term studies
Estramustine phosphate	Added cytotoxic effects (?)	Added cytotoxic effects (?); estrogenic side effects; more nausea than estrogens
LHRH agonists	Equivalent efficacy to estrogens; can be discontinued	Frequent medical visits; requires injection; initial testosterone surge; less toxic than estrogens
LHRH antagonists	Effective; no testosterone surge	Medical visits; requires injection; unproven in long-term studies

primary effect of estrogens is suppression of LH production, with a consequent decrease in testosterone production. Estrogens may also directly inhibit the function of Leydig cells [29]. Some of the most definitive studies of hormonal suppression of prostate cancer were carried out by the Veterans Administration Cooperative Urological Research Group (VACURG), demonstrating that improvements in outcome from prostate cancer were offset by losses due to cardiovascular toxicity [7, 8].

Another major therapeutic option introduced more recently has been the use of LHRH analogues,which act by impeding the release of LH and thus inhibiting testosterone production. These agents produce equivalent response rates and survival to other front-line hormonal therapies [35]. However, LHRH analogues have but a transient agonist effect, often causing a rebound surge of testosterone 1–7 days after initiation of therapy, and thus can cause transient worsening of symptoms. To avoid this effect, most clinicians have used peripheral inhibitors, such as flutamide or bicalutamide, to inhibit the effects of the testosterone surge.

An alternative approach currently being tested is the use of LHRH antagonists, which simply block the function of LHRH, and thus can bring about suppression of testosterone production without an initial surge. Preliminary randomized trials have suggested that LHRH agonists used without peripheral blockers have equivalent anticancer efficacy to the LHRH antagonists, but that the antagonists are associated with fewer symptom flare reactions.

26.3 Intermittent Hormonal Therapy

At present, a major change in the paradigm of systemic hormonal therapy is being assessed – specifically, the potential role of intermittently interrupting treatment with hormones. Preliminary data from Canada have suggested that intermittent interruption of hormones can improve quality of life (based on a return of sexual function and an improved sense of well-being associated with the return of normal circulating androgen levels) [21]. Perhaps of more fundamental importance has been the suggestion from these workers that the return of androgenic function may actually provide a longer duration of cancer control by overcoming the development of resistance to the effects of hormonal deprivation. It has been postulated that this could occur either:

(a) By blocking the occurrence of spontaneous mutations of the androgen receptor associated with the hormone-deprived environment
(b) By impeding the evolution of up-regulation of androgen receptor expression, a phenomenon also thought to occur in the androgen-deprived environment

While promising data have been reported from Canada and elsewhere, this concept is currently being tested in a randomized clinical trial by the Southwest Oncology Group, with survival as the primary endpoint. It appears that intermittent androgen blockade has gained considerable popularity in the community, because of the associated improvement in quality of life, but should still be regarded as investigational until the survival figures from randomized clinical trials are available.

26.4 Combined Androgenic Blockade

Combined androgenic blockade (CAB) involves the addition of central inhibition of androgen production (i.e., medical or surgical orchiectomy) to peripheral blockade of circulating androgens (e.g., the use of flutamide, bicalutamide, or cyproterone acetate). This concept has arisen largely from the work of Labrie and colleagues, who have reported objective tumor regression in nearly 100% of cases of prostate cancer in preclinical models and then in clinical trials [33, 34]. While extremely important in concept, some aspects of this work have been questioned subsequently because of the inability of other investigators to duplicate the very high reported response rates. Nevertheless, these studies have given rise to a generation of subsequent studies of combined androgenic blockade.

Perhaps one of the most important early studies to test this concept, and certainly the most widely cited in the literature, was reported by Crawford and colleagues [13] for the North American Intergroup. In this randomized clinical trial, 300 patients with metastatic prostate cancer were treated with leuprolide and placebo and 303 received leuprolide and flutamide. Progression-free survival was 13.8 and 16.9 months, respectively, and the median survival times were 28.3 and 35.6 months. When viewed in the context of the overall life expectancy of patients with advanced prostate cancer, this result, despite being statistically significant, is not viewed as clinically of great importance. However, of interest, in a retrospective subset analysis it was noted that a more substantial difference in outcome was seen among patients with good performance status and minimal metastatic disease (i.e., bone metastases confined to the axial skeleton and/or only lymph node involvement). In this small subgroup, at 96 months of follow-up, there was a 29-month difference in progression free survival and a 19-month difference in median total survival in favor of the CAB arm [15]. In addition to the small numbers in this subset, it should also be noted that in the whole trial the complete response rate to CAB was 7.9%, compared to 7.1% after monotherapy. This suggests that the major biological impact was achieved among the patients who sustained partial objective responses (35.7% with CAB; 28.2% after monotherapy). In fact, it seems unlikely that, with similar complete response rates, a difference in the frequency of partial remission would have had a particularly important biological impact on any disease.

Notwithstanding the above, Crawford and others interpreted the results of the Intergroup study as supporting the importance of the role of CAB and launched another randomized trial, in this instance assessing the utility of bilateral orchiectomy with or without flutamide in patients stratified for the extent of disease. The results of this trial are discussed below, with the results of other similarly structured studies.

Several randomized trials have been reported in which the authors have interpreted their data to show no significant role for CAB. For example, in the first report of a trial conducted by the European Organization for the Research and Treatment of Cancer, Keuppens et al. [30] found no difference in outcome for patients randomized to receive orchiectomy alone versus those who received goserelin plus flutamide. However, of interest, a later analysis of this study suggested a survival advantage for CAB, particularly in a subset analysis of patients with minimal disease [16]. In my view, substantially different results of a randomized trial in two closely spaced consecutive reports, in a disease with a relatively long natural history, calls into question the power and accuracy of that study.

Similar studies have been completed by the Danish Prostatic Cancer Group (orchiectomy vs. goserelin vs. goserelin plus flutamide) [27], the International Prostate Cancer Study Group (goserelin vs. goserelin plus flutamide) [65], and the Italian Prostatic Cancer Project Study Group (goserelin vs. goserelin plus flutamide) [4]. None of these has shown a large difference in outcome between monotherapy and combined androgen blockade, especially when total survival was considered as the primary endpoint. Less clearly defined are differences in disease-free survival, although this endpoint can be influenced substantially by the methodology employed to detect relapse [51].

The Australian Prostate Cancer Study Group compared the use of bilateral orchiectomy plus flutamide vs. bilateral orchiectomy plus placebo [69]. Although this trial accrued only 222 patients and was interpreted as showing no significant difference in response rate (45% and 56%, respectively) or relapse-free survival, the patients treated with bilateral orchiectomy plus flutamide had a shorter median overall survival (23 months) than those treated by combined androgenic blockade (31 months). However, this did not achieve statistical significance. Similarly, the time points at which 25% and 75% of deaths had occurred were not significantly different in this trial.

The results of this study were duplicated by the second Intergroup trial [17]. To the surprise of the members of the Intergroup, there was no overall survival difference between orchiectomy plus placebo and orchiectomy plus flutamide. Of greatest importance, combined androgenic blockade showed no benefit even in patients with limited extent metastases. Although no definitive explanation has been provided for differences between the two Intergroup studies, it has been speculated that combined androgenic blockade with LHRH agonists provides a benefit through inhibition of the initial agonist effects of these agents.

Perhaps one of the most strident arguments against the impact of CAB is the recent meta-analysis published by the international Prostate Trialists' Collaborative Group [46, 47]. In these analyses of all of the registered randomized clinical trials comparing CAB with monotherapy, more than 6000 deaths had occurred. Dalesio and colleagues [46, 47] reported only a very small difference in end results when the whole group was considered, despite small differences in favor of CAB in some of the constituent trials.

Finally, in considering whether to recommend CAB, the toxicity of the regimen should be considered. Although many patients in the various clinical trials were able to tolerate this treatment for periods measured in years, it should not be forgotten that flutamide can cause gastrointestinal side effects, including nausea, diarrhea, and occasionally hepatitis. It has been suggested that some of the newer analogues, such as bicalutamide (Casodex) and nilutamide (Nilandron), will be better tolerated and will thus allow the true impact of CAB to be realized (as a function of improved patient compliance). If it is found that bicalutamide is more active than flutamide, it is possible that an improved outcome will be achieved by this approach. However, it seems unlikely that amelioration of a relatively modest profile of toxicity, in the absence of enhanced anticancer activity, will have a major impact on survival.

Another consideration is cost effectiveness. The annual cost of flutamide was reported as $2,500 per patient [38]. If one considers the major "positive" trial [13], with a median survival of just under 3 years from CAB compared to 28 months for monotherapy, the cost per year of life saved was more than $12,000 [38]. While it is difficult to place a specific value on human life, we must be aware of the reduction in health resources available caused by such expenditure, and it will become increasingly important to define the presence or absence of real, quantifiable benefit when additional therapies are being considered for routine use.

Finally, it is not surprising to find only a modest impact from CAB, compared to monotherapy, when one considers the broader context of prostate cancer, a malignancy that is composed of diverse constitutive elements that include hormonally sensitive and nonresponsive elements.

26.5 Timing of Hormone Therapy for Advanced Disease

One of the major issues today is the optimal timing for the introduction of hormonal therapy for advanced or metastatic disease. With the widespread use of PSA monitoring after completion of definitive radiotherapy or radical prostatectomy, patients are increasingly being faced with the problem of a rising PSA in the absence of symptoms. In addition, up to 20%–25% of new cases have advanced disease at initial presentation. Because of the toxicity of hormonal therapy, patients are faced with conflicting pressures – the desire to receive the best anticancer therapy with the longest duration of remission and survival versus the wish to avoid unnecessary toxicity for as long as possible.

The British Medical Research Council (1997) attempted to address this issue in a randomized trial that compared the use of early hormonal intervention at the time of initial diagnosis of asymptomatic, advanced, or metastatic disease versus delayed use of hormones at the time of symptomatic progression. More than 900 patients were randomly allocated to the treatment arms between 1985 and 1993. At the time of reporting, 51 patients on the deferred therapy arm had died from causes other than prostate cancer before treatment was started. However, pathological fractures, spinal cord compression, ureteric obstruction, and the development of extraskeletal metastases were twice as common in deferred patients. On the deferred arm, 361 patients died, compared with 328 in the immediate therapy arm (P=0.02). The major difference in deaths from prostate cancer occurred in the M0 patients. However, it is important to note that this study was somewhat flawed. Not all patients underwent bone scanning as part of initial staging, and there was an imbalance in the nature of follow-up between the two groups. The trial was designed as a pragmatic study, and follow-up was left to the discretion of the investigator. This clearly would have biased the study in favor of the early-therapy group. Thus, it is not clear that a survival benefit would have been achieved in two cohorts of patients uniformly staged and undergoing identical follow-up protocols.

26.6 Heterogeneity of Prostate Cancer: Impact on Hormone Therapy

There is clear evidence from preclinical models and some clinicopathological studies that diverse populations of tumor cells, with different morphological and functional characteristics, are present within individual deposits of cancer at the time of first presentation. This is further manifest by the range of histologic, ultrastructural, hormone receptor, growth factor receptor, and flow cytometric features present in human biopsy specimens [3, 24, 56].

Of particular importance is the demonstration of coincidental subpopulations of cells with classical adenocarcinomatous features intermingled with cells that exhibit neuroendocrine differentiation [14, 28, 52], features of small cell undifferentiated carcinoma [52, 57], and even cells that actually represent transitional cell carcinoma [40]. It thus has seemed unlikely that any one procedure would permanently control these disparate tumor cell populations, at least in the setting of advanced disease [48].

The factors that regulate growth, differentiation, tumor progression, and response to treatment in prostate cancer have not been defined, although candidate genes being studied include Rb, ras, p53, bcl, neu, erbB-2 and those governing expression of the androgen receptor, TGF-β, and other growth factors [6, 10, 23, 39, 42, 55, 63]. The ability to identify these more accurately and to define prognostic determinants with greater specificity will allow more appropriate selection of aggressive therapy for localized disease with greater metastatic potential as well as more precise management of patients with advanced disease.

Thus, the broad range of genetic anomalies associated with prostate cancer appears likely to be intimately involved in the constitutive heterogeneity of function of prostate cancer and in turn to create a more complex target for therapeutic endeavors.

Because of the demonstration of elements that are apparently not responsive to hormonal manipulation *ab initio*, alternative strategies have been explored, including the use of first-line cytotoxic chemotherapy [59] and the combination of cytotoxic chemotherapy with endocrine treatment (chemoendocrine therapy) [12, 59]. To date, the use of first-line cytotoxic chemotherapy has not been successful in improving survival for patients with metastatic prostate cancer. Despite encouraging objective response rates with chemoendocrine therapy, randomized clinical trials have either demonstrated no survival benefit [43] or, in one study without clearly defined randomization, only a modest difference in outcome in favor of chemoendocrine treatment [31]. The problem may also be that the traditionally available cytotoxic agents are simply not very active against prostate cancer. Recently, several innovative cytotoxic treatments have been assessed for advanced prostate cancer, including suramin [41], mitoxantrone [53, 62], and oral cyclophosphamide [54], each of which appears to be demonstrating substantial anticancer activity. It may be that the incorporation of such agents into the treatment of advanced cancer may make significant contributions to the prolongation of patient survival.

26.7 Adjunctive Hormones for Stage C Prostate Cancer

Our current concepts regarding tumor progression are consistent with differences in tumor characteristics between early stage and advanced disease. Because of a greater level of tumor heterogeneity in advanced disease, it appears quite possible that systemic therapy could be much more effective in the treatment of early stage disease than in metastatic disease. This lends support to the concept of the early introduction of systemic therapy into the management of prostate cancer.

A provocative trial was reported from the British Medical Research Council [20], in which radical radiotherapy, systemic hormonal treatment, and a combination of the two were compared for patients with locally extensive prostate cancer. Although the study may have been somewhat under-powered to detect small differences in survival, there was no clear evidence of superiority from any arm, raising an interesting question regarding the timing and respective roles of each component of treatment in this context.

By contrast, Messing et al. [39a] reported an important randomized trial in which 98 men were randomly allocated to early adjuvant castration versus observation (and delayed treatment) after radical prostatectomy for node-positive prostate cancer. In this preliminary report of an under-powered trial, there were seven deaths among 47 men who received immediate castration, compared with 18 of 51 men in the delayed therapy arm (p=0.02). This was strong evidence in favor of early hormonal intervention; but is in strong contrast to the lack of survival benefit documented in a Scandinavian trial that assessed the use of early estrogen therapy after prostatectomy [36a].

To date, several randomized trials have assessed the impact of initial hormonal therapy on the results of treatment of stage C prostate cancer, as reviewed in detail previously [49]. Patients with stage C disease have been invited to participate in such trials because the likely cure rate with conventional local treatment (radical radiotherapy, radical prostatectomy) is less than 40%. One of the major problems in interpreting this literature is the very substantial difference in what constitutes "standard" hormone therapy in the various trials. Substantial variations in the type, duration, and sequencing of systemic hormonal therapies employed could easily have contributed to dramatic differences in outcome.

At present, the major defined role for initial hormone therapy appears to be in combination with radiotherapy. The Radiation Therapy Oncology Group (RTOG) has completed an important trial, in which hormonal therapy was combined with definitive radiotherapy for stage C prostate cancer. Pilepich et al. [44] have demonstrated a statistically significant disease-free survival benefit from neoadjuvant systemic hormonal therapy plus radical radiotherapy, compared with radiotherapy alone for stage C disease. Of importance, an overall survival benefit has not been demonstrated in this study. However, Bolla et al. [5], reporting for the European Organization for the Research and Treatment of Cancer, have recorded an overall survival benefit from the use of the combination of hormones and radiotherapy for stage C disease.

Another RTOG trial (no. 85-31) has suggested a disease-free survival benefit for patients treated with adjuvant hormones after definitive radiotherapy, compared to radiotherapy alone [45]; once again, no overall survival benefit was documented, although a retrospective subset analysis suggested a survival benefit for patients with high-grade tumors. It is widely believed that retrospective subset analyses may be heavily flawed statistically, introducing a range of analytical biases, and this limits the importance of this observation.

The role of initial hormonal therapy followed by radical prostatectomy is less clearly defined. Although several studies have reported down-staging of the primary tumor after initial hormonal therapy, overall survival benefit has not been recorded in randomized trials to date. At least one trial has reported a high failure rate after the combination of neoadjuvant hormonal therapy and radical prostatectomy [11]. One potentially important difference between the combined modality trials of radiotherapy and of prostatectomy is the shorter duration of hormonal therapy in most of the surgical trials. This may have contributed to the lack of impact of systemic hormones prior to surgery on ultimate survival.

26.8 Future Strategies for Treatment of Advanced Prostate Cancer

For the future, there are two situations in which CAB is likely to have a continued role in routine management:

1. For patients who are about to commence treatment with LHRH agonists (to avoid the phenomenon of tumor flare that arises from the transient agonist phase of testosterone production after the initial administration of the LHRH agonist)

2. For cases of documented production of significant androgenic steroids from the adrenal glands, where either peripheral blockade (with flutamide or bicalutamide) or central reduction of steroid production (by aminoglutethimide or ketoconazole) may have a role. Otherwise, it seems unlikely that CAB will have any major role in the routine management of advanced prostate cancer in the future.

The provocative report by the Southwest Oncology Group [43] of a possible survival benefit from estrogens compared to orchiectomy in an assessment of chemoendocrine therapy requires further testing. The use of estrogens appears to be reappraised generally in view of the presentation of data showing the efficacy of the commercial preparation, PC-SPES, which appears to be composed predominantly of natural phyto-estrogens [16a]. Of interest, preliminary data suggest that this preparation appears to have fewer cardiovascular side effects than conventional estrogens. This is being tested formally in a randomized clinical trial by Small et al. (personal communication). Interestingly, in a recent study of a novel 5α-reductase inhibitor for initial management of prostate cancer, investigators at Johns Hopkins Oncology Center, the University of Chicago, and the University of Southern California showed a paradoxical elevation of endogenous circulating estrogens that appeared to correlate with suppression of PSA levels [61].

Finally, the exploration, in well-structured clinical trials, of the combination of modern cytotoxic chemotherapy and hormonal manipulation may produce a real improvement in the results of treatment of prostate cancer. Although cytotoxic chemotherapy did not appear particularly promising in early studies, more recent regimens have shown greater anticancer efficacy [2]. This strategy may be especially useful if focused on patients with early stage disease with adverse prognostic factors, such as high grade, aneuploidy, or local tumor extension.

References

1. Aragona C, Friesen H (1975) Specific prolactin binding sites in the prostate and testis of rats. Endocrinology 97:677–684
2. Beer T, Raghavan D (2000) Chemotherapy for hormone-refractory prostate cancer: beauty is in the eye of the beholder. Prostate 45:184–193
3. Bichel P, Frederiksen P, Kjaer T, et al (1977) Flow microfluorometry and transrectal fine needle biopsy in the classification of human prostatic carcinoma. Cancer 40:1206–1211
4. Boccardo F, Pace M, Rubagotti A, et al (1993) Goserelin acetate with or without flutamide in the treatment of patients with locally advanced or metastatic prostate cancer. Eur J Cancer 29A: 1088–1093
5. Bolla M, Gonzalez D, Warde P, et al (1996) Immediate hormonal therapy improves locoregional control and survival in patients with locally advanced prostate cancer. Results of a randomized phase III clinical trial of the EORTC Radiotherapy and Genitourinary Tract Cancer Cooperative Groups. Proc Am Soc Clin Oncol 15:238
6. Brooks JD, Bova GS, Isaacs WB (1995) Allelic loss of the retinoblastoma gene in primary human prostatic adenocarcinomas. Prostate 26:35–39
7. Byar DP (1973) The Veterans' Administration Cooperative Urological Research Group's studies of cancer of the prostate. Cancer 32:1126–1130
8. Byar DP (1980) VACURG studies of conservative treatment. Scand J Urol Nephrol [Suppl 55]: 99–102
9. Cabot AT (1896) The question of castration for enlarged prostate. Ann Surg 24:265–309
10. Carter BS, Epstein JI, Isaacs WB (1990) Ras gene mutations in human prostate cancer. Cancer Res 50:6830–6832
11. Cher ML, Shinohara K, Breslin S, Vapnek J, Carroll PR (1995) High failure rate associated with long-term follow-up of neoadjuvant androgen deprivation followed by radical prostatectomy for stage C prostatic cancer. Br J Urol 75:771–777
12. Citrin DL, Hogan TF, Davis TE (1983) Chemohormonal therapy of metastatic prostate cancer: a pilot study. Cancer 52:410–414

13. Crawford ED, Eisenberger MA, McLeod DG, et al (1989) A controlled trial of leuprolide with and without flutamide in prostatic carcinoma. N Engl J Med 321:419–424
14. Davis NS, diSant'Agnese PA, Ewing JF, Mooney RA (1989) The neuroendocrine prostate: characterization and quantitation of calcitonin in the human prostate gland. J Urol 142:884–888
15. Denis L, Murphy GP (1993) Overview of phase III trials in combined androgenic treatment in patients treated with metastatic prostate cancer. Cancer [Suppl 12]:3888–3895
16. Denis L, Carneiro de Moura JL, Bono A, et al (1992) Goserelin acetate and flutamide versus bilateral orchiectomy: a phase III EORTC trial (30853). Urology 42:119–130
16a. DiPaola RS, Zhang H, Lambert GH, et al (1998) Clinical and biologic activity of an estrogenic herbal combination (PC-SPES) in prostate cancer. N Engl J Med 339:785–791
17. Eisenberger MA, Crawford ED, McLeod D, et al (1997) A comparison of bilateral orchiectomy (orch) with or without flutamide in stage D2 prostate cancer (PC) (NCI INT-0105). Proc Am Soc Clin Oncol 16:2a
18. Eisenkraft S, Huben RP, Pontes JE (1984) Orchiectomy and chemotherapy with estramustine, cis-platinum, cyclophosphamide, and 5-fluorouracil in newly diagnosed prostate cancer with bone metastases. Urology [Suppl 23]:51–53
19. Farnsworth WE, Slaunwhite WR Jr, Sharma M, et al (1981) Interaction of prolactin and testosterone in the human prostate. Urol Res 9:79–88
20. Fellowes GJ, Clark PB, Beynon LL, et al (1992) Treatment of advanced localised prostate cancer by orchiectomy, radiotherapy, or combined treatment. Br J Urol 70:304–309
21. Goldenberg SL, Bruchovsky N (1997) Hormonal manipulation for advanced prostate cancer – conventional approaches. In: Raghavan D, Scher HI, Leibel S, Lange PH (eds) Principles and practice of genitourinary oncology. Lippincott-Raven, Philadelphia, pp 591–597
22. Grayhack JT, Bunce PL, Kearns JW, Scott WW (1955) Influence of the pituitary on prostatic response to androgen in the rat. Bull Johns Hopkins Hosp 96:154–163
23. Harper ME, Goddard L, Glynne-Jones E, et al (1993) An immunocytochemical analysis of TGF-α expression in benign and malignant prostatic tumors. Prostate 23:9–23
24. Horoszewicz JS, Leong SS, Kawinski E, et al (1977) LNCaP model of human prostatic carcinoma. Cancer Res 43:4049–4058
25. Huggins C, Hodges CV (1941) Studies on prostatic cancer. I. The effect of castration, of estrogen and of androgen injection on serum phosphatases in metastatic carcinoma of the prostate. Cancer Res 1:293–297
26. Hunter J (1786) Observations on certain parts of the animal oeconomy. Bibliotheca osteriana, London
27. Iversen P, Christensen MG, Friis E, et al (1990) A phase III trial of zoladex and flutamide versus orchiectomy in the treatment of patients with advanced carcinoma of the prostate. Cancer 66: 1058–1066
28. Jelbart ME, Russell PJ, Russell P, Raghavan D (1988) The biology and management of small cell undifferentiated carcinoma of the prostate. In: Williams CJ, Krikorian J, Raghavan D (eds) Textbook of uncommon cancer, Wiley-Liss, London, pp 249–262
29. Jones TM, Fang VS, Landau RL, Rosenfield R (1978) Direct inhibition of Leydig cell function by estradiol. J Clin Endocrinol Metab 47:1368–1373
30. Keuppens F, Denis L, Smith P, et al (1990) Zoladex and flutamide versus bilateral orchiectomy. A randomized phase III EORTC 30853 study. Cancer 66:1045–1057
31. Kubota Y, Nakada T, Imai K, et al (1995) Chemo-endocrine therapy in patients with stage D2 prostate cancer. Prostate 26:50–54
32. Kyprianou N, English HF, Isaacs JT (1990) Programmed cell death during regression of PC-82 human prostate cancer following androgen ablation. Cancer Res 50:3748–3752
33. Labrie F, Dupont A, Belanger A, et al (1982) New hormonal therapy in prostatic carcinoma: combined therapy with LHRH agonist and antiandrogen. Clin Invest Med, 5:267–275
34. Labrie F, Dupont A, Belanger A, et al (1985) Combination therapy with flutamide and castration (LHRH agonist or orchiectomy) in advanced prostate cancer: a marked improvement in response and survival. J Steroid Biochem 23:833–841
35. Leuprolide Study Group (1984) Leuprolide versus diethylstilbestrol for metastatic prostate cancer. N Engl J Med 311:1281–1286
36. Linja MJ, Savinainen KJ, Saramaki OR, et al (2001) Amplification and overexpression of androgen receptor gene in hormone-refractory prostate cancer. Cancer Res 61:3550–3555
36a. Lundgren R, Nordle O, Josefsson K (1995) Immediate estrogen or estramustine phosphate therapy versus deferred endocrine treatment in nonmetastatic prostate cancer: a randomized multicenter study with 15 years of followup. The South Sweden Prostate Cancer Study Group. J Urol 153:1580–1586
37. Makrdakis N, Ross RK, Pike MC, et al (1997) A prevalent missense substitution that modulates activity of prostatic steroid 5a-reductase. Cancer Res 57:1020–1022
38. McLeod DG, Moul JW (1995) Controversies in the treatment of prostate cancer with maximal androgen deprivation. Surg Clin North Am 4:345–359
39. Mellon K, Thompson S, Charlton RG, et al (1992) p53, c-erbB-2 and the epidermal growth factor receptor in the benign and malignant prostate. J Urol 147:496–499

39a. Messing EM, Manola J, Sarosdy M, et al (1999) Immediate hormonal therapy compared with observation after radical prostatectomy and pelvic lymphadenectomy in men with node-positive prostate cancer. N Engl J Med 341:1781–1788
40. Montie JE, Wood DP Jr, Venderburg S, et al (1990) The significance and management of transitional cell carcinoma of the prostate. Semin Urol 7:262–268
41. Myers C, Cooper M, Stein C, et al (1992) Suramin: a novel growth factor antagonist with activity in hormone-refractory metastatic prostate cancer. J Clin Oncol 10:881–889
42. Myers RB, Oelschlager D, Srivastava S, Grizzle WE (1994) Accumulation of the p53 protein occurs more frequently in metastatic than in localized prostatic adenocarcinomas. Prostate 25:243–248
43. Osborne CK, Blumenstein B, Crawford ED, et al (1990) Combined versus sequential chemo-endocrine therapy in advanced prostate cancer: final results of a Southwest Oncology Group Study. J Clin Oncol 8:1675–1682
44. Pilepich MV, Sause WT, Shipley WU, et al (1995) Androgen deprivation with radiation therapy compared with radiation therapy alone for locally advanced prostatic carcinoma: a randomized comparative trial of the Radiation Therapy Oncology Group. Urology 45:616–623
45. Pilepich MV, Caplan R, Byhardt RW, et al (1997) Phase III trial of androgen suppression using goserelin in unfavorable-prognosis carcinoma of the prostate treated with definitive radiotherapy: report of Radiation Therapy Oncology Group Protocol 85–31. J Clin Oncol 15:1013–1021
46. Prostate Cancer Trialists' Collaborative Group (1995) Maximum androgen blockade in advanced prostate cancer: an overview of 22 randomised trials with 3283 deaths in 5710 patients. Lancet 346:265–269
47. Prostate Cancer Trialists' Collaborative Group (2000) Maximum androgen blockade in advanced prostate cancer: an overview of the randomised trials. Lancet 355:1491–1498
48. Raghavan D (1988) Non-hormone chemotherapy for prostate cancer: principles of treatment and application to the testing of new drugs. Semin Oncol 15:371–389
49. Raghavan D (1996) Adjuvant systemic therapy of prostate cancer. Semin Oncol 22:633–640
50. Raghavan D, Lange PH (1985) Endocrine aspects of genito-urinary neoplasia. In: Shearman RP (ed) Clinical reproductive endocrinology. Churchill Livingstone, Edinburgh, pp 727–752
51. Raghavan D, Tannock IF (1989) Clinical trials in genitourinary oncology: what have they achieved? In: Smith PH (ed) Combination therapy in urological malignancy. Springer, London Berlin Heidelberg New York, pp 225–253
52. Raghavan D, Russell P (1999) Small cell undifferentiated (neuroendocrine) carcinoma of the prostate. In: Raghavan D, Brecher M, Johnson D, et al (eds) Textbook of uncommon cancer, Wiley-Liss, New York pp 63–73
53. Raghavan D, Pearson B, Coorey G, et al (1989) Management of hormone-resistant prostate cancer: experience at Royal Prince Alfred Hospital. In: Johnson DE, Logothetis CJ, von Eschenbach AC (eds) Systemic therapy for genitourinary cancers. Year Book Medical Publishers, Chicago, pp 245–250
54. Raghavan D, Cox K, Pearson B, et al (1993) Oral cyclophosphamide for the management of hormone refractory prostate cancer. Br J Urol 72:625–628
55. Rinker-Schaeffer CW, Partin AW, Isaacs WB, Coffey DS, Isaacs JT (1994) Molecular and cellular changes associated with the acquisition of metastatic ability by prostatic cancer cells. Prostate 25:249–265
56. Ronstrom L, Tribukait B, Esposti PL (1981) DNA pattern and cytological findings in fine-needle aspirates of untreated prostatic tumors. A flow-cytofluorometric study. Prostate 2: 79–88
57. Scher HI, Logothetis CJ (1997) Chemotherapy of advanced prostate cancer. In: Raghavan D, Scher HI, Leibel S, Lange PH (eds) Principles and practice of genitourinary oncology. Lippincott-Raven, Philadelphia, pp 599–612
58. Scott WW, Menon M, Walsh PC (1980) Hormonal therapy of prostatic cancer. Cancer 45:1929–1936
59. Seifter EJ, Bunn PA, Cohen MH, et al (1986) A trial of combination chemotherapy followed by hormonal therapy for previously untreated metastatic carcinoma of the prostate. J Clin Oncol 4:1365–1373
60. Shearer RJ, Hendry WF, Sommerville IF, Fergusson JD (1973) Plasma testosterone: an accurate monitor of hormone treatment in prostate cancer. Br J Urol 45:668–677
61. Sinibaldi V, Laufer M, Eisenberger M, Raghavan D (2001) Proc Am Soc Clin Oncol 20:
62. Tannock IF (1985) Is there evidence that chemotherapy is of benefit to patients with carcinoma of the prostate? J Clin Oncol 3:1013–1021
63. Taplin M-E, Bubley GJ, Shuster TD, et al (1995) Mutation of the androgen-receptor gene in metastatic androgen-independent prostate cancer. N Engl J Med 332:1393–1398
64. Thigpen AE, Davis DL, Milatovitch A, et al (1992) Molecular genetics of steroid 5 alpha-reductase 2 deficiency. J Clin Invest 90:799–809
65. Tyrell C, Altwein J, Klippel F, et al (1991) A multicenter randomized trial comparing the luteinizing hormone-releasing hormone analogue goserelin acetate alone and with flutamide in the treatment of advanced prostate cancer. J Urol 146:1321–1326

66. Vermeulen A, Reubens R, Verdonck L (1972) Testosterone secretion and metabolism in male senescence. J Clin Endocrinol 34:7340–735
67. Visakorpi T, Hyytinen E, Koivisto P, et al (1995) In vivo amplification of the androgen receptor gene and progression of human prostate cancer. Nat Genet 9:401–406
68. White JW (1895) The results of double castration in hypertrophy of the prostate. Ann Surg 22:1–80
69. Zalcberg J, Raghavan D, Marshall V, Thompson P (1996) Bilateral orchiectomy and flutamide versus orchiectomy alone in newly diagnosed patients with metastatic carcinoma of the prostate – an Australian multicentre trial. Br J Urol 77:865–869

27 Therapeutic Options in Hormone Refractory Prostate Cancer

A. Heidenreich

27.1 Introduction

Adenocarcinoma of the prostate is the most prevalent tumor in men, a major cause of morbidity and mortality mainly because of the hormone refractory component. Hormone refractory prostate cancer (HRPCA) causes about 42,000 deaths annually [58, 98].

HRPCA is to be diagnosed when a continuous rise of prostate-specific antigen (PSA) occurs despite androgen deprivation down to castrate levels of testosterone [70]. The clinical situation of patients with HRPCA is dominated by bone metastases which may be accompanied by bone pain, pathological fractures, weight loss, spinal cord compression, anemia, and thrombocytopenia, not surprisingly resulting in a significant reduction in performance status [70, 96]. Although a number of systemic treatment options such as narcotics, non-steroidal antiinflammatory drugs, bisphosphonates, and local radiation are available to HRPCA patients, the goal of therapeutic efforts should be to identify single agents or combinations that increase life expectancy, reduce suffering, and maintain an adequate quality of life [96].

In the recent past, several new chemotherapeutic and biological agents have been evaluated in clinical phase-I and phase-II trials with promising results. However, we have to keep in mind that HRPCA is a heterogenous disease, and varied patient cohorts have been studied . The median survival time of these groups differs significantly (Table 27.1) and must be considered when analyzing and designing trials in HRPCA [53, 70, 96].

Lack of consensus on response criteria is another problem associated with clinical phase-II trials in HRPCA, making comparisons between treat-

Table 27.1. Clinical characteristics of patients with hormone refractory prostate cancer potentially influencing preference and outcome of treatment

Patient characteristics	Estimated median survival
Rising PSA levels only, no measurable disease	52 weeks
Rising PSA levels, measurable low volume metastatic disease, no symptoms	41–52 weeks
Rising PSA levels, measurable high volume metastatic disease, no symptoms	10–28 weeks
Rising PSA levels, measurable low volume metastatic disease, symptoms	32–41 weeks
Rising PSA levels, measurable high volume metastatic disease, symptoms	10–28 weeks

PSA, prostate-specific antigen.

ment modalities impossible and impeding the identification of agents appropriate for progress into randomized clinical phase-III trials. It will be necessary to adhere to practical guidelines when designing and analyzing new phase-II trials [5].

The task of this chapter is to introduce the biology of HRPCA, to identify prognostic markers in HRPCA, and to discuss the rational use of second line hormonal therapy and chemotherapy.

27.1.1 Biology of Hormone Refractory Prostate Cancer

It is a well known clinical observation that patients with metastatic disease treated with androgen deprivation either by the use of antiandrogens, luteinizing hormone releasing hormone (LHRH) analogues, or surgical castration will develop progressive disease usually after a mean time of 18–36 months [53].

Based on the stem cell model of the prostate, it has become clear that there are multiple pathways for the development of hormone resistance resulting from the emergence of androgen-independent or androgen-sensitive cells [35].

The normal prostate is composed of a limited number of androgen-independent stem cells, maintaining their limited number by cell division and giving rise to androgen-sensitive cells. In the presence of physiologic serum levels of testosterone these cells differentiate into glandular epithelial cells until their normal number of cells is reached and their proliferation rate equals their rate of cell death so that no glandular overgrowth occurs. Based on this clonally expansive growth, the normal prostate is mainly composed of androgen-dependent glandular epithelial cells, lower numbers of androgen-sensitive basal cells, and very few androgen-independent basal stem cells.

Although the exact mechanism has not been resolved, a number of events such as genetic instability due to changes in the microenvironment, deactivation of detoxifying enzymes (GST-?), activation of oncogenes, and amplification of androgen receptors might result in androgen independence.

27.1.2 Prognostic Risk Factors in Hormone Refractory Prostate Cancer

As stated, HRPCA is a heterogenous disease (Table 27.1) and survival time and response to chemotherapy will be different between these different groups; prognosticators in HRPCA – identified as existing when relapse follows multiple hormonal manipulations – might therefore be clinically useful in order to identify patients who may benefit from different therapeutic approaches. In addition, the clinical identification of reliable prognosticators might enable the definition of subgroups of HRPCA, and thus facilitate the comparison of various clinical trials based on specific patient characteristics. Unfortunately, only a few parameters (to be discussed) have been tested and analyzed by multivariate analysis (MVA) in well designed trials [10, 11, 21].

Performance status is an important reproducible prognostic marker that independently predicts both response to therapy and survival time when submitted to multivariate analysis. A Karnofsky index of ≤80% versus a Karnofsky index of >80% may be used as indicating significant prognostic differences.

Although a 15% reduction of hemoglobin levels occurs in patients undergoing androgen deprivation [86], plasma levels of hemoglobin have been demonstrated by MVA to independently predict outcome. In some studies, the combination of low hemoglobin levels with other predictors of negative outcome, such as high PSA serum levels, low performance status, and/or fatigue, confirmed an even worse prognosis. The negative prognostic impact of low hemoglobin levels reflects the fact that bone metastases of PCA predominantly involve the red bone marrow; the degree of anemia roughly parallels the extent of bone disease, which by itself is a poor prognosticator.

PSA has been validated as the most clinically useful tumor marker of treatment failure and tumor response following local therapy, as well as of tumor progression following hormonal treatment. However, although PSA has evolved as a good marker of tumor volume, no threshold levels reproducibly predicting survival have been identified.

A number of studies have evaluated changes in pretreatment PSA levels following therapy in order to predict therapeutic response. It has reproducibly turned out that a ≥50% decline in pretreatment PSA following chemotherapy is associated with a significant survival advantage. The study of Smith et al. [83] even suggests that the 8-week time point might be the most significant one: median survival from that landmark was 91 weeks in patients with a decline in PSA of 50% or greater versus 38 weeks in patients with a PSA decline of less than 50%.

Molecular markers are just starting to be evaluated as prognostic in HRPCA. In one promising study, Ghossein et al. [22] investigated the use of the reverse transcriptase polymerase chain reaction (RTPCR) to detect mRNA of PSA in the peripheral blood, observing a poor survival in the presence of positive RTPCR findings. These data have to be corroborated in other trials before recommendations can be made on their routine clinical use. At the moment, RTPCR for PSA is not useful for the clinical differentiation of responders and non-responders to chemotherapy in HRPCA.

27.2 Second Line Hormonal Therapy

27.2.1 Addition of Antiandrogens

As pointed out, PSA progression following initial androgen deprivation usually results from the clonal expansion of androgen-independent prostate cancer cells, mutations of androgen receptors [89], and amplification of the androgen receptors with a consequent increase in receptor density, all of which results in cancer growth stimulation even in the presence of low levels of circulating androgens [89]. Finally, in addition, amplification of the bcl-2 oncogene inhibits cellular apoptosis [25, 52].

However, it has been shown that prostate cancer cells resistant to androgen deprivation might be inhibited by estrogens and by additional blockage of circulating testicular or adrenal androgens. Since about 10%–20% of all patients who undergo subcapsular orchiectomy or pharmacological castration still demonstrate normal testosterone serum levels, these levels should be measured [43]. If elevated testosterone levels are found, additional androgen deprivation either by orchiectomy or by addition of an antiandrogen should be performed.

Currently, there is no uniform opinion as to whether continuous androgen deprivation is necessary in patients with disease progression despite castrate levels of testosterone. The conclusion of a retrospective analysis of four Eastern Cooperative Oncology Group clinical trials that identified 55 patients with discontinued androgen suppression was that continued androgen suppression is an independent predictor of survival [90]. However, a review of patients treated by the Southwest Oncology Group [34] did not demonstrate any survival benefit from continuous androgen suppression among the 173 patients as compared to 34 patients with discontinued androgen ablation. Evidence-based medicine criteria suggesting that continuation of androgen ablation really benefits the patient thus appears to be lacking. Accordingly, the continuation of gonadal testosterone ablation should be discussed with the patient.

Patients with antiandrogenic monotherapy either by medical castration or by subcapsular orchiectomy might benefit from the additional application of LHRH analogs, as has been demonstrated by Ornstein et al. [55] who observed a significant PSA decrease in 67% of their patients over a mean interval of 20 months. In another study, Fowler et al. [19] treated 90 patients with rising PSA after subcapsular orchiectomy with flutamide and noted a PSA response in 80%. The authors noted that the extent of disease at time of deferred flutamide treatment held prognostic impact: patients with localized disease responded better (80% vs. 54%) than patients with metastatic disease. While a PSA response can be achieved in a subset of patients, the impact of deferred flutamide treatment on survival is unknown.

27.2.2 Antiandrogen Withdrawal

Regardless of whether therapy is begun as complete androgen blockade (CAB) or antiandrogens are added subsequently, withdrawal of antiandrogens (AAW) might result in both clinical and serum PSA responses. This phenomenon has initially been reported in four patients of Kelly and Scher [39]. Subsequent studies in more than 300 patients with serum PSA progression demonstrated a PSA response in about 30% in a mean time of about 4 months (Table 27.2); PSA decrease after AAW is found to be first experienced within the first 6 weeks. AAW has been observed following discontinuation of flutamide, biclutamide, and nilutamide [23, 29, 54, 76].

The mechanism underlying the AAW has not yet been identified, although pathogenetic possibilities have been discussed: (1) mutations of the

Table 27.2. Summary of published reports on antiandrogen withdrawal in patients with prostate-specific antigen (*PSA*) progression following initial hormonal therapy

Author	Antiandrogen	*n*	PSA↓ >50%	Duration
Scher et al. 1995 [2]	Flutamide	57	28%	4 months
Small and Srinivas 1995 [77]	Flutamide	82	15%	3.5 months
Figg et al. 1995 [18]	Flutamide	21	33%	3.7 months
Herrada et al. 1996 [27]	Flutamide	39	28%	3.3 months
Dupont et al. 1993 [15]	Flutamide	40	80%	14.5 months
Sartor et al. 1994 [39]	Flutamide	29	48%	8 months
Breul et al. 1998 [4]	Flutamide	12	16%	5 months
Schellhammer et al. 1997 [69]	Flutamide	8	50%	n. d.
	Biclutamide	14	29%	n. d.
Nieh, 1995 [29]	Biclutamide	3	33%	6 months
Small and Carroll, 1994 [30]	Biclutamide	1	100%	1 month
Huan et al. 1997 [32]	Nilutamide	2	100%	6 months
Total		308	34.4%	5.5 months

hormone-binding domain of the androgen receptor (AR) resulting in stimulation by antiandrogens [89, 92]; (2) amplification of the wild-type AR gene conferring exquisite sensitivity to even low levels of testosterone or antiandrogens [95].

The identification of the AAW syndrome has had a significant impact on the clinical management of patients with primary androgen ablation since: (a) from a clinical standpoint, AAW has to be the mandatory first intervention in patients with progressive disease; (b) AAW is nontoxic and might benefit a significant subset of patients for a limited period; and (c) it is mandatory that AAW has been completed at least 4–6 weeks before beginning a trial of chemotherapy.

27.2.3 Secondary Antiandrogens

It has been suggested that different antiandrogens have different functional interactions with the AR, resulting in different response rates. This hypothesis has been tested in clinical trials applying high dose biclutamide therapy in 51 patients (150 mg/day) [71] and 31 patients (200 mg/day [37], who demonstrated PSA progression following flutamide therapy. Response rates were 38% and 22.5% in all patients with a significantly better response in patients with AAW. Joyce et al. [37] noted further that only patients having undergone primary flutamide-based androgen deprivation responded to secondary antiandrogenic therapy; only 6% of those patients having undergone other hormonal manipulations exhibited a PSA decline of over 50%.

27.2.4 Adrenal Androgen Inhibitors

Five to ten percent of peripheral testosterone is produced in the adrenal glands, and it has been suggested that the inhibition of adrenal testosterone synthesis might result in clinical and/or PSA responses in patients failing initial antiandrogen therapy.

Aminoglutethimide (AG) has been reported to produce response rates of about 30% when combined with steroid replacement in HRPCA; however, randomized clinical trials suggest that the response rates are primarily due to the corticoids [143]. The combination of AG and hydrocortisone (HC) together with AAW results in encouraging response rates of 48%–80% [14, 64, 68]. It is not clear, however, that AG plus HC has more clinical efficacy than HC alone, as has been questioned by Dowsett et al. [14] These investigators showed that HC results in a significant suppression of testicular and adrenal androgen synthesis in patients with HRPCA, whereas the application of AG leads to an increase in serum testosterone and androstendione. Concomitant AAW appears to be an important cofactor in the response, as has been demonstrated in a clinical trial giving suramin and aminoglutethimide simultaneously with or without AAW [68]. When AAW was added, response rates of 44% were realized, as compared to a rate of only 14% in the group without AAW.

Ketoconazole effectively inhibits testicular and adrenal testosterone production and might even exert direct cytotoxic effects on prostate cancer cells. Monotherapy with this agent is associated with response rates of about 20% [36] in HRPCA. Combining high-dose ketoconazole (1200 mg/day) with hydrocortisone has been shown to result in a >50% PSA decrease in 62% of the patients for a median duration of 3.5 months [79]. A second trial of high-dose ketoconazole combined with hydrocortisone and AAW reported identical response rates, but median duration of response was now 8.5 months [80]. The clinical significance of newer generation adrenal inhibitors such as liarozole remains unclear since recent prospective trials have been halted [12].

27.2.5 Estrogen-Based Therapy

Diethylbestrol single agent therapy might have a role in the management of HRPCA, as demonstrated by the study of Smith et al. [84] in which diethylstilbestrol (DES) was given at 1 mg/day in 21 patients following antiandrogen withdrawal. Interestingly, 43% of them experienced a PSA decline of more than 50% and the estimated survival at 2 years was 63%. Single agent DES would thus appear to be an effective alternative in patients with HRPCA.

In a second study, Klotz et al. [42] compared the therapeutic efficacy of oral DES at either 3 mg daily, or 2 mg daily combined with 1 mg warfarin, in a total of 32 patients with hormone-refractory prostate cancer. Although the mean pretreatment PSA decreased from 95.4 to 1.5 µg/l after 3 months of therapy, 31% of the patients developed proximal deep venous thrombosis, 7% developed myocardial infarction, and another 7% experienced transient ischemic attacks, so that the clinical application of single agent DES at higher doses than 1 mg/day does not seem to be justified in the management of HRPCA.

27.2.6 PC-SPES

PC-SPES is a herbal therapeutic that has been commercially available since 1996. It is a combination of eight different herbs, each with some antitumoral effectivity [13]. PC-SPES has been shown to exert significant apoptotic effects on prostate cancer cell lines LNCaP, PC3, and DU145 [13], whereas suppression of tumor growth in xenografts could only be documented when therapy was initiated at the same day of tumor cell injection. Apparently, PC-SPES has potent estrogenic activity as has been demonstrated in in vitro studies with estrogen-dependent yeast and bacteria strains [13]. In their initial study on eight patients, DiPaola et al. [13] observed a PSA response in five who additionally experienced "estrogenic" side effects such as breast tenderness and loss of libido due to significant decrease in serum testosterone levels.

With regard to clinical trials, only three studies published recently have evaluated the efficacy of PC-SPES in HRPCA. In the first, DeLa Taille et al. [8] assessed patients with progressive PSA levels who had undergone hormone therapy. They found a significant PSA response at 2 months in 27/31 (87%). Only 18 patients could be followed after 6 months of therapy and although all of them had lower PSA serum concentrations than at the initiation of therapy, the majority of them already exhibited an increase in PSA serum levels. In another study, DeLa Taille et al. [9] observed 22 patients who experienced PSA progression following prior hormonal therapy; unfortunately, the type of hormonal treatment and the status as to AAW were not reported. Two months after initiation of therapy, 14/22 (66%) of patients demonstrated a decrease in serum PSA ≥50%. However, at 12 months of follow-up none of the patients had maintained their lowered PSA levels. Side effects included nipple tenderness in 42%, gynecomastia in 8%, hot flashes in 7%, and deep venous thrombosis in 2%. Recently, Small et al. [81] reported on 37 patients with androgen-independent prostate cancer with PSA progression who received 320 mg capsules tid for 3 weeks. Although 19/37 (54%) of them experienced a >50% PSA decrease, the median duration of PSA decline was only 18 weeks and the median time to progression was only 16 weeks. Furthermore, six patients (16.2%) stopped therapy because of significant grade 4 toxicities. Included were grade 4 thromboembolic events in 4.3%, other grade 3/4 toxicities in 10%, leg cramps in 69%, gastrointestinal discomfort in 53%, breast tenderness in 93%, and (non grade 4 thromboembolic) cardiovascular events in 5.7%.

In conclusion, PC-SPES has a significant estrogenic activity resulting in a short-term PSA decline in HRPCA. While response rates do not differ from classical DES therapy, duration of response after PC-SPES is significantly lower than with DES treatment. A problem with PC-SPES appears to be difficulty in controlling the application. Concentrations of the active compounds vary from vial to vial, and therefore cardiovascular side effects are apt to crop up even to rates as high as after high-dose estrogen therapy. The administration of PC-SPES should only be pursued in large scale, detailed clinical trials.

27.2.7
Other Hormonal Manipulations

Glucocorticoids have been used in the palliative management of HRPCA for years. Hydrocortisone (40 mg/day) following PSA progression after AAW will result in a 20% PSA response [40]. In addition, this response rate has to be considered as a solitary steroid effect when analyzing trials combining corticosteroids with antineoplastic agents. Prednisolone alone exerts a palliative effect in terms of improvement of quality-of-life or significant reduction of bone pain in about 40% of the patients, as has been shown in recent prospective randomized clinical trials [87]; identical data have been obtained with hydrocortisone [88].

27.3
Rationale Use of Chemotherapy in HRPCA

Chemotherapy of HRPCA with both single agents and drug combinations has been studied since the early 1970s with the depressing result of a low response rate and a high frequency of treatment-related toxicities. Yagoda and Petrylak [99] reviewed 26 chemotherapeutic studies that had been performed between 1988 and 1991 and found on overall response rate of only 8.7% without any survival benefits for the patients. This negative experience has led to much scepticism regarding chemotherapy in HRPCA. Recently this view has been challenged with the development of new agents and combinations specifically targeting cellular mechanisms.

Chemotherapy can be integrated into the therapeutic management of HRPCA after antiandrogens and other hormonal therapies have failed (Fig. 27.1). Whenever chemotherapy is started, the clinical issue remains as to the further application of endocrine treatment. Most authors recommend continuing androgen deprivation, a position primarily based on the data of Manni et al. [47] who demonstrated that survival rates were significantly lower in patients without continuous androgen deprivation. However, two recently published trials challenge these data by showing only a marginal survival benefit for patients staying on LHRH analogues throughout treatment [34, 90]. Unfortunately, there are no prospective-randomized trials answering this important issue – one that also bears an important socioeconomic factor considering the high treatment costs.

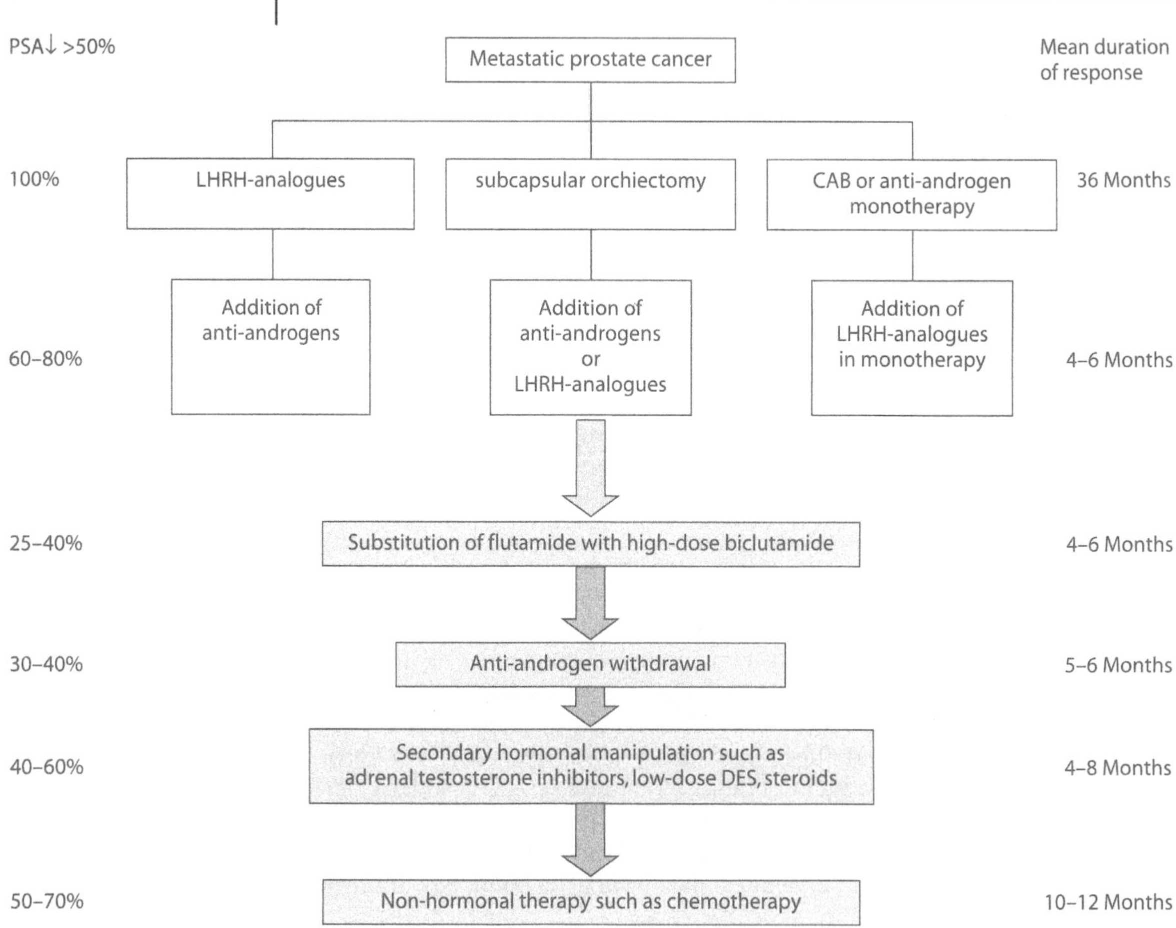

Fig. 27.1. Flowsheet of the potential therapeutic options after prostate-specific antigen (*PSA*) progression following initial hormonal therapy

Antiandrogens and secondary hormonal manipulations, however, should be stopped 4–6 weeks prior to the use of chemotherapy, allowing the anti-androgen withdrawal effect to become effective as recommended by the PSA working group [6, 50, 53, 59, 65, 66, 67].

27.3.1 Estramustine-Based Chemotherapy

Estramustine phosphate (EMP) is a combination of nornitrogen mustard and estradiol and was originally designed for the treatment of estrogen receptor-positive cancer cells. Initial studies by the National Cancer Institute (NCI) using EMP as a single agent demonstrated only modest response rates of around 20%. However, it has been shown in recent preclinical trials that EMP depolymerizes cytoplasmic microtubules and microfilaments, binds to microtubule-associated proteins, inhibits P-glycoprotein function and disrupts the nuclear matrix. In addition, EMP demonstrated an additive antitumor effect when combined with vinca alkaloids, taxanes, and polypodopyotoxines [2, 26, 91].

Based on these preclinical experience a number of clinical trials combining EMP with vinblastine (VBL), etoposide, paclitaxel, and docetaxel have been conducted [72, 32, 1]. Hudes et al. [32] initiated a randomized phase-III trial of vinblastine versus EMP/vinblastine in 203 patients. VBL was administered weekly at 4 mg/m^2 body surface area for 6 consecutive weeks followed by 2 weeks off. Combination therapy consisted of the identical schedule and dose for VBL and EMP at 600 mg/m^2 per day on days 1–42 of each 8-week cycle.

Although a statistically significant improvement in time to progression (3.7 versus 2.2 months) and in frequency of ≥50% PSA decrease (25% versus 5.2%) for the EMP/VBL arm was noted, median survival did not differ significantly (VBL 9.2 months; EMP/VBL 11.9 months).

Treatment-related hematological side effects such as grade III/IV granulocytopenia occurred more frequently in the VBL arm (27.8% vs 10%), whereas nonhematological toxicities such as nausea (27% vs 7%) and leg edema (11% vs 3%) developed more often in those taking EMP/VBL. The reason for the higher frequency of hematotoxicity in the VBL arm remains unclear, but it has been shown in EMP single agent studies that patients experience increased white blood cell and granulocyte counts consistent with enhanced mobilization or synthesis of granulocytes.

Another European Organization for Research and Treatment of Cancer (EORTC) trial evaluating EMP versus EMP/VBL [1] reported much less favorable results with a median survival of 93.5 weeks and 46.6 weeks, respectively, in 92 patients with HRPCA.

It appears in conclusion that combination therapy of EMP and VBL improves time to progression by 6 weeks, but has no impact on survival as compared to EMP monotherapy.

The rationale of combining EMP and taxanes is based on the hypothesis of achieving greater inhibition of microtubule function and cytotoxicity by combining drugs that bind to different, but complementary protein targets in the microtubules [2, 26, 91].

Paclitaxel at a dose of 120 mg/m^2 over 96 h in combination with EMP at a dose of 600 mg/m^2 per day resulted in a >50% PSA decrease in 65% of patients in one study, and an overall objective response in 44%. Median survival time, however, was only 7 months [33].

Two phase-I trials evaluated the therapeutic efficacy of EMP in combination with docetaxel in patients with HRPCA who had been exposed to a variety of prior chemotherapies. Petrylak et al. [59] found docetaxel at 70 mg/m^2 on day 2 and EMP 840 mg/day from day 1 through day 5 to be the maximum tolerated dose in 34 minimally pretreated patients (MPT); in 17 heavily pretreated patients (EPT) docetaxel at 60 mg/m^2 on day 2 was found to be the maximum tolerated dose. Seventy percent of the MPT patients and 50% of the EPT patients manifested a ≥50% PSA decrease. Most interestingly, the median survival of all patients was 22.8 months with no difference between the MPT and the EPT group. Kreis et al. [44] treated 17 patients with EMP at 14 mg/kg per day on days 1 through 21 and docetaxel at 40 to 80 mg/m^2 on day 1 of a 21-day cycle. As in the study by Petrylak et al. [59], docetaxel at 70 mg/m^2 was found to be the maximum tolerated dose, with grade 3 and 4 hematotoxicity developing in 30% of the patients; alopecia and fluid retention was found in all patients at all dosages. Diarrhea grades 1–3 was the most compelling side effect occurring in basically all patients. Although response to therapy was not the primary end point of the study, 82% of these patients received a ≥50% decrease in PSA lasting for 1–11 months.

Recently, a number of phase-II trials combining EMP and docetaxel have been conducted on 70 patients [20, 75, 97]. A PSA decrease of 50% or more was observed in 31%–84% of the patients, with a median duration of PSA nadir of 22 weeks. Dose-limiting side effects were grade 3 and 4 hematotoxicity developing in 13%–42% of the patients, and three (5.5%) treatment-related deaths were reported.

In summary, the combination of EMP with taxanes appears to be an effective chemotherapeutic regime with tolerable and reversible side effects. However, to draw any conclusions from these phase-I and phase-II trials, large, prospectively randomized clinical trials should be initiated.

To achieve a maximum therapeutic effect of combination therapy, Smith et al. combined etoposide (100 mg/day) with EMP (280 mg tid) and paclitaxel (135 mg/m^2 IV over 1 h, day 2) in 40 patients with HRPCA [85]. The overall response rate (complete response [CR]/partial response [PR]) was 45%, and 65% of the patients demonstrated a PSA decrease of more than 50%. The median duration of response was 3.2 months with a maximum of 8.7 months; the estimated median survival was 12.8 months. Major toxicity in this group of heavily pretreated patients with HRPCA was grade 4 leukopenia and anemia in eight patients (20%). Prior chemotherapy did not seem to influence the outcome of therapy, but only was a predictor of toxicity.

27.3.2 Anthracyclines

Anthracyclines have been studied extensively in HRPCA, single agent therapy resulting in an overall response rate of measurable disease in 0%–33% of patients; most agents have demonstrated a significant palliative effect but have lacked an objective therapeutic response.

Besides its use as a single agent, doxorubicin has been applied in polychemotherapy regimes in combination with 5-flourouracil and mitomycin [3, 45, 46]; combined with ketoconazole [74]; and in combination with ketoconazole, EMP, and VBL [16] (Table 27.3). The latter schedule yielded a response in patients with measurable disease in 75% and a PSA decrease of greater than 50% in 67% [16]. Median duration of response was 8.4 months, and median survival time for the entire group was 19 months. Since side effects were modest

Table 27.3. Outcome of different EMP-based chemotherapeutic regimes

Author	*n*	CR/PR	PSA↓ >50%	Survival
EMP and VBL				
Seidman [68]	25	40%	54%	7 months[a]
Hudes [32]	201	20%	25%	12 months[b]
Albrecht [71]	92	No data	37%	11 months[b]
EMP and etoposide				
Pienta [61]	62	53%	39%	13 months
Pienta [62]	42	50%	52%	44 (38 vs 91 wks)[c]
EMP and taxanes				
Hudes [32]	34	44%	53%	69 weeks
Petrylak [60]	34	28%	63%	23 months
Kreis [75]	17	16%	82%	No data
Weitzman [76]	19	75%	84%	22 weeks[b]
Friedland [78]	19	8%	42%	5 months[b]
Sinibaldi [79]	16	28%	31%	No data
Smith [85]	40	45%	65%	13 months

EMP, estramustine phosphate; VBL, vinblastine; CR/PR, overall response rate.
[a] Median duration of response.
[b] Median survival for the EMP/VBL group was better than for the VBL alone group (9 month and 10 months).
[c] Median survival in PSA-responders was significantly better than in PSA-nonresponders.

and could be managed without growth factor support, this alternating regime of chemohormonal therapy is worthy of being evaluated in prospective randomized clinical phase-III trials.

In two other studies, combinations of doxorubicin with EMP [7] and with dose-escalating cyclophosphamide [78] were investigated. Whereas the therapeutic efficacy of the first regime was minimal, the latter one providing doxorubicin at 40 mg/m^2 and cyclophosphamide at 800 to 2,000 mg/m^2 every 21 days demonstrated an objective response in 33% and a PSA decline of >50% in 46% of the patients. Median survival of the entire group was 11 months, but median survival of patients with a PSA response was significantly longer than in nonresponders (23 vs. 7 months, p=0.02). Hematotoxicity occurred in 33% of the patients, with only 8% developing febrile neutropenia; nonhematologic toxicity was minimal.

Recently, Doxil, a doxorubicin formulation of polyethylene glycol-coated liposomes, has demonstrated significant antitumor effects in Kaposi's sarcoma and cisplatin-resistant ovarian cancer. Experimental animal studies using Doxil against human prostate cancer xenografts (PC3) in nude mice showed a 25-fold increase in intratumoral Doxil concentrations as compared to free doxorubicin, indicating potential therapeutic effects in humans [93]. Clinical experiences with Doxil in HRPCA are limited: Hubert et al. [31] performed an exploratory study with pharmacokinetics using either 45 mg/m^2 every 3 weeks or 60 mg/m^2 every 4 weeks – two regimes of equal dose intensity. Although the latter regime appeared to be active against HRPCA, severe mucocutaneous side effects prevented further investigations. Our own group initiated a three-arm prospective, randomized clinical phase-II trial in HRPCA, giving Doxil at 25 mg/m^2 every 2 weeks, 50 mg/m^2 every 4 weeks, and at 50 mg/m^2 every 4 weeks for three cycles followed by Doxil at 40 mg/m^2 every 4 weeks for another three cycles in 60 patients. Whereas the palliative effect with significant reduction of bone pain on the day of application was impressive, none of the patients with measurable disease experienced an objective response rate, and only a minority of the patients developed a greater than 50% PSA decrease. Treatment-related side effects, on the other hand, were significant, with severe stomatitis and hand-and-foot syndrome requiring prolongation of the cycles, reduction of doses, or discontinuation of therapy. Based on these experiences, Doxil does not seem to be a candidate for a major role in the future treatment of HRPCA.

Epirubicin, another anthracycline, has been used in a limited number of combination studies (Table 27.4). Overall, the combination of epirubicin and cisplatin has not been very successful, with a marginal antitumor effect and a high frequency of side effects [30]. Combining cisplatin, epirubicin, and EMP led to an objective response rate of 39% and a median survival of 15 months [94]. Combinations of suramin with epirubicin demonstrated limited therapeutic efficacy in HRPCA [17, 48], with a high frequency of treatment-related side effects. None of these regimes appears to be a clinically useful improvement in the therapy of HRPCA.

The anthracenedione mitoxantrone has a chemical structure similar to doxorubicin but a significantly lower toxicity profile. Initial studies demonstrated limited overall response rates of only 12% in patients with HRPCA [56], but most studies showed beneficial effects on disease-related symptoms and quality of life. After a first study [49] achieved a palliative response in 36% of patients, two prospective randomized clinical phase-III studies were performed comparing mitoxantrone/prednisone versus prednisone alone in 161 and 242 HRPCA patients, respectively [38, 87, 88]. In both studies mitoxantrone was given at 12 mg/m^2 intravenously at 3-week intervals and 10 mg oral prednisone was taken daily. Pain relief as the major indicator of palliation was the primary

Table 27.4. Outcome of anthracycline-based chemotherapy for hormone refractory prostate cancer

Author	*n*	CR/PR	PSA↓ >50%	Survival
Doxorubicin, CDDP, 5-FU				
Logothetis [85]	62	48%	Not done	47.5/23.8 weeks[b]
Blumenstein [83]	68	16.2%	Not done	9 months
Laurie [84]	144	14%	Not done	9 months
Doxorubicin, ketoconazole				
Sella [82]	12	55%	55%	No data given
Doxorubicin, EMP, ketoconazole, VBL				
Ellerhorst [81]	46	75%	67%	13 months
Doxorubicin, EMP				
Culine [86]	31	45%	58%	12 months
Doxorubicin, cyclophosphamide				
Small [76, 78]	35	33%	46%	23 vs 7 months[a]
Epirubicin, CDDP, EMP				
Huan [30]	21	14%	32%	?
Veronesi [91]	28	39%	Not done	15 months
Epirubicin, Suramin				
Falcone [92]	26	27%	33%	8 months
Miglietta [93]	10	0%	0%	?

EMP, estramustine phosphate; VBL, vinblastine; CR/PR, overall response rate; 5-FU, 5-fluoruracil; PSA, prostate-specific antigen.
[a] Responders/nonresponders to therapy.
[b] PSA responders showed a significantly better survival than PSA nonresponders.

endpoint of the first study by Tannock et al. [87, 88], whereas PSA decrease and survival were secondary goals. Primary response criteria were met by 23/80 (29%) patients receiving mitoxantrone/prednisone and by 10/81 (12%) patients receiving prednisone alone (p=0.01). Also, the duration of response was significantly longer in patients receiving chemotherapy (43 weeks) as compared to the prednisone alone group (18 weeks, p<0.0001). Although there was no difference in survival between the groups, the reduction in serum PSA correlated with a positive palliative response. Changes in serum PSA did not, however, provide clinically useful information for discriminating between these groups of patients. Treatment-related toxicity included hematologic toxicity of grade 3 and 4 in 32%, however, febrile neutropenia developed in only 1.1%.

A similar study comparing mitoxantrone/hydrocortisone versus hydrocortisone alone was conducted by the Cancer and Leukemia Group [38]. Hydrocortisone was administered orally at 40 mg daily and mitoxantrone was given intravenously at 14 mg/m^2 every 3 weeks to 119 (mitoxanreone+hydrocortisone) and 123 (hydrocortisone) patients. The primary endpoint of the study was survival, while secondary concerns were with time to disease progression, time to treatment failure, best response, quality of life, and decrease in serum PSA. There were no significant differences in survival (12.3 vs 12.6 months) and progression (31% vs 27%); no complete responses were found in either treatment arm and only 14% and 19% of the patients achieved a >50% PSA decrease in the in the respective groups. However, after 56 days of treatment 38% of 112 patients of the mitoxatrone/hydrocortisone group and only 22% of the 116 patients of the hydrocortisone group achieved a PSA decrease of over 50%. Finally, no statistically significant difference was found between the groups in a variety of quality of life factors.

In another study, Osoba et al. [57] assessed the effects of mitoxantrone/prednisone versus prednisone alone on quality of life in men with HRPCA using the EORTC QLQ-30 and the prostate-specific quality of life module 14 (QOLM-P14). Although the two groups experienced a similar improvement at 6 weeks after initiation of therapy, only the mitoxantrone/prednisone group showed significant improvements in quality of life over four functioning domains and nine symptoms. In addition, improvement in quality of life lasted longer in the combination group (11 to 19 weeks vs 3 to 7 weeks).

The combination of mitoxantrone with corticosteroids can be viewed as a palliative option of choice and is currently regarded as standard treatment in the USA. However, benefits of the mitoxantrone-based therapy have to be balanced against treatment-related side effects and alternative options of palliative therapy in HRPCA. For instance, bisphosphonates. which have been reported as bringing significant pain relief to 75% of treated patients [28], have to be considered.

27.3.3 Suramin

Suramin is a polysulfonated naphthylurea that acts as a competitive inhibitor for a variety of cellular enzymes and growth factors being used in the treatment of HRPCA [51]. In-vitro studies have demonstrated a concentration-dependent activity against prostate cancer cell lines.

In studies performed so far, objective response rates varied between 35% and 50% whereas a PSA decline >50% was observed in approximately 75% of the patients [40, 41, 51, 82]. Treatment-related toxicities such as fatigue, malaise, weakness, anorexia, wasting, and neurotoxicity resulted in discontinuation of therapy in nearly half of the patients – and clearly indicated the major problem associated with suramin [40, 41, 51, 82].

In a recent multicenter, randomized, double-blind trial, suramin and hydrocortisone were compared with placebo and hydrocortisone in 458 patients with HRPCA and symptomatic skeletal disease [82]. Patients who progressed on the placebo arm could cross over to the combination arm. Primary endpoints of the study were quality of life and pain relief. The suramin/hydrocortisone arm showed a significant improvement in bone pain (43% vs 28%, p=0.01), in median duration of pain response (240 vs 69 days, p=0.0027), and in the risk of disease progression (1.0 vs 1.5, p=0.0003). Survival, however, was similar in both groups, perhaps the result of the cross-over study design. In contrast to other suramin-based studies published so far, adverse events were mild with less than 10% of the patients experiencing WHO grade 3 and 4 toxicity.

Still, the future of suramin in the treatment of patients with HRPCA remains unclear mainly because of the prolonged half-life of 56 days and the narrow therapeutic window with regard to the optimal dose schedule.

Table 28.5. Suramin-based chemotherapy in patients with hormone refractory prostate cancer

Author	*n*	PSA ↓ ≥50%	CR/PR
Myers [99]	38	34%	35%
Kelly [40]	61	79%	50%
Kelly [41]	28	18%	0%
Small [82]	458	33%	No data

CR/PR, overall response rate; PSA, prostate-specific antigen.

27.4 Oral Chemotherapy

The rationale for oral chemotherapy in HRPCA is that the delivery of drugs at a lower dose over an extended period of time reduces adverse side effects while killing cancer cells despite low proliferation rates. In the past, a variety of combinations such as EMP and etoposide, cyclophosphamide, diethylbestrol, and prednisone, as well as single agent diethylbestrol, have been used in HRPCA.

Pienta et al. [60, 61] performed two trials and administered EMP (15 mg/kg per day) and etoposide (50 mg/m^2 per day) orally for 21 of 28 days in 42 patients in his first trial; in the second trial EMP (10 mg/kg per day) and etoposide (50 mg/m^2 per day) were administered orally for 21 of 28 days to 62 patients. In both trials, patients were followed for a minimum of 26 weeks. Toxicity was moderate with 10% of the patients requiring dose reduction due to grade III/IV leukopenia and thrombocytopenia, and approximately 25% developed significant gastrointestinal side effects. Therapeutic activity of the regimes was quite high with an overall response rate of 53% and a ≥50% PSA decrease in 39%. Mean duration of PSA nadir was 8 weeks, median survivals of the two treatment groups were 44 weeks and 56 weeks, respectively, with no differences between patients with measurable soft tissue disease and those with skeletal metastases only. However, patients responding with a ≥50% PSA decrease demonstrated a significantly longer survival of 91 weeks as compared only 38 weeks in non-responders (p=0.0005).

EMP and etoposide were given at doses of 15 mg/kg per day and 50 mg/m^2, respectively, in 42 patients in a first study [61]; in a second study 62 patients were enrolled and EMP was given at 10 mg/kg per day for 21 days of a 28-day cycle. In the second trial antiandrogens had been discontinued at least 4 weeks prior to initiation of oral chemotherapy. Objective response rates in patients with soft-tissue lesions were 53% and 50%, respectively; a PSA decline of at least 50% from baseline was seen in 52% and in 39% of the patients in the first and the second trial, respectively. Median overall survival in both groups was 44 and 56 weeks, respectively, with PSA responders demonstrating a significantly longer survival of 91 weeks as compared to the non-responders with 38 weeks (p=0.0005). Side effects of therapy were well tolerated, with leg edema (48% and 35%) and nausea (25%) being the most frequent toxicities. Dose reduction of etoposide due to cytopenia was necessary in 25% and 18% of the patients in trial one and two, respectively, whereas episodes of neutropenic fever occurred in only 5 and 1 instances, making the dual drug regime a safe and well tolerated schedule with favorable response rates.

In another oral protocol involving 58 patients, DES at 1 mg/day was combined with prednisone at 20 mg/day for 20 days and then at 10 mg/day; finally, 100 mg cyclophosphamide was administered on days 1–20 of a 30-day treatment schedule [61]. With regard to soft-tissue lesions, 43% of the patients experienced a partial response and 36% of the patients had a PSA decline of more than 50%. The median overall survival was 62 weeks, with a significantly longer survival in PSA responders vs. non-responders (120 weeks vs. 48 weeks). Treatment-related side effects were minimal, with none of the patients developing substantial neutropenia or thrombocytopenia; one patient sustained a deep venous thrombosis during therapy.

27.5 Conclusion

HRPCA includes a heterogeneous group of patients with variable rates of tumor growth. It is evident that survival rates of these different groups differ significantly and that these facts have to be accounted for when designing and analyzing future trials in HRPCA. When dealing with HRPCA it is therefore of utmost importance to use a generally binding definition:

1. Consecutive PSA rise on three consecutive measurements occurring at a minimum of 1 week from the reference value
2. Serum testosterone at castrate levels (<50 ng/ml)
3. PSA rise following antiandrogen withdrawal or the addition of secondary hormonal manipulations.

Furthermore, it is of major importance that generally binding response criteria be applied in determining which of the agents tested in clinical phase-II trials should progress to randomized phase-III trials. A PSA decline ≥50% (confirmed by a second PSA value 4 weeks later) represents such a marker for measuring outcome.

The first therapeutic step should be to withdraw antiandrogens. Alternatively, secondary hormonal measures such as the addition of inhibitors of adrenal testosterone synthesis and application of low-dose estrogens might be pursued. In patients having undergone subcapsular orchiectomy, the addition of antiandrogen might be successful. Only when secondary hormonal manipulations have failed should chemotherapy be tried.

Currently, chemotherapy does not cure these patients. It has been shown, however, that chemotherapy can be effective in prolonging life and providing palliation. For patients with advanced symptomatic HRPCA, mitoxantrone/ prednisone or bisphosphonates result in significant improvements with regard to pain reduction and the need for narcotics. Improvement in quality of life, and pain and fatigue reduction would seem to be clinically appropriate endpoints for palliative clinical trials.

For those patients with HRPCA characterized by rising PSA levels or by measurable asymptomatic disease, prospective randomized clinical phase-III studies are needed to define the role of the different effective chemotherapeutic approaches which have been tested in phase-II studies.

References

1. Albrecht W, Horenblas S, Marechal JM, Mikisch G, Horwich A, Seretta V, Cassetta G, van Poppel H, Kalman S, Sylvester R (1998) EMP versus EMP/VBL Chemotherapie beim hormonrefraktären Prostatakarzinom. Urologe A 37:32
2. Benson R, Hartley-Asp B (1990) Mechanisms of action and clinical uses of estramustine. Cancer Invest 8:375
3. Blumenstein B, Crawford ED, Saiers JH, Stephens RL, Rivkin SE, Coltman CA Jr (1993) Doxorubicin, mitomycin C and 5-flourouracil in the treatment of hormone refractory adenocarcinoma of the prostate: a Southwest Oncology Group study. J Urol 150:411–413
4. Breul J, Paul R (1998) Das Antiandrogen-Entzugssyndrom. Urologe A 37:156–158
5. Bubley GJ, Carducci M, Dahut W, Dawson N, Daliani D, Eisenberger M, et al (1999) Eligibility and response guidelines for phase II clinical trials in androgen-independent prostate cancer: recommendations from the prostate-specific antigen working group. J Clin Oncol 17:3461–3467
6. Crawford ED, Rosenblum M, Ziada AM, Lange PH (1999) Overview: hormone refractory prostate cancer. Urology 54 [Suppl 6A]:1–7
7. Culine S, Kattan J, Zanetta S, Theodore C, Fizazi K, Droz JP (1998) Evaluation of estramustine phosphate combined with weekly doxorubicin in patients with androgen-independent prostate cancer. Am J Clin Oncol 21:470–474

8. DeLa Taille A, Hayek OR, Buttyan R, et al (1999) Effects of a phytotherapeutic agent, PC-SPES, on prostate cancer: preliminary investigation on human cell lines and patients. Br J Urol 84: 845–850
9. DeLa Taille A, Buttyan R, Hayek O, et al (2000) Herbal therapy PC-SPES: in vitro effects and evaluation of its efficacy in 69 patients with prostate cancer. J Urol 164:1229–1234
10. Denis L (1998) European organization for research and treatment of cancer (EORTC) prostate cancer trials, 1976–1996. Urology 51 [Suppl 5A]:50–57
11. De Voogt HJ, Sucuiu S, Sylvester R (1989) Univariate analysis of prognostic factors in patients with advanced prostatic carcinoma: results from two European organizations for research on treatment of cancer trials. J Urol 141:883–888
12. Dijkman GA, van Moorseiaar RJ, van Ginckel R, van Stratum P, Wouters L, Debruyne F, Schalken JA, de Coster R (1994) Antitumoral effects of liarozole in in androgen dependent and independent prostate cancer. J Urol 151:217–222
13. DiPaola RS, Zhang H, Lambert GH, et al (1998) Clinical and biologic activity of an estrogen herbal combination (PC-SPES) in prostate cancer. N Engl J Med 339:785–791
14. Dowsett M, Shearer RJ, Ponder BAJ, et al (1988) The effects of aminogluthetimide and hydrocortisone, alone and combined, on androgen levels in prost-orchiectomy prostate cancer patients. Br J Cancer 57:190–192
15. Dupont A, Gomez JL, Cusan L, Koutselieris M, Labrie F (1993) Response to flutamide withdrawal in advanced prostate cancer in progression under combination therapy. J Urol 150:908–913
16. Ellerhorst JS, Tu SM, Amato RJ (1997) A phase II trial of alternating weekly chemohormonal therapy for patients with androgen-independent prostate cancer. Clin Cancer Res 3:2371
17. Falcone A, Antonuzzo A, Danesi R, Allegrini G, Monica L, Pfanner E, Masi G, Ricci S, Del Tacca M, Conte P (1999) Suramin in combination with weekly epirubicin for patients with advanced hormone-refractory prostate carcinoma. Cancer 86:470–476
18. Figg WD, Sartor O, Cooper MR (1995) Prostate specific antigen decline following the discontinuation of flutamide in patients with stage D2 prostate cancer. Am J Med 98:412–414
19. Fowler JE, Pandey P, Seaver LE, et al (1995) Prostate specific antigen after gonadal androgen withdrawal and deferred flutamide treatment. J Urol 154:448–453
20. Friedland D, Cohen J, Miller R, Gluckamn R, Zidar B, Lembersky B, Keating M, Voloshin M, Balaban E, Pinkerton R, Reilly N, Dimitt P, Kinney C (1999) A phase II trial in hormone refractory prostate cancer: correlation of antitumor activity to phosphorylation of bcl-2. Proc Am Soc Clin Oncol 18:322a
21. George DJ, Kanthoff PW (1999) Prognostic indicators in hormone refractory prostate cancer. Urol Clin North Am 26:303–309
22. Ghossein RA, Rosai J, Scher HI (1997) Prognostic significance of detection of prostate-specific antigen transcripts in the peripheral blood of patients with metastatic androgen-independent prostatic carcinoma. Urology 50:100–105
23. Gomella LG, Ismail M, Nathan FE (19970 Antiandrogen withdrawal syndrome with nilutamide. J Urol 157:1366
24. Graefen M, Hammerer P, Haese A, Huland H (2000) Therapieoptionen des hormonrefraktären Prostatakarzinoms. Urologe A 39:267–273
25. Haldar S, Basu A, Croce CM (1996) Bcl-2 is the guardian of the microtubule. Cancer Res 2:389–395
26. Hartley-Asp B, Kruse E (1986) Nuclear protein matrix as a target for estramustine induced cell death. Prostate 9:387
27. Herrada J, Dieringer P, Logothetis CJ (1996) Characterization of patients with androgen-independent prostatic carcinoma whose serum prostate specific antigen decreased following flutamide withdrawal. J Urol 1996; 155:620–623
28. Heidenreich A, Engelmann UH, Hofmann R (2001) The use of bisphosphonates for the palliative treatment of painful bone metastases due to hormone refractory prostate cancer. J Urol 165:136–140
29. Huan SD, Gerridzen RG, Yau JC, et al (1997) Antiandrogen withdrawal syndrome with nilutamide. Urology 49:632–634
30. Huan SD, Stewart DJ, Aitken SE, Segal R, Yau JC (1999) Combination of epirubicin and cisplatin in hormone-refractory metastatic prostate cancer. Am J Clin Oncol 22:471–474
31. Hubert A, Lyass O, Pode D, Gabizon A (2000) Doxil (Caelyx): an exploratory study with pharmacokinetics in patients with hormone-refractory prostate cancer. Anticancer Drugs 11:123– 127
32. Hudes G, Einhorn L, Ross E, Balsham A, Loehrer P, Ramsey H, Sprandio J, Entmacher M, Dugan W, Ansari R, Monaco F, Hanna M, Roth B (1999) Vinblastine versus vinblastine plus oral estramustine phosphate for patients with hormone-refractory prostate cancer: a Hoosier Oncology Group and Fox Chase Network phase III trial. J Clin Oncol 17:3160–3166
33. Hudes GR, Nathan F, Khater C (1997) Phase II trial of 96-hour paclitaxel plus oral estramustine phosphate in metastatic hormone refractory prostate cancer. J Clin Oncol 15:3156
34. Hussain M, Wolf M, Marshall E, et al (1994) Effects of continued androgen-deprived therapy and other prognostic factors on response and survival in phase II chemotherapy trials for hormone-refractory prostate cancer: a Southwest Oncology Group Report. J Clin Oncol 12: 1868–1875

35. Isaacs JT (1999) The biology of hormone refractory prostate cancer. Why does it develop? Urol Clin North Am 26:263–273
36. Johnson DE, Babaian RJ, von Eschenbach AC, et al (1988) Ketoconazole therapy for hormonally refractive metastatic prostate cancer. Urology 31:132–134
37. Joyce R, Fenton MA, Rode P, et al (1998) High dose biclutamide for androgen independent prostate cancer: effect of prior hormonal therapy. J Urol 159:149–153
38. Kanthoff PW, Halabi S, Conaway M, Picus J, Kirshner J, Hars V, Trump D, Winer EP, Vogelzang NJ (1999) Hydrocortisone with or without mitoxantrone in men with hormone-refractory prostate cancer: results of the Cancer and Leukemia Group B 9182 study. J Clin Oncol 17:2506–2513
39. Kelly WK, Scher H (1993) Prostate specific antigen decline after androgen withdrawal syndrome. J Urol 149:607–613
40. Kelly WK, Curley T, Leibertz C, et al (1995) Prospective evaluation of hydrocortisone and suramin in patients with androgen-independent prostate cancer. J Clin Oncol 13:2208–2213
41. Kelly WK, Scher HI, Mazumdar M (1995) Suramin and hydrocortisone: determining the efficacy in androgen-independent prostate cancer. J Clin Oncol 13:2214
42. Klotz L, McNeill I, Fleshner N (1999) A phase 1–2 trial of diethylstilbestrol plus low dose warfarin in advanced prostate carcinoma. J Urol 161:169–172
43. Kluog RC, Farah RN, Cerny JC (1981) Bilateral orchiectomy for carcinoma of the prostate: response of serum testosterone and clinical response to estrogen therapy. Urology 17:49–54
44. Kreis W, Budman DR, Fetten J, Gonzales AL, Barile B, Vinciguerra V (1999) Phase I trial of the combination of daily estramustine phosphate and intermittent docetaxel in patients with metastatic hormone refractory prostate carcinoma. Ann Oncol 10:33–38
45. Laurie JA, Hahn RG, Therneau TM (1992) Chemotherapy for hormonally refractory advanced prostate carcinoma: a comparison of combined versus sequential treatment with mitomycin C, doxorubicin and 5-flourouracil. Cancer 69:1440
46. Logothetis CJ, Samuels ML, von Eschenbach AC (1983) Doxorubicin, mitomycin C and 5-flourouracil in the treatment of metastatic hormonal refractory adenocarcinoma of the prostate, with a note on the staging of metastatic prostate cancer. J Clin Oncol 1:368
47. Manni A, Bartholomew M, Caplan R, Boucher A, Santen R, Lipton A, Harvey H, Simmonds M, White-Hersey D, Gordon R, Rohner T, Drago J, Wettlaufer J, Glode L (1988) Androgen priming and chemotherapy in advanced prostate cancer: evaluation of determinants of clinical outcome. J Clin Oncol 6:1456–1466
48. Miglietta L, Canobbio L, Grabetto C, Vannozzi MO, Esposito M, Boccardo F (1997) Suramin/epidoxorubicin association in hormone-refractory prostate cancer: preliminary results of a pilot phase II study. J Cancer Res Clin Oncol 123:407–410
49. Moore MJ, Osoba D, Murphy K, Tannock IF, Armitage A, Findlay B, Coppin C, Neville A, Venner P, Wilson J (1994) Use of palliative end points to evaluate the effects of mitoxantrone and low-dose prednisone in patients with hormonally resistant prostate cancer. J Clin Oncol 12:689–694
50. Murphy GP (1999) Review of phase II hormone refractory prostate cancer trials. Urology 54 [Suppl 6A]:19–21
51. Myers CE, Cooper MR, Stein C (1992) Suramin: a novel growth factor antagonist with activity in hormone-refractory metastatic prostate cancer. J Clin Oncol 10:881
52. Navone NM, Troncoso P, Pisters LL, et al (1993) p53 protein accumulation and gene mutation in the progression of human prostate carcinoma. J Natl Cancer Inst 85:1657–1663
53. Newling DW, Dennis L, Vermeylen K (1993) Orchiectomy versus goserelin and flutamide in the treatment of newly diagnosed metastatic prostate cancer. Cancer 72:3793–3798
54. Nieh PT (1995) Withdrawal phenomenon with the antiandrogen Casodex. J Urol 153:1070–1073
55. Ornstein DK, Smith DS, Andriole GL (1998) Biochemical response to testicular androgen ablation among patients with prostate cancer for whom flutamide and/or finasteride therapy failed. Urology 52:1094–1097
56. Osborne CK, Blumenstein BA, Crawford ED, Weiss GR, Bukowski RM, Larrimer NR (1992) Phase II study of platinum and mitoxantrone in metastatic prostate cancer: a Southwest Oncology Group study. Eur J Cancer 28:477–478
57. Osoba D, Tannock IF, Ernst SD, Neville AJ (1999) Health related quality of life in men with metastatic prostate cancer treated with prednisone alone or mitoxantrone and prednisone. J Clin Oncol 17:1654–1663
58. Parker SL, Tong T, Bolden S, Wingo PA (1996) Cancer statistics, 1997. CA Cancer J Clin 46: 5–27
59. Petrylak DP (1999) Chemotherapy for advanced hormone refractory prostate cancer. Urology 54 [Suppl 6A]:31–35
60. Petrylak DP, Macarthur RB, O'Connor J, Shelton G, Judge T, Balog J, Pfaff C, Bagiella E, Heitjan D, Fine R, Zuech N, Sawczuk I, Benson M, Olsson CA (1999) Phase I trial of docetaxel with estramustine in androgen-independent prostate cancer. J Clin Oncol 17:958–967
61. Pienta KJ, Redman B, Hussain M (1994) Phase II evaluation of oral estramustine and oral etoposide in hormone-refractory adenocarcinoma of the prostate. J Clin Oncol 12:2005–2012

62. Pienta KJ, Esper PS, Smith DC (1997) The oral regimen of cytoxan, prednisone, and diethylbestrol is an active, non-toxic treatment for patients with hormone refractory prostate cancer. Proc Annu Meet Am Soc Clin Oncol 16:1104
63. Pienta KJ, Redman BG, Bandekar R, Strawderman MA, Cease K, Esper PS, Naik H, Smith DC (1997) A phase II trial of oral estramustine and oral etoposide in hormone refractory prostate cancer. Urology 50:401–407
64. Plowman PN, Perry LA, Chard T (1987) Androgen suppression by hydrocortisone without aminogluthetmide in orchiectomised men with prostatic cancer. Br J Urol 59:255–257
65. Presti JC (1999) The role of the urologist in adjuvant chemotherapy trials for prostate cancer. Urology 54 [Suppl 6A]:47–50
66. Reese DM, Small EJ (1999) Secondary hormonal manipulations in hormone refractory prostate cancer. Urol Clin North Am 26:311–319
67. Richie JP (1999) Anti-androgens and other hormonal therapies for prostate cancer. Urol Clin North Am 26:15–18
68. Sartor O, Cooper M, Weinberger M, et al (1994) Surprising activity of flutamide withdrawal, when combined with aminogluthetimide, in treatment of "hormone-refractory" prostate cancer. J Natl Cancer Inst 86:222–227
69. Schellhammer P, Venner P, Haas G (1997) Prostate specific antigen decreases after withdrawal of antiandrogen therapy with biclutamid or flutamide in patients receiving combined androgen blockade. J Urol 157:1731–1735
70. Scher H, Steinneck G, Kelly WK (1995) Hormone-refractory (D3) prostate cancer: refining the concept. Urology 46:142–148
71. Scher H, Liebertz C, Kelly WK, et al (1997) Biclutamide for advanced prostate cancer: the natural versus treated history of disease. J Clin Oncol 15:2928–2938
72. Seidman AD, Scher HI, Petrylak D, Dershaw DD, Curley T (1992) Estramustine and vinblastine: use of prostate specific antigen as a clinical trial and point for hormone refractory prostatic cancer. J Urol 147:931–934
73. Seidmon EJ, Trump DL, Kreis W, et al (1995) Phase I/II dose-escalation study of liarazole in patients with stage D hormone-refractory carcinoma of the prostate. Ann Surg Oncol 2:550–556
74. Sella A, Kilbourn R, Amato R (1994) Phase II study of ketoconazole combined with weekly doxorubicin in patients with androgen-independent prostate cancer. J Clin Oncol 12:683
75. Sinibaldi VJ, Carduci MA, Moore-Cooper S, Enger C, Laufer M, Wolff C, Eisenberger MA (1999) A phase II study evaluating a one day course of estramustine phosphate and docetaxel in patients with hormone refractory prostate cancer. Proc Am Soc Clin Oncol 18:322a
76. Small EJ, Carroll PR (1994) Prostate specific antigen decline after Casodex withdrawal: evidence for an antiandrogen withdrawal syndrome. Urology 43:408–410
77. Small EJ, Srinivas S (1995) The antiandrogen withdrawal syndrome: experience in a large cohort of unselected patients with advanced prostate cancer. Cancer 76:1428–1434
78. Small EJ, Srinivas S, Egan B, McMillan A, Rearden TP (1996) Doxorubicin and dose-escalating cyclophophamide with granulocyte colony-stimulating factor for the treatment of hormone-resistant prostate cancer. J Clin Oncol 14:1617–1625
79. Small EJ, Baron AD, Fippin L, et al (1997) Ketoconazole retains activity in advanced prostate cancer patients with progression despite flutamide withdrawal. J Urol 157:1204–1207
80. Small EJ, Baron AD, Bok R, et al (1997) Simultaneous anitandrogen withdrawal and treatment with ketoconazole and hydrocortisone in patients with advanced prostate carcinoma. Cancer 80:1755–1759
81. Small EJ, Frohlich MW, Bok R, et al (2000) Prospective trial of the herbal supplement PC-SPES in patients with progressive prostate cancer. J Clin Oncol 18:3595–3603
82. Small EJ, Meyer M, Marshall ME, Reyno LM, Meyers FJ, Natale RB, Lenehan PF, Chen L, Slichemeyer WJ, Eisenberger M (2000) Suramin therapy for patients with symptomatic hormone-refractory prostate cancer: results of a randomized phase III trial comparing suramin plus hydrocortisone to placebo plus hydrocortisone. J Clin Oncol 18:1440–1450
83. Smith DC, Dunn RL, Strawderman MS, Pienta KJ (1998) Change in serum prostate-specific antigen as a marker of response to cytotoxic therapy for hormone-refractory prostate cancer. J Clin Oncol 16:1835–1843
84. Smith DC, Redman BG, Flaherty LE, Li L, Strawderman M, Pienta KJ (1998) A phase II trial of oral diethylbestrol as a second line hormonal agent in advanced prostate cancer. Urology 52:257–260
85. Smith DC, Esper P, Strawderman M, Redman B, Pienta KJ (1999) Phase II trial of oral estramustine, oral etoposide, and intravenous paclitaxel in hormone-refractory prostate cancer. J Clin Oncol 17:1664–1671
86. Strum SB, McDermed JE, Scholz MC, Johnson H, Tisman G (1997) Anaemia associated with androgen deprivation in patients with prostate cancer receiving combined hormone blockade. Br J Urol 79:933–941
87. Tannock IF, Gospodarowicz M, Meakin W, et al (1989) Treatment of metastatic prostate cancer with low-dose prednisone: evaluation of pain and quality of life as pragmatic indices of response. J Clin Oncol 7:590–597

88. Tannock IF, Osoba D, Stockler MR, Ernst DS, Neville AJ, Moore MJ, Armitage GR, Wilson JJ, Venner PM, Coppin CML, Murphy KC (1996) Chemotherapy with mitoxantrone plus prednisone or prednisone alone for symptomatic hormone-resistant prostate cancer: a Canadian randomized trial with palliative end points. J Clin Oncol 14:1756–1764
89. Taplin ME, Bubley GJ, Shuster TD, et al (1995) Mutation of the androgen-receptor gene in metastatic androgen-independent prostate cancer. N Engl J Med 332:1393–1398
90. Taylor CD, Elson P, Trump DL (1993) Importance of continued testicular suppression in hormone refractory prostate cancer. J Clin Oncol 11:2167–2172
91. Tew KD, Stearns ME (1987) Hormone-independent, non-alkylating mechanism of cytotoxicity for estramustine. Urol Res 15:155
92. Tilley WD, Buchanan G, Hickey TE, et al (1996) Mutations in the androgen receptor gene are associated with progression of human prostate cancer to androgen independence. Clin Cancer Res 2:277–285
93. Vaage J, Barbera-Guillem E, Abra R, Huang A, Working P (1994) Tissue distribution and therapeutic effect of intravenous free or encapsulated liposomal doxorubicin on human prostate carcinoma xenografts. Cancer 73:1478–1484
94. Veronesi A, Re GL, Foladore S, Merlo A, Giuliotto N, Talamini R, Monfradini S (1996) Multidrug chemotherapy in the treatment of non-elderly patients with hormone-refractory prostatic carcinoma. A phase II study. North Eastern Italian Oncology Group. Eur Urol 29:434–438
95. Visakorpi T, Hyytinen E, Kovisto P, et al (1995) In vivo amplification of the androgen receptor and progression of prostate cancer. Nat Genet 9:401–409
96. Vogelzang NJ, Crawford ED, Zietman A (1998) Current clinical trial design issues in hormone-refractory prostate cancer. Cancer 82:2093–2101
97. Weitzman A, Shelton G, Zuech N, Englnad-Owen C, Newhouse J, Bagiella E, Katz A, Sawczuk I, Benson M, Olsson C, Petrylak DP (1999) Phase II study of estramustine combined with docetaxel in patients with androgen-independent prostate cancer. Proc Am Soc Clin Oncol 18: 355a
98. Wingo PA, Landis S, Ries LAG (1997) An adjustment to the 1997 estimate for new prostate cancer. CA Cancer J Clin 47:239–242
99. Yagoda A, Petrylak D (1993) Cytotoxic chemotherapy for advanced hormone resistant prostate cancer. Cancer 1098–1109

Subject Index